Cardiovascular Physiology

Questions for Self Assessment With Illustrated Answers

J Rodney Levick DSc DPhil MA MRCP BM BCh (Oxon)
Professor of Physiology
St George's Hospital Medical School
University of London, UK

CRC Press
Taylor & Francis Group
Boca Raton London New York

CRC Press is an imprint of the
Taylor & Francis Group, an **informa** business

CRC Press
Taylor & Francis Group
6000 Broken Sound Parkway NW, Suite 300
Boca Raton, FL 33487-2742

First issued in hardback 2017

Version Date: 20161215

ISBN-13: 978-0-340-98511-3 (pbk)
ISBN-13: 978-1-138-45145-2 (hbk)

Visit the Taylor & Francis Web site at
http://www.taylorandfrancis.com

and the CRC Press Web site at
http://www.crcpress.com

Contents

Introduction

The questions in this little book are intended primarily as an accompaniment to the fifth edition of the textbook, *An Introduction to Cardiovascular Physiology* (JR Levick, Hodder Arnold, 2010) – though the explanations and the numerous diagrams should help make this a useful 'stand-alone' volume if desired. The companion volume has a small, 'taster' selection of the questions on its website. The aim of this collection of over 230 questions is to offer students an element of self-assessment, as they progress through the companion book or revise for examinations. Lecturers may find some of the questions useful as a template when setting questions of their own, but should note that the questions are primarily educational in intent; their discriminatory power has not been tested. The questions are grouped under the same headings as the chapters of the companion textbook, so they become progressively more advanced (see Contents). Occasional statements call for information from later chapters. Medically relevant questions are introduced wherever they are appropriate. I have set at least one question on each learning objective given at the start of the chapter in the companion volume, to help you assess your achievement of the learning objectives. Some questions require you to integrate information from other chapters too. The questions aim to test basic understanding, fundamental principles and medical relevance. Hopefully they avoid excessive detail – always the examiner's easy option!

The questions. Most of the questions are multiple choice questions (MCQs), generally with five true/false statements, but occasionally more or less than five. Although some 'educationalists' now demand single correct answer questions (SAQs, one correct answer out of four or five options), these test less knowledge, so the MCQ style has been retained here. To add variety, there is a sprinkling of other styles of question, such as 'extended matching questions' (i.e. choose the best answer from a list), data interpretation problems, and little numerical problems that test reasoning power and ability to do simple calculations.

The answers. Each answer is accompanied by a brief explanation, and very often an illustrative figure, which should help if you got the answer wrong. Most of the figures are from the accompanying textbook, but there are also new, explanatory diagrams after some questions. It is sometimes difficult to avoid ambiguity in MCQ questions; so use your common sense – choose the answer that will be right most of the time, rather than a remote, rare possibility. Nevertheless, if you disagree with the 'official' answer, do let me know.

Your score. What score represents a good performance? There are roughly equal numbers of T and F answers. Therefore, if +1 is allotted for each correct answer and none subtracted for a wrong answer, a score of 50% could be achieved simply by responding True (or False) to every question. Around 65% (two-thirds) correct answers would probably be a 'pass' under this marking scheme. Many universities use a negative marking scheme, namely −1 for an incorrect answer, 0 for no answer and +1 for a correct answer. On this scheme, guessing True (or False) for every answer would score roughly zero, and the pass mark is therefore usually set at a little below 50%. Over 60% would be good, and over 70% excellent. Good luck!

Rodney Levick
Physiology
St George's Hospital Medical School,
University of London, UK

CHAPTER 1

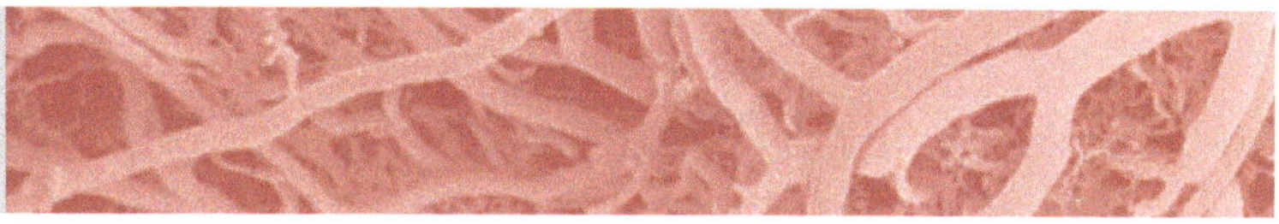

Overview of the cardiovascular system

T F

1.1 Concerning transport by the cardiovascular system,

a. the transport of glucose by the circulation is convective rather than diffusive.
b. diffusion depends on transport up a concentration gradient.
c. the time taken for O_2 to diffuse a certain distance is directly proportional to the distance.
d. O_2 is carried from capillary blood to the tissue cells mainly by fluid filtration.
e. if coronary perfusion were halted, O_2 would take about 15 hours to diffuse from the cavity of the left ventricle to the subepicardial muscle fibres.

1.2 Regarding the distribution of cardiac output (CO) to the tissues of a resting human,

a. about 20% goes to skeletal muscle, which accounts for ~20% of resting O_2 consumption.
b. about 20% goes to the kidneys, which account for ~6% of resting O_2 consumption.
c. about 10% goes to the myocardium, which accounts for ~10% of resting O_2 consumption.
d. the proportion of the CO going to a given organ is regulated mainly by the conduit arteries feeding the organ.
e. about 50% goes to the lungs, due to their low vascular resistance.

1.3 Regarding the flow of blood,

a. flow is proportional to the pressure difference between the inlet and outlet of the blood vessel.
b. Darcy's law states that flow equals pressure times resistance.
c. the flow per unit pressure drop along a vessel is called the hydraulic conductance of the vessel.
d. the units for hydraulic resistance are mmHg per unit flow or equivalent.
e. the flow resistance of the pulmonary circulation is about two-thirds that of the systemic circulation.

1.4 As blood flows around the systemic circulation,

a. its mean pressure falls markedly from the aorta to small, named arteries, such as the radial artery.
b. the systolic pressure is higher in the brachial artery than the aorta.
c. the biggest fall in pressure occurs in the resistance arteries.
d. the greatest net, cross-sectional vascular area is encountered in the capillaries.
e. its velocity decreases in microvessels, yet the total flow does not.
f. its pressure falls to ~30 mmHg in the antecubital vein at heart level.

T F

1.5 The conclusion that terminal arteries and arterioles offer more resistance to blood flow than other vessels stems from the observation that

a. they have the thickest walls, relative to lumen width.
b. they have a rich sympathetic vasomotor innervation.
c. they have the smallest internal radius of all blood vessels.
d. they have the biggest pressure drop across them.
e. they are less numerous than venules.

1.6 Blood vessels classified as

a. elastic vessels expand to receive the stroke volume of the heart.
b. conduit vessels conduct venous blood back to the heart.
c. resistance vessels can actively regulate the blood flow through a tissue.
d. exchange vessels include some venules as well as capillaries.
e. capacitance vessels have the capacity to alter blood pressure directly.

1.7 The wall of a blood vessel

a. is lined internally by cells that secretes anti-thrombotic agents.
b. is divided into two layers (tunica) by a sheet of elastin.
c. always contains tension-resisting collagen.
d. has a higher proportion of elastin in the aorta than in distal arteries.
e. always contains contractile smooth muscle, except in capillaries.
f. has the lowest proportion of smooth muscle in the arterioles.
g. rarely contains efferent nerve fibres.

1.8 The proximal aorta gives off arteries to the brain; the abdominal aorta gives off arteries to the intestine; and the distal aorta gives off arteries to the leg; but the liver is supplied chiefly by venous blood from the intestine. Therefore,

a. the blood supply to the brain and intestine are in parallel.
b. the blood supply to the intestine and leg are in series.
c. the pressure of arterial blood supplying the leg is substantially lower than that supplying the brain.
d. the blood supply to the liver is in series with the intestinal supply.
e. the blood supply to the liver is an example of a portal circulation.

1.9 Roles of different classes of systemic blood vessel

(Here is a different style of question, the extended matching question (EMQ). If you succeeded with questions 1–8, you will find this one easy.)

Regarding the various systemic blood vessels, enter the code from the list below to answer questions (i) to (vii). A code can be used more than once, or not at all.

a. proximal aorta
b. conduit arteries
c. arterioles
d. capillaries
e. venules
f. peripheral veins
g. central vein

(i) This vessel has the largest radius.
(ii) If all the vessels in parallel are added together, this class of vessel has the greatest net cross-sectional area.

(iii) This vessel has the slowest velocity of blood flow. ☐
(iv) This vessel has the highest velocity of blood flow. ☐
(v) This category of vessel has the greatest pressure drop across it. ☐
(vi) These *three* types of vessel together contain around two-thirds of the circulating blood volume. ☐
(vii) This vessel actively regulates the blood flow through a tissue. ☐

Answers

1.1 a. **T** – The circulation evolved because convective transport (wash-along) is faster than diffusion over long distances.

b. **F** – Diffusion is a passive transport process *down* a concentration gradient **(Figure 1.1)**.

c. **F** – Einstein showed that the time increases as the *square* of distance. This is why diffusion is so slow over distances of over a millimetre **(Table 1.1)**.

d. **F** – Transport from blood to tissue is by passive diffusion down the concentration gradient, not fluid filtration down a pressure gradient **(Figure 1.2)**.

e. **T** – This is why the coronary circulation evolved **(Table 1.1)**.

1.2 a. **T** – Organ blood flow is, as a broad generalization, related to the organ's O_2 consumption **(Figure 1.3)**.

b. **T** – The high flow is 'excessive' relative to renal O_2 demand, but is needed for adequate renal excretion and urine production **(Figure 1.3)**.

c. **F** – The myocardium receives only ~4% of the cardiac output, despite the fact that it consumes 10% of the oxygen **(Figure 1.3)**.

d. **F** – It is not the wide, low-resistance conduit arteries that primarily regulate blood flow. It is the fine arterioles and terminal arterial twigs – the resistance vessels. Dilatation of conduit arteries prevents their resistance becoming a flow-limiting factor during exercise.

e. **F** – What a silly question! The lungs of course receive the *entire* cardiac output of the right ventricle **(Figure 1.4)**.

1.3 a. **T** – The difference in pressure, ΔP, provides the energy gradient driving the flow.

b. **F** – Darcy's law states the flow $\dot{Q}$ equals pressure *difference*, *divided* by resistance; $\dot{Q} = \Delta P/R$, or equivalently $\dot{Q} = \Delta P \times$ conductance K **(Figure 1.5)**.

c. **T** – From Darcy's law, conductance K is $\dot{Q}/\Delta P$ **(Figure 1.5)**.

d. **T** – From Darcy's law, resistance R is $\Delta P/\dot{Q}$; so the units of resistance are pressure difference required to drive unit flow.

e. **F** – The pulmonary circulation has a much lower resistance, namely ~15% of systemic resistance. This is proved by the low pulmonary artery pressure required to drive the cardiac output through the lungs.

1.4 a. **F** – Mean pressure falls by only a few mmHg in the named arteries, because they are wide and offer little resistance to flow. This is evident from the pressure profile of the circulation **(Figure 1.6)**.

b. **T** – Although the mean brachial arterial pressure is slightly lower than mean aortic pressure, brachial artery systolic pressure is actually higher than aortic systolic pressure, because the shape of the pressure wave changes as it travels distally **(Figure 1.6)**.

c. **T** – Darcy's law tell us that resistance is pressure drop per unit flow. The resistance vessels are the terminal arteries and arterioles, as is evident from the large pressure drop across them **(Figure 1.6)**.

d. **T** – Though narrow individually, there are millions of capillaries in parallel. This creates a very large total cross-sectional area, much bigger than that of the aorta **(Figure 1.6)**.

e. **T** – The entire cardiac output (cm^3/min) flows through the microcirculation, but its velocity (cm/min) is slowed by the very large, net cross-sectional area (cm^2) of the microvessels **(Figure 1.6)**. Note that velocity (cm/min) = flow (cm^3/min) / area cm^2.

f. **F** – Peripheral venous pressure at heart level is much lower, namely ~8–10 mmHg **(Figure 1.6)**.

1.5 a. **F** – The high wall/lumen ratio is true, but this does not prove that resistance is high. Resistance is pressure drop required to produce unit flow.
b. **F** – Again, the fact is true but it does not prove that resistance is high.
c. **F** – Capillaries are even narrower, ~5 μm wide.
d. **T** – Resistance is by definition the pressure drop required to produce unit flow (Darcy's law). The biggest pressure drop is across the terminal arteries and arterioles **(Figure 1.6)**.
e. **F** – Again the fact is true, but it does not prove their high resistance.

1.6 a. **T** – The aorta and major branches are elastin rich and expand to accommodate the stroke volume **(Figure 1.7)**.
b. **F** – Conduit vessels are arteries with abundant smooth muscle that conduct blood to the tissues. Examples include the coronary arteries, cerebral arteries and popliteal artery.
c. **T** – Dilatation reduces their resistance and thus increases local perfusion (blood flow). Contraction increases resistance and thus reduces local blood flow.
d. **T** – Post-capillary venules, as well as capillaries, are permeable to water and respiratory gases.
e. **F** – Capacitance vessels are veins. They serve as contractile, adjustable blood reservoirs. Any effect on blood pressure is mediated indirectly, by changing the volume of blood in the heart (Starling's law of the heart).

1.7 a. **T** – The endothelium secretes the anti-thrombotic agents nitric oxide and prostaglandins.
b. **F** – There are *three* layers (tunica intima, tunica media, tunica adventitia), as defined by *two* elastin sheets, the internal and external elastic laminae **(Figure 1.8)**.
c. **T** – Even the capillary has collagen (type IV) in its basal lamina; all other vessels also have type I-III collagen fibrils throughout the wall.
d. **T** – See **Table 1.2**. Elastin allows the aorta to stretch readily to accommodate the stroke volume of the left ventricle.
e. **T** – Smooth muscle makes up most of the tunica media in most vessels **(Figure 1.8)**.
f. **F** – Arterioles have the *highest* proportion of smooth muscle **(Table 1.2)**. This enables them to act as contractile 'taps' that regulate local blood flow and blood pressure.
g. **F** – Most blood vessels, except capillaries, are innervated by sympathetic vasoconstrictor fibres **(Figure 1.8)**. Some also have afferent fibres, e.g. nociceptor (pain) fibres.

1.8 a. **T** – The plumbing is 'in parallel', by analogy with electrical circuits **(Figure 1.4)**.
b. **F** – These two circulations are again in parallel, as are most circulations **(Figure 1.4)**.
c. **F** – The arterial pressure is virtually identical in all parallel arteries, so the tissues are all perfused by the same pressure head and receive blood with the same O_2 content. This is the big advantage of parallel plumbing.
d. **T** – Almost three-quarters of the liver's blood supply comes from the portal vein, which drains the intestine **(Figure 1.4)**.
e. **T** – A portal circulation delivers material directly from one organ to another without mixing in the general circulation.

1.9 (i) g (ii) d (iii) d (iv) a (v) c (vi) e, f, g. (vii) c

CHAPTER 2

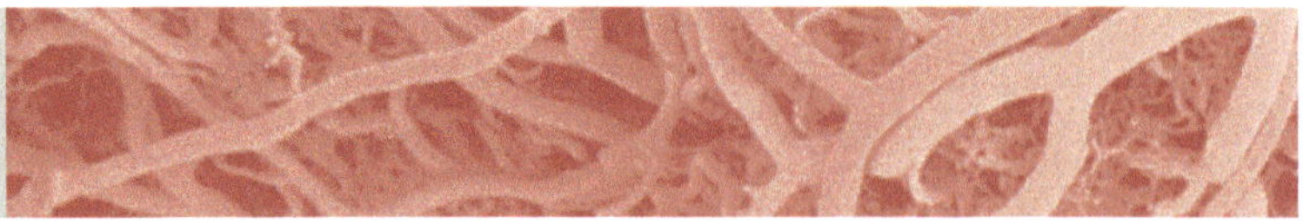

The cardiac cycle

T F

2.1 During cardiac development in the fetus,

a. the ductus arteriosus shunts blood from the aorta into pulmonary trunk.
b. the foramen ovale remains open until birth.
c. the coronary sinus does not open until birth.
d. failure of the atrial or ventricular septum to close causes cyanosis after birth.
e. transposition of the major vessels occurs in Fallot's tetralogy.

2.2 During the cardiac cycle of a human adult,

a. pressure is higher in the left atrium than right atrium.
b. ventricular filling depends mainly on atrial contraction.
c. the ventricle fills fastest during early diastole.
d. the atria and ventricles contract simultaneously during systole.
e. systole is initiated in the left atrium.

2.3 With reference to the cardiac cycle,

a. right atrial pressure is typically 3–5 mmHg.
b. the work of the right ventricle is greater than the work of the left ventricle.
c. the first heart sound occurs at the end of the isovolumetric contraction phase.
d. two-thirds of the blood in the ventricle is ejected during systole in a resting human.
e. the QRS complex of the ECG immediately precedes the isovolumetric contraction phase.

2.4 Ventricular filling

a. begins as soon as the aortic valve closes.
b. is increasingly dependent on atrial contraction during exercise.
c. can cause a third heart sound in some healthy people.
d. is boosted initially by the elastic recoil of the ventricle wall.
e. influences the force of the next heart beat.

2.5 The right ventricle

a. receives blood through the mitral valve.
b. ejects less blood than the left ventricle because its wall is thinner.
c. blood has an O_2 content which is approximately three-quarters that of aortic blood in a resting human.
d. raises pulmonary blood pressure to ~100 mmHg during ejection.
e. is connected to the left atrium by the ductus arteriosus before birth.

2.6. Isovolumetric contraction is closely associated with

a. the first heart sound.
b. the P wave of the ECG.

T F

c. a falling pressure in the aorta.
d. a 'c' wave in the right atrium
e. a closed tricuspid, mitral, pulmonary and aortic valve.

2.7 During the ventricular ejection phase of the normal human cardiac cycle,
a. ejection takes less time than filling, in a resting human.
b. the left ventricle diameter decreases *and* the ventricle shortens from base to apex.
c. papillary muscles close the atrioventricular valves.
d. the apex beat is best felt in the anterior axillary line, fifth intercostal space.
e. the chordae tendineae are tensed.

2.8. Regarding cardiac ejection,
a. the opening of the aortic and pulmonary valves causes the first heart sound.
b. ventricular pressure rises more quickly during early ejection than during isovolumetric contraction.
c. the aortic valve stays open for some time after ventricular pressure has fallen below aortic pressure.
d. aortic valve incompetence creates a mid-systolic murmur.

2.9 During the human cardiac cycle,
a. the 'a' wave of atrial pressure coincides with the arterial pulse.
b. the 'v' wave of the jugular pulse coincides with the P wave of the ECG.
c. ejection reduces ventricular blood volume by more than 90% at rest.
d. ventricular pressure falls soon after the T wave of the ECG.
e. the first heart sound follows immediately after the arterial pulse.

2.10 In the human neck the jugular venous
a. pressure increases on standing up.
b. pulse is exaggerated if tricuspid incompetence develops.
c. pressure is raised in right ventricular failure.
d. 'a' wave is exaggerated in atrial fibrillation.
e. pulse is exaggerated in patients with complete heart block when a P wave occurs between the QRS and T wave.

2.11 In the classic pressure–volume loop of the left ventricle,
a. the right-hand vertical line represents isovolumetric relaxation.
b. the top left corner represents aortic valve closure.
c. the bottom right corner represents tricuspid valve closure.
d. the width of the loop represents stroke work.
e. the area of the loop represents cardiac output.

2.12 With respect to the cardiac valves,
a. the mitral valve closes at the end of isovolumetric contraction.
b. mitral valve incompetence produces a pansystolic murmur.
c. the aortic valve closes at the onset of isovolumetric relaxation.
d. the aortic valve usually has two cusps.
e. the tricuspid valve opens during the rapid filling phase of the cycle.

T F

2.13 The aortic valve

a. cusps comprise vascular myocytes covered by endothelium. ☐ ☐
b. is just superior to the openings of the coronary arteries. ☐ ☐
c. is prevented from collapsing by chordae tendineae. ☐ ☐
d. provides the first component of a split second heart sound. ☐ ☐
e. when stenosed creates a systolic crescendo–decrescendo murmur. ☐ ☐

2.14 During cardiac auscultation,

a. the second heart sound marks closure of the tricuspid and mitral valve. ☐ ☐
b. the first heart sound is associated with the opening of the aortic and pulmonary valves. ☐ ☐
c. tricuspid murmurs are heard best at the lower left sternal border. ☐ ☐
d. the aortic area is the second right intercostal space adjacent to the sternum. ☐ ☐
e. murmurs heard best at the cardiac apex typically arise from the pulmonary valve. ☐ ☐

2.15 The second heart sound

a. is caused in part by the mitral valve opening. ☐ ☐
b. occurs at the end of atrial systole. ☐ ☐
c. is closely followed by a fall in ventricular pressure. ☐ ☐
d. shows splitting that is increased by inspiration. ☐ ☐
e. immediately precedes the T wave of the ECG. ☐ ☐

2.16 In the clinical assessment of the cardiovascular system

a. radial artery palpation during sphygmomanometry provides an initial estimate of diastolic pressure. ☐ ☐
b. a highly irregular radial pulse may indicate atrial fibrillation. ☐ ☐
c. a pulse rate of 40 beats/min may indicate complete heart block. ☐ ☐
d. the jugular venous pulse is normally visible in the neck of a human sitting upright. ☐ ☐
e. an early diastolic murmur may indicate mitral valve incompetence. ☐ ☐

For a change, here is a simple numerical problem.

2.17 The pressure–volume loop of a human left ventricle had end-systolic and end-diastolic volumes of 42 and 120 ml, respectively, the mean diastolic and mean systolic pressures were 8 and 88 mmHg, respectively, and aortic pressure was 119/79 mmHg.

a. What was the subject's stroke volume?
b. How much did systole raise the mean left ventricular pressure?
c. What, approximately, was the subject's stroke work?
d. What was the arterial pulse pressure?

Answers

2.1 a. **F** – The ductus arteriosus shunts blood *from* the pulmonary trunk *into* the aorta, to bypass the lungs.
b. **T** – The foramen ovale in the interatrial wall shunts blood from the right to left atrium, thus bypassing the unused fetal lungs.
c. **F** – The coronary sinus **(Figure 2.1)** is the main drainage vessel for coronary blood; it develops very early in the embryo.
d. **F** – A septal defect alone does not cause cyanosis. Pressures are higher on the left side than the right **(Table 2.1)**. Consequently, blood flow through the defect is from left (oxygenated) to right.
e. **T** – Fallot's tetralogy comprise the aortic orifice overlying the ventricular septum, a ventricular septal defect, a narrow pulmonary trunk and a hypertrophied right ventricle.

2.2 a. **T** – The left atrium has to fill the thick-walled, relatively stiff left ventricle, so it has to exert a higher pressure than the right atrium **(Table 2.1)**.
b. **F** – Most filling is passive and occurs before atrial contraction **(Figures 2.2 and 2.3)**.
c. **T** – Rapid filling occurs in early diastole **(Figures 2.2)**. This is important because, as heart rate increases (exercise), diastolic interval shortens **(Figure 2.4)**.
d. **F** – The atria contract first to boost the filling of the still-relaxed ventricles **(Figure 2.2)**.
e. **F** – The pacemaker (SA node) is in the right atrium.

2.3 a. **T** – Since the right ventricle has a thin, compliant wall, the right atrium only needs to exert a low pressure to fill it **(Table 2.1)**.
b. **F** – Work = increase in pressure × volume displaced. The right side pumps to a lower pressure than the left, so it does less work.
c. **F** – The first heart sound is made by the closure of the mitral and tricuspid valves as pressure begins to rise in the ventricles. This happens at the *start* of the isovolumetric contraction phase **(Figure 2.2)**.
d. **T** – The ejection fraction in a healthy human is 67% at rest and more during exercise.
e. **T** – The QRS complex, created by the action potential upstroke in the excited ventricles, must precede contraction **(Figure 2.2)**.

2.4 a. **F** – Filling does not start until the atrioventricular valves open at the end of the next phase, the isovolumetric relaxation phase **(Figure 2.2)**.
b. **T** – As heart rate increases, diastole shortens **(Figure 2.4)**. Consequently, the atrial 'boost' to filling becomes increasingly important.
c. **T** – The initial rapid filling phase in diastole can cause a low third sound, especially in young people.
d. **T** – The recoil has a sucking effect during early diastole.
e. **T** – Increased filling stretches the ventricular myocytes, which raises their contractile energy. This is Starling's law of the heart.

2.5 a. **F** – The *tricuspid* valve connects the right atrium to the right ventricle **(Figure 2.1)**.
b. **F** – Each ventricle ejects the same stroke volume on average.
c. **T** – Mixed venous blood is about three-quarters saturated with O_2 in a resting human.
d. **F** – Systolic pressure in the low-resistance pulmonary circulation is only ~25 mmHg in a resting human **(Figure 1.6)**.
e. **F** – The ductus arteriosus connects the pulmonary trunk to the aorta before birth, diverting the right ventricular output away from the unused lungs.

2.6 a. **T** – The sharp rise in ventricular pressure closes the mitral and tricuspid valves **(Figure 2.2)**.
b. **F** – The P wave marks atrial depolarization, which long precedes ventricular contraction. **(Figure 2.2)**.
c. **T** – At this point in the cycle, blood is leaving the aorta for the periphery and not entering it from the ventricle, so aortic pressure is falling **(Figure 2.2)**.
d. **T** – The atrial 'c' wave is created by the bulging of the tricuspid valve back into the right atrium as right ventricle pressure rises **(Figure 2.2)**.
e. **T** – This is why each ventricle is isovolumetric – both the inlet and outlet valves are closed.

2.7 a. **T** – Systole occupies only a third of the cycle at rest **(Figure 2.4)**.
b. **T** – The ventricle contracts in all three dimensions.
c. **F** – Pressure closes the valves; the papillary contraction tenses the chordae tendineae to prevent valve inversion **(Figure 2.1)**.
d. **F** – The apex beat is normally best felt in the *mid-clavicular* line, fifth interspace **(Figure 2.5)**.
e. **T** – Tension in the chordae prevents valve eversion during systolic shortening **(Figure 2.1)**.

2.8 a. **F** – The opening of healthy valves is silent. The first heart sound is caused by mitral and tricuspid valve closure **(Figure 2.2)**.
b. **F** – Pressure rises fastest when no blood can escape, i.e. during isovolumetric contraction. dP/dt_{max} serves as a cardiological index of contractility **(Figure 2.2)**.
c. **T** – This is because the escaping blood has to be decelerated to zero velocity by a reversed pressure gradient before the valve leaflets can close **(Figure 2.2)**.
d. **F** – The murmur of aortic regurgitation occurs in early diastole **(Figure 2.6, bottom)**.

2.9 a. **F** – The 'a' is for atrial contraction, which long precedes the arterial pulse **(Figure 2.2)**.
b. **F** – The 'v' is for ventricular contraction, which coincides with the ST segment of the ECG **(Figure 2.2)**. The P wave denotes atrial contraction and is closely followed by the 'a' wave.
c. **F** – About two-thirds (67%) is ejected at rest. The ejection fraction only reaches 90% during heavy exercise.
d. **T** – The T wave marks ventricular repolarization, hence relaxation and a fall in ventricular pressure **(Figure 2.2)**.
e. **F** – The first heart sound, i.e. mitral and tricuspid closure, immediately *precedes* the arterial pulse **(Figure 2.2)**.

2.10 a. **F** – Jugular venous pressure falls on standing, due to the effect of gravity.
b. **T** – Regurgitation from the right ventricle into the right atrium and central veins creates a pathological 'v' wave that is visible in the neck.
c. **T** – This is key diagnostic sign. The raised jugular venous pressure is brought about by reduced pumping out of venous blood by the ventricle, coupled with peripheral venoconstriction and fluid retention by the kidneys.
d. **F** – The 'a' stands for atrial systole. There is no longer a co-ordinated, discrete atrial systole during atrial fibrillation, so the 'a' wave disappears.
e. **T** – The P wave marks the onset of atrial contraction. If the atria contract, yet the atrioventricular valves remain closed (as during the ST period when the ventricle is contracting), a wave of raised pressure shoots up the jugular veins.

2.11 a. **F** – The right, vertical side denotes isovolumetric contraction **(Figure 2.7)**.
b. **T** – The top left corner marks the end of ejection as the aortic valve closes **(Figure 2.7)**.

c. **F** – The bottom right corner marks *mitral* valve closure, because the loop depicts the *left* ventricle.
d. **F** – The width of the loop equals the stroke volume **(Figure 2.7)**.
e. **F** – Cardiac output is heart rate × stroke volume. The area of the loop, pressure × volume, is called the stroke work.

2.12 a. **F** – The mitral valve closes at the *onset* of isovolumetric contraction **(Figure 2.2)**.
b. **T** – The pansystolic murmur is due to regurgitation into the left atrium throughout systole **(Figure 2.6, middle)**.
c. **T** – This produces a notch, the incisura, in the arterial pressure trace **(Figure 2.2)**.
d. **F** – The aortic valve usually has three cusps. Occasional individuals with two cusps are more prone to aortic valve stenosis.
e. **T** – This allows blood to enter from the right atrium.

2.13 a. **F** – All valves consist of *fibrous tissue* covered by endothelium.
b. **F** – The coronary ostia are just superior to the valve, in the sinuses of Valsalva **(Figure 2.1)**.
c. **F** – The aortic valve has no chordae tendineae or associated papillary muscle **(Figure 2.1)**.
d. **T** – The aortic valve closes slightly before the pulmonary valve **(Figure 2.2)**.
e. **T** – The turbulence waxes and wanes as ejection waxes and wanes **(Figure 2.6, top)**.

2.14 a. **F** – Heart sound 2 marks closure of aortic and pulmonary valves **(Figure 2.2)**.
b. **F** – Heart sound 1 marks closure of the atrioventricular valves. The aortic and pulmonary valve are already closed **(Figure 2.2)**.
c. **T** – This is because the sound projects into the chamber that the valve feeds – the right ventricle in the case of the tricuspid valve **(Figure 2.8)**.
d. **T** – For similar reasons to 'c', see **Figure 2.8**.
e. **F** – The apex region is actually the mitral valve auscultation area **(Figure 2.8)**.

2.15 a. **F** – Heart sound 2 is caused by the closure of the aortic and pulmonary valves **(Figure 2.2)**.
b. **F** – Atrial systole long precedes ventricular ejection and heart sound 2 **(Figure 2.2)**.
c. **T** – The fall in pressure occurs during the isovolumetric relaxation phase **(Figure 2.2)**.
d. **T** – Inspiration boosts right ventricular filling, prolonging its ejection duration. Inspiration also reduces left ventricle filling due to pulmonary vascular expansion, shortening left ventricle ejection duration.
e. **F** – Repolarization (the T wave) precedes the cessation of ejection and therefore the T wave precedes valve closure and the second sound **(Figure 2.2)**.

2.16 a. **F** – The radial pulse is first detected when cuff pressure is lowered just below *systolic* pressure.
b. **T** – When the atria are in fibrillation, transmission through the AV node is very irregular. Consequently, the pulse is 'irregularly irregular' **(Figure 4.3f)**.
c. **T** – When conduction from the atria to ventricles fails (heart block), the atrial pacemaker can no longer activate the ventricle. A much slower pacemaker located in the ventricular conduction system then takes over **(Figure 4.3e)**. In athletes, a slow heart rate can be due to vagal inhibition of the pacemaker.
d. **F** – The jugular vein is normally collapsed in an upright subject, due to the action of gravity **(Figure 8.24)**.
e. **F** – Mitral valve incompetence causes backflow throughout systole, creating a pansystolic murmur **(Figure 2.6, middle)**.

2.17 a. 78 ml. Stroke volume is end-diastolic volume (120 ml) minus end-systolic volume (42 ml) **(Figure 2.7)**.

b. 80 mmHg – i.e. mean systolic pressures 88 mmHg minus mean diastolic pressure 8 mmHg **(Figure 2.7)**.

c. 6240 ml.mmHg. Stroke work is increase in pressure × volume ejected, i.e. 80 mmHg × 78 ml. Stroke work is the area inside the pressure–volume loop.

d. 40 mmHg. Pulse pressure is systolic pressure, 119 mmHg, minus diastolic pressure, 79 mmHg **(Figure 8.7)**.

CHAPTER 3

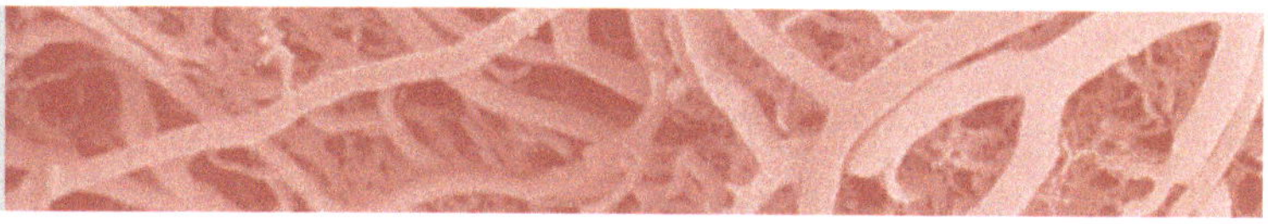

Cardiac myocyte excitation and contraction

T F

3.1 The myocardium

a. contains myocytes that depolarize spontaneously.
b. contains myocytes that do not depolarize spontaneously.
c. is excited fractionally earlier in the right atrium than the left atrium.
d. conducts propagating currents directly from atrial to ventricular myocytes.
e. exhibits the phenomenon of 'dominance'.

3.2 Ventricular myocytes

a. are non-striated muscle fibres.
b. comprise approximately one-third mitochondria by volume, due to a dependence on aerobic metabolism.
c. are electrically insulated from one another by gap junctions.
d. are bound together by cadherin molecules at desmosomes junctions.
e. differ from skeletal muscle fibres by lacking a transverse tubular system.

3.3 Concerning myocardial contractile proteins,

a. the thick filament is a polymer of actin molecules.
b. the filaments between two Z lines make up a sarcomere.
c. myosin-binding sites on actin are blocked during diastole by K^+ ions.
d. myosin-binding sites on actin are indirectly activated in systole by Ca^{2+} ions.
e. the force of contraction is independent of the number of crossbridges formed.

3.4 The sarcoplasm of a resting cardiac myocyte

a. has a K^+ concentration 30–40 times higher than that of extracellular fluid.
b. has a high Na^+ concentration, due to the sarcolemmal Na-K pump.
c. has a low Ca^{2+} concentration in diastole, due partly to a sarcolemmal Na^+–Ca^{2+} exchanger.
d. is in ionic equilibrium with the sarcoplasmic reticulum.
e. has a raised Na^+ concentration in the presence of digoxin.

3.5 The resting membrane potential of a ventricular myocyte

a. is around −80 volts.
b. is generated chiefly by the electrogenic effect of the $3Na^+$–$2K^+$ pump.
c. is nearly, but not quite, a Nernst equilibrium potential for K^+.
d. is made less negative by a background inward current of Na^+ ions.
e. is reduced by hyperkalaemia.

T F

3.6 The action potential of a human ventricular myocyte

a. has a duration of 20–30 milliseconds.
b. has a long duration due mainly to the prolonged activation of Na^+ channels.
c. exhibits a plateau, during which the ventricle is already contracting.
d. is associated with an early fall in sarcolemmal permeability to K^+ ions.
e. has a shorter duration in subepicardial than subendocardial myocytes.

3.7. The action potential of an atrial or ventricular myocyte

a. reaches +20–30 mV, due to the opening of voltage-sensitive sodium channels.
b. is triggered by sympathetic nerve fibres.
c. is associated with an influx of extracellular Ca^{2+} ions into the myocyte.
d. causes a release of Ca^{2+} ions from a store within the myocyte.
e. is prolonged by β_1-adrenoceptor stimulation.

3.8. Concerning the excitation of a cardiac ventricular myocyte,

a. Na^+ influx during the action potential raise the intracellular Na^+ concentration by ~10%.
b. a very slow depolarization closes many Na^+ channels.
c. the plateau inward current is increased by sympathetic stimulation.
d. the absolute refractory period is approximately as long as active contraction.
e. repolarization is brought about mainly by the $3Na^+$–$2K^+$ pump.

3.9 During cardiac excitation–contraction coupling,

a. extracellular Ca^{2+} entry triggers the contractile process.
b. the contractile force is proportional to the amount of Ca^{2+} released from the sarcoplasmic reticulum.
c. the re-uptake of Ca^{2+} into the SR store is brought about chiefly by the Na^+–Ca^{2+} exchanger.
d. the sarcoplasmic store of Ca^{2+} can be enhanced by sympathetic stimulation.
e. the sarcoplasmic store of Ca^{2+} can be reduced by digoxin.

3.10. The force of cardiac contraction can be raised by

a. caffeine, which raises intracellular cyclic AMP.
b. shortening the sarcomere during diastole.
c. adrenaline, which increases sarcolemmal Ca^{2+} channel activity.
d. the phosphodiesterase inhibitor milrinone, which reduce intracellular cyclic AMP.
e. verapamil and diltiazem, which inhibit potassium channels.

3.11 A delayed after-depolarization (DAD) is

a. a premature depolarization during repolarization (phase 3).
b. often associated with a high cardiac sympathetic activity.
c. triggered by a sudden uptake of Ca^{2+} by the sarcoplasmic reticulum
d. mediated by an increased turnover of the sarcolemmal Na^+–Ca^{2+} exchanger.
e. a common trigger for arrhythmia in an ischaemic heart.

Here is a little numerical problem to round off this section. You will need a pocket calculator.

3.12 Regarding cardiac membrane potentials and electrolyte concentrations, the following table summarizes ion concentrations in the resting cardiac myocyte cytosol and in the surrounding interstitial fluid.

	Intracellular C_i (mM)	Extracellular C_o (mM)
K^+	130	3.5
Na^+	10	140
Ca^{2+}	0.0001	1.2

a. What intracellular potential would just prevent K^+ diffusion out of the cell, yet not draw K^+ ions into the cell? (Hint: what is the K^+ equilibrium potential for this cell?) If the potential is actually −80 mV, which direction will K^+ ions move through K^+-conducting sarcolemmal channels?

b. If the patient experienced hyperkalaemia, namely a plasma K^+ concentration of 10 mM, how would this affect the K^+ equilibrium potential and cardiac resting membrane potential?

c. During the action potential, the membrane potential was +5 mV shortly after the initial spike, and the cytosolic Ca^{2+} concentration increased 20-fold to 0.002 mM. Would the positive intracellular potential result in Ca^{2+} ions moving into or out of the cell, through the open Ca^{2+}-conducting channels?

Answers

3.1 a. **T** – Pacemaker cells and Purkinje fibres **(Figure 3.1)** depolarize spontaneously albeit at different rates. Both are specialized types of cardiac myocytes.
b. **T** – The vast majority of cardiac myocytes do not depolarize spontaneously. The ventricular myocyte is an example **(Figure 3.1)**.
c. **T** – The pacemaker (sino-atrial node) is in the right atrium, near the superior vena cava junction **(Figure 3.2)**. Consequently, the right atrial myocytes are activated earliest.
d. **F** – The fibrotendinous ring (annulus fibrosus) blocks direct conduction **(Figure 2.5)**. The only electrically conductive connection is the bundle of His **(Figure 3.2)**.
e. **T** – The SA pacemaker dominates myocytes with a lower depolarization rate, such as the Purkinje fibres. The slower pacemakers are revealed in heart block.

3.2 a. **F** – The sarcomeres are aligned in register by Z lines, so cardiac myocytes appear striated **(Figure 3.3)**.
b. **T** – The abundance of mitochondria is shown in **Figure 3.3**. Myocyte contractility is tightly coupled to mitochondrial ATP generation by oxidative phosphorylation.
c. **F** – Gap junctions are formed by connexons. Connexons link the cytoplasm of adjacent myocytes. Consequently, myocardium behaves like an electrically continuous sheet – an 'electrical syncytium' **(Figure 3.3)**.
d. **T** – The desmosomes rivet the cells together in the intercalated disc **(Figure 3.3)**.
e. **F** – The invaginating, transverse tubular system is well developed in ventricular myocytes, though not in atrial myocytes **(Figure 3.3)**.

3.3 a. **F** – The thick filament consists of ~400 myosin molecules **(Figure 3.4)**.
b. **T** – The thin actin filaments on either side of the thick filament are rooted in the Z lines, making up a sarcomere **(Figure 3.3)**.
c. **F** – They are blocked by tropomyosin **(Figure 3.4)**.
d. **T** – The blocking tropomyosin is shifted out of the way when the troponin complex is activated by Ca^{2+} ions **(Figure 3.4)**.
e. **F** – Force is directly proportional to the number of crossbridges.

3.4 a. **T** – Intracellular [K^+] is typically 140 mM, extracellular concentration is ~4 mM K^+, and the ratio is ~35 **(Table 3.1)**.
b. **F** – The pump extrudes Na^+ from the cell, so intracellular Na^+ is only ~10 mM, compared with 140 mM in extracellular fluid **(Figure 3.5)**.
c. **T** – In its usual 'forward' mode, the exchanger transfers Ca^{2+} outwards, driven by a Na^+ influx down the Na^+ concentration gradient **(Figure 3.5)**.
d. **F** – The SR stores Ca^{2+} at a far higher concentration (~1 mM) than in the sarcoplasm (0.1 µM at rest) **(Figure 3.6)**.
e. **T** – Digoxin's primary action is to inhibit the Na^+–K^+ pump. The resulting rise in intracellular Na^+ reduces the Na^+ gradient driving the Na–Ca exchanger, so intracellular Ca^{2+} levels increase too **(Figure 3.6)**.

3.5 a. **F** – Membrane potential is around −80 *milli*volts **(Figure 3.1)**.
b. **F** – The pump contributes only a few mV. The potential is set up mainly by the diffusion of K^+ ions out of the cell through inward rectifier K^+ channels, K_{ir} **(Figure 3.5)**.
c. **T** – At the Nernst equilibrium potential, the outward diffusion tendency is exactly offset by the inward electrical attraction for the cation. For K^+, this would happen at around −94 mV.

d. **T** – An inward Na^+ 'leak' reduces the membrane potential to below the Nernst value **(Figure 3.5)**.
e. **T** – Hyperkalaemia depolarizes the myocyte **(Figure 3.7)**. This follows from the Nernst equation, which states that the potential depends on the logarithm of the ratio of ion concentration inside and outside the membrane **(Figure 3.8)**. The logarithm of 1 (equal concentrations) is zero.

3.6 a. **F** – A cardiac action potential lasts much longer, 200–300 ms **(Figure 3.1)**.
b. **F** – The long plateau is caused by Ca^{2+}-channel activation, and later the $3Na^+$–Ca^{2+} exchanger current.
c. **T** – Contraction begins soon after the initial depolarization; ejection has already peaked by the end of the plateau **(Figure 3.9)**.
d. **T** – The reduced open-state of the inward rectifier channel K_{ir} reduces K^+ ion loss during the long cardiac action potential **(Figure 3.10)**.
e. **T** – This determines the QT interval of an ECG and accounts for the fact that the T wave is upright, even though repolarization is the reverse of depolarization **(Figure 5.2)**.

3.7 a. **T** – The peak of the action potential approaches, but does not quite reach, the Nernst Na^+ equilibrium potential of +70 mV **(Figure 3.1)**.
b. **F** – Unlike skeletal muscle, cardiac contraction is not initiated by external motor nerves. It is initiated by an internal pacemaker, the SA node.
c. **T** – Depolarization activates voltage-dependent L-type Ca^{2+} channels in the T-tubules and surface sarcolemma, allowing extracellular Ca^{2+} ions to move down the steep concentration gradient **(Figure 3.6)**.
d. **T** – Although extracellular Ca^{2+} influx accounts for 10–25% of the rise in intracellular Ca^{2+}, three-quarters or more comes from the partial discharge of the sarcoplasmic reticulum store, triggered by calcium-induced calcium release **(Figure 3.6)**.
e. **F** – Sympathetic noradrenaline and circulating adrenaline activate β_1-adrenoceptors on the myocytes. This shortens the action potential, so that more can be fitted into each minute as the heart rate increases **(Figure 3.11)**.

3.8 a. **F** – The number of Na^+ ions entering the cell per action potential is very small relative to the number present – around 0.02% – so intracellular Na^+ concentration is not materially altered by a single action potential.
b. **T** – Although rapid depolarization activates voltage-gated Na^+ channels, slow depolarization (e.g. by chronic hyperkalaemia) allows time for the inactivation gates to close **(Figure 3.12)**.
c. **T** – Beta-adrenergic stimulation increase the inward Ca^{2+} current, leading to a dome-shaped plateau and increased contractility **(Figure 3.11)**.
d. **T** – The absolute refractory period extends from the onset of depolarization to mid-repolarization, by which time relaxation is just beginning **(Figure 3.9)**.
e. **F** – Repolarization is brought about mainly by a passive outward K^+ current through K_v and K_{ir} channels **(Figure 3.13)**.

3.9 a. **T** – Ca^{2+} influx through L-type Ca^{2+} channels activates Ca^{2+}-release channels (ryanodine receptors) on the sarcoplasmic reticulum. This raises cytosolic Ca^{2+} concentration sufficiently to initiate contraction **(Figure 3.6)**.
b. **T** – The number of crossbridges formed is proportional to cytosolic Ca^{2+} concentration.
c. **F** – Ca^{2+} re-uptake into the SR store is due chiefly to an energy-dependent Ca^{2+}-ATPase pump **(Figure 3.6)**.

d. **T** – Beta-adrenoceptor activation by the sympathetic neurotransmitter noradrenaline (1) stimulates the SR Ca^{2+} pump (by reducing the tonic inhibition of the pump by phospholamban) and (2) increases extracellular Ca^{2+} influx through sarcolemmal L-type Ca^{2+} channels **(Figure 3.14)**.

e. **F** – Digoxin increases the SR Ca^{2+} store and thus the size of the systolic Ca^{2+} transient **(Figure 3.15)**. The primary action of digoxin is to inhibit, partially, the sarcolemmal Na–K pump **(Figure 3.6)**. The ensuing rise in intracellular Na^+ reduces the gradient driving the sarcolemmal Na^+–Ca^{2+} exchanger, so less Ca^{2+} is expelled from the cell.

3.10 a. **T** – Caffeine inhibits phosphodiesterase III, the enzyme that normally breaks down cAMP **(Figure 3.14)**. Caffeine therefore raises cAMP, just like adrenaline and noradrenaline.

b. **F** – *Stretch* increases contractile force, by increasing the sensitivity of the actin-myosin to Ca^{2+}. This is the cellular basis of Starling's law of the heart.

c. **T** – In addition, adrenaline disinhibits the SR Ca^{2+} pump to increase store size **(Figure 3.14)**. Adrenaline acts by activating the β-adrenoceptor-cAMP pathway.

d. **F** – Inhibitors of phosphodiesterase III (milrinone and amrinone) *raise* cAMP levels and hence contractile force **(Figure 3.14)**. They are sometimes used to support the acutely failing heart.

e. **F** – These drugs are cardiac Ca^{2+} channel blockers, so they weaken the heart beat.

3.11 a. **F** – This would be an *early* after-depolarization (EAD). A DAD occurs during diastole **(Figure 3.16)**.

b. **T** – Excessive β-adrenoceptor stimulation by high sympathetic activity can overload the SR store with Ca^{2+}. Store release in diastole causes the DAD.

c. **F** – A DAD is initiated by a sudden spontaneous *discharge* of the SR Ca^{2+} store **(Figure 3.16)**.

d. **T** – The rise in sarcoplasmic Ca^{2+} increases the forward-mode turnover of the $3Na^+$–Ca^{2+} exchanger to expel Ca^{2+}. The turnover carries a net depolarizing positive charge (Na^+) into the cell.

e. **T** – The DAD is a common cause of arrhythmia in chronic cardiac failure and heart attacks.

3.12 To answer these questions, you need the Nernst equation, which states that no net exchange of a particular ion (X) will occur when the intracellular potential has a particular value, called the equilibrium potential (E, in mV), that is given by:

$$E_X = (61.5/z_x)\log_{10}(C_o/C_i)$$

where z_x is the ion valency.

a. For the given K^+ concentrations, E_K equals $(61.5/1)\log_{10}(3.5/130)$. This is 96.5 mV. In other words, an intracellular potential of −96.5 mV would just prevent net K^+ loss or entry through K^+-conducting channels. Since the membrane potential (−80 mV) is not that big, K^+ ions will diffuse out of the cell down the concentration gradient.

b. Substituting C_o = 10 mM into the Nernst equation, we get E_K = −68.5 mV. Since the membrane potential depends primarily on E_K, the cell will depolarize, from its normal value of −80 mV to some value less than −68.5 mV. This can trigger arrhythmia.

c. At this instant during the action potential, the equilibrium potential for Ca^{2+} (valency +2) would be $(61.5/2)\log_{10}(1.2/0.002) = +85$ mV. Since the intracellular potential is actually only +5 mV, there is no equilibrium for the Ca^{2+}; Ca^{2+} ions will enter the cell down the steep concentration gradient.

CHAPTER 4 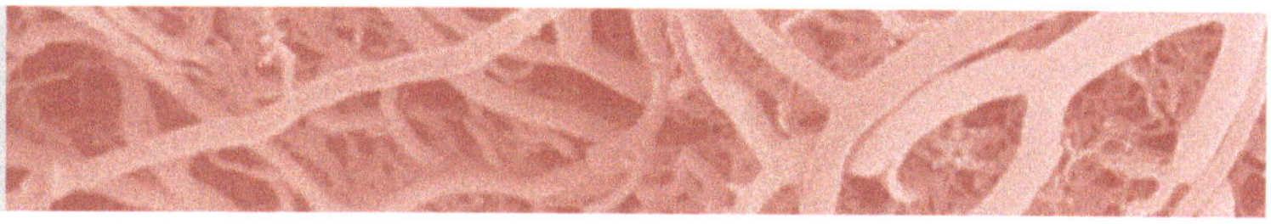

Initiation and nervous control of heart beat

T F

4.1 The sino-atrial node

a. cells depolarize faster at 39°C than 37°C. ☐ ☐
b. is connected electrically to the AV node by Purkinje fibres. ☐ ☐
c. has a parasympathetic innervation whereas the AV node does not. ☐ ☐
d. cells depolarize faster in the presence of acetylcholine. ☐ ☐
e. is the only pacemaking tissue in the mammalian heart. ☐ ☐

4.2 The membrane of a human sino-atrial node cell (pacemaker)

a. has an intracellular potential of -80 to -90 mV during diastole. ☐ ☐
b. can be hyperpolarized by acetylcholine during diastole. ☐ ☐
c. has a greater permeability to Na^+ than to K^+ during diastole. ☐ ☐
d. is well endowed with β_1-adrenoceptors. ☐ ☐
e. depolarizes spontaneously in under 1 second in most humans. ☐ ☐

For a change, try this 'choose the best answer' style of question (extended matching question, EMQ). Any word from the list can be used once, more than once, or not at all, to fill in the blanks in the text.

4.3 Concerning the cardiac pacemaker,

The decay of the pacemaker potential is, in the early stages, due to decay in sarcolemmal permeability to ______ as the ______ (K_v) slowly inactivates. This causes the polarizing current, ______, to decay with time and allows several inward ______ currents to dominate. Many pacemaker cells have a specialized, inward current of ______ called the ______, which is peculiar in that it is activated by ______, not ______ – in contrast to the ______ of ventricular mycocytes. Since ______, a recently introduced i_f blocker, does not stop the pacemaker decay completely, there are clearly additional pacemaking currents. Two such ______-directed currents are the ______ and, as the potential decays beyond -55 mV, an inward current of ______ passing through voltage operated ______ and ______. When the pacemaker potential reaches ______, it triggers an ______. The nodal action potential is small and sluggish, because the node has few functional ______. The nodal action potential is generated solely by an inward ______, which can be inhibited by ______. Repolarization is brought about by an ______ current of ______ through the ______, a voltage-gated channel that is activated very slowly by depolarization.

Choose from:

sodium ions	outward	hyperpolarization	voltage-operated Na^+ channels
potassium ions	inward	depolarization	delayed rectifier K^+ channel
calcium ions	outward current i_K	action potential	chloride channels
'funny' current, i_f	depolarizing	threshold	acetylcholine
Ca^{2+} current	hyperpolarizing	verapamil	T-type Ca^{2+} channels
3Na + $-1Ca^{2+}$ exchanger current	propanolol	ivabradine	L-type Ca^{2+} channels

T F

4.4 The atrioventricular node

a. is located in the upper interventricular septum.
b. delays the transmission of electrical excitation to the ventricles.
c. is connected to the left and right bundle branches via the bundle of His.
d. is normally one of several electrical connections across the annulus fibrosus.
e. transmits excitation more quickly during sympathetic stimulation.

4.5 The Purkinje fibres of the heart

a. are nerve fibres that conduct excitation rapidly to the ventricles.
b. are the narrowest cells in the ventricles.
c. can conduct impulses as fast as some sensory nerves.
d. excite the subendocardial myocytes before the subepicardial myocytes.
e. excite the interventricular septum last.

4.6 The propagation of electrical excitation across the heart

a. requires the transmission of intracellular ions from one myocyte into its neighbour.
b. generates the clinical electrocardiogram.
c. is mediated by the desmosomes joining adjacent myocytes.
d. is faster for rapidly depolarizing, large action potentials than for slowly depolarizing, small action potentials.
e. is speeded up by myocardial ischaemia.

4.7 An increase in the activity of cardiac sympathetic fibres

a. increases the heart rate.
b. reduces the slope of the pacemaker potential.
c. lengthens the myocardial action potential.
d. increases contractile force and stroke volume.
e. increase the rate of relaxation during diastole.

4.8 The stimulation of cardiac β-adrenoceptors by sympathetic fibres

a. inhibits adenylate cyclase via β_1-receptor activated G_s protein.
b. activates protein kinase A via a change in intracellular cAMP concentration.
c. increases the plateau current carried by L-type Ca^{2+} channels.
d. cause early repolarization via phosphorylation of delayed rectifier K^+ channels.
e. increases the sarcoplasmic reticulum Ca^{2+} store by inhibiting phospholamban.

4.9 The rate of beating of the human heart

a. is controlled by motor nerves innervating the ventricular muscle.
b. increases when the bundle of His is blocked.
c. commonly increases during inspiration in young people.
d. is increased by atropine.
e. can reach 250 beats per min during maximal exercise.

4.10 Increased activity of the postganglionic parasympathetic fibres to the heart

a. causes bradycardia.
b. stimulates myocardial nicotinic receptors.
c. markedly weakens ventricular contraction.

T F

d. reduces the membrane potential of sino-atrial node cells.
e. is a normal accompaniment to expiration.

4.11 Regarding the effect of the ionic composition of body fluids on the heart,

a. hypocalcaemia weakens the heart beat.
b. hyperkalaemia is a rise in plasma K^+ concentration above 3.5 mM.
c. hyperkalaemia reduces the amplitude of the cardiac action potential.
d. hyperkalaemia causes flattened T waves in the ECG.
e. intracellular acidosis increases cardiac contractility.

4.12 Cardiac performance can be manipulated pharmacologically by

a. propranolol and atenolol, which are β-blockers used to treat angina.
b. verapamil and diltiazem, which have a positive inotropic effect.
c. lignocaine, which is used as an anti-arrhythmia drug.
d. adenosine, which slows the heart by activating nodal K^+ channels.
e. ivabradine, which increases the heart rate.

Answers

4.1 a. **T** – A fever causes a fast pulse rate.

b. **F** – Atrial muscle conducts excitation from the pacemaker to the AV node. Purkinje fibres are found in the ventricles **(Figure 3.2)**.

c. **F** – Both nodes have a parasympathetic vagal innervation and a sympathetic innervation **(Figure 4.1)**.

d. **F** – Acetylcholine, the vagal parasympathetic neurotransmitter, *slows* the rate of pacemaker depolarization, causing a bradycardia **(Figure 4.2)**.

e. **F** – Cells in the AV node, bundles and Purkinje system can all pacemake, but they do so at a lower rate than the SA node. The SA node, therefore, dominates the slower pacemakers normally, but the slower pacemakers keep the ventricles beating slowly during complete heart block **(Figure 4.3e)**.

4.2 a. **F** – The SA node resting potential is relatively depolarized, namely −70 to −60 mV **(Figure 4.4)**. This is because the cells lack inward rectifier K^+ channels, K_{ir}. K_{ir} are abundant in atrial and ventricular myocytes and are mainly responsible for their very negative potentials, close to the Nernst equilibrium potential.

b. **T** – ACh, the vagal parasympathetic neurotransmitter, activates nodal K_{ACh} (K_G) channels. This increases the membrane K^+ permeability, which shifts the potential closer to the Nernst equilibrium potential of −94 mV. The resulting hyperpolarization causes a sudden bradycardia **(Figure 4.2)**.

c. **F** – A negative intracellular potential means that the cell is closer to the Nernst K^+ equilibrium potential (−94 mV) than the Na^+ equilibrium potential (+70 mV). This can only be the case if the membrane is more permeable to K^+ than Na^+.

d. **T** –Beta$_1$-adrenoceptors mediate the chronotropic effect of noradrenaline, the sympathetic neurotransmitter, and of circulating adrenaline.

e. **T** – The gradual diastolic depolarization is due initially to a 'funny' inward Na^+ current i_f coupled with a declining K^+ permeability due to K_v inactivation. A Ca^{2+} influx and $3Na^+$–$1Ca^{2+}$ exchanger current contribute to the later stages **(Figure 4.4)**. When threshold is reached, the node action potential is triggered. The decaying diastolic potential normally takes <1 s to reach the threshold, except in bradycardic athletes.

4.3 The decay of the pacemaker potential is at first due to decay in sarcolemmal permeability to **potassium ions** as the **delayed rectifier K^+ channel** (K_v) slowly inactivates. This causes the polarizing current, **outward current i_K**, to decay with time and allows several inward **depolarizing** currents to dominate. Many pacemaker cells have a specialized inward current of **sodium ions** called the **'funny' current, i_f**, which is peculiar in that it is activated by **hyperpolarization**, not **depolarization**, in contrast to the **voltage-operated Na^+ channels** of ventricular mycocytes. Since **ivabradine**, a recently introduced i_f blocker, does not stop the pacemaker decay completely, there are clearly additional pacemaking currents. Two such **inward** currents are the **3Na–1Ca^{2+} exchanger current** and, as the potential decays beyond −55 mV, an inward current of **calcium ions** passing through voltage operated **T-type Ca^{2+} channels** and **L-type Ca^{2+} channels**. When the pacemaker potential reaches **threshold**, it triggers an **action potential**. The nodal action potential is small and sluggish, because the node has few functional **voltage-operated Na^+ channels**. The nodal action potential is generated solely by an inward Ca^{2+} current, which can be inhibited by verapamil. Repolarization is brought about by an outward current of potassium ions through the delayed rectifier K^+ channel, a voltage-gated channel that is activated very slowly by depolarization.

4.4 a. F – The AV node is located in the atrial septum, close to the top of the interventricular septum (Figure 3.2).
b. T – The delay is vital, because it allows the atria time to contract before the ventricles, and thus boost ventricular filling.
c. T – The bundle of His provides a high-speed excitation pathway into the ventricles (Figure 3.2).
d. F – The AV node – His pathway is normally the sole electrical connection across the annulus fibrosus.
e. T – This is called the 'dromotropic' effect of sympathetic activity.

4.5 a. F – Purkinje fibres are specialized cardiac muscle fibres, not nerve fibres.
b. F – Purkinje fibres are the *widest* cells in the heart, enabling them to conduct very rapidly.
c. T – With a conduction velocity of 3–5 $m s^{-1}$, Purkinje fibres actually conduct faster than nociceptor C fibres (0.6–2.5 $m s^{-1}$).
d. T – This sequence of activation determines the shape of the QRS complex of the ECG.
e. F – They excite the septum first. This influences the shape of the QRS complex.

4.6 a. T – Gap junction composed of connexons provide cytoplasmic continuity between adjacent myocytes (Figures 3.3). This establishes the electrical circuit needed to transmit excitation (Figure 4.5).
b. T – The ECG is an external recording of the wave of electrical excitation and repolarization that sweeps across the heart.
c. F – Desmosomes are the non-conducting 'rivets' that hold adjacent myocytes together at the intercalated junctions. Gap junctions composed of connexons provide the electrically conducting pathway (Figure 3.3).
d. T – Large, rapid depolarizations create big currents that can extend well ahead of the active region (Figure 4.5). Hyperkalaemia causes a small, slow depolarization, and therefore slow transmission of excitation (Figure 3.7).
e. F – Ischaemia slows conduction, because it reduces the size and rate of depolarization of action potentials. It does so partly by raising the local extracellular K^+ concentration.

4.7 a. T – The activation of β_1-adrenoceptors by the sympathetic mediator, noradrenaline, increases the heart rate – the chronotropic effect (Figure 4.6).
b. F – The pacemaker slope is *increased*, so that threshold is reached in a shorter time (Figure 4.6).
c. F – The action potential duration is *shortened*, so that more beats can be fitted into each minute (Figure 3.11).
d. T – This is called the positive inotropic effect (Figure 3.11). The mechanism involves the β_1-adrenoceptor – cAMP – protein kinase A pathway, which increases the size of the Ca^{2+} store and systolic Ca^{2+} transient (Figure 3.14).
e. T – This effect is called the lusitropic effect (Figure 3.11). It is brought about by the β-adrenoceptor–cAMP–PKA pathway, which phosphorylates phospholamban, and thereby disinhibits the SR Ca^{2+} pump (Figure 3.14). Increased pump activity lowers cytosolic $[Ca^{2+}]$ faster.

4.8 a. **F** – $Beta_1$-receptors activate G_s protein, which *activates* adenylate cyclase **(Figure 3.14)**.

b. **T** – cAMP is raised through the β_1–G_s–adenylate cyclase pathway. cAMP in turn activates PKA **(Figure 3.14)**.

c. **T** – The increase is brought about by the phosphorylation of L-type Ca^{2+} channels by protein kinase A **(Figure 3.14)**. The increased Ca^{2+} current causes a 'humping' of the plateau **(Figure 3.11)** and raises contractility.

d. **T** – The activated G_s – cAMP–PKA pathway phosphorylates the K_v channels **(Figure 3.14)**. The resulting increase in repolarizing current shortens the action potential, e.g. during exercise **(Figure 3.11)**.

e. **T** – Phospholamban normally acts as a brake on the Ca^{2+}-ATPase pump of the sarcoplasmic reticulum membrane. The inhibiting of phospholamban speeds up the pump (disinhibition, **Figure 3.14**).

4.9 a. **F** – The heart rate is controlled by the autonomic nerves that innervate the SA node.

b. **F** – This condition, heart block, is associated with a very low heart rate, because a slow pacemaker in the Purkinje system takes over the excitation of the ventricles **(Figure 4.3e)**.

c. **T** – This is called sinus arrhythmia **(Figure 4.3a)**. It is caused mainly by the activity of inspiratory neurons in the brainstem, which inhibit the cardiac vagal neurons.

d. **T** – Atropine blocks muscarinic M_2 receptors, so it abolishes the tonic inhibitory action of the vagal parasympathetic transmitter, acetylcholine, on the pacemaker **(Figure 3.14)**.

e. **F** – The maximum normal human heart rate is $\sim 200\,min^{-1}$. Higher rates constitute a pathological tachycardia. They cause a decline in output, due to the curtailment of filling time as the cardiac cycle becomes excessively brief.

4.10 a. **T** – The parasympathetic neurotransmitter, acetylcholine, reduces the slope of the pacemaker potential, and also hyperpolarizes it **(Figure 4.2)**. These changes causes bradycardia – and can even arrest the heart for many seconds at the onset of a faint **(Figure 4.7)**.

b. **F** – Cardiac myocytes express *muscarinic* M_2 receptors **(Figure 3.14)**. Nicotinic receptors occur on the postganglionic sympathetic neurons in the sympathetic ganglia, where neurotransmission is cholinergic.

c. **F** – The ventricles are only sparsely innervated by parasympathetic fibres **(Figure 4.1)**.

d. **F** – Acetylcholine rapidly hyperpolarizes the SA node cells, causing rapid-onset bradycardia **(Figure 4.2)**. Hyperpolarization is due to activation of a type of inward rectifier K^+ channel called the K_{ACh} or K_G channel. This channel is activated by G_i protein linked to the M_2 receptor **(Figure 3.14)**.

e. **T** – Cardiac vagal neuron activity in the brainstem is modulated by the neurons controlling breathing. Consequently, the heart rate slows during expiration (sinus arrhythmia, **Figure 4.3a**).

4.11 a. **T** – Hypocalcaemia reduces Ca^{2+} influx, and thus weakens the heart beat, as discovered by Sidney Ringer in 1883.

b. **F** – The normal range for human plasma $[K^+]$ is 3.5–5.5 mM.

c. **T** – Hyperkalaemia reduces the Nernst potential **(Figure 3.8)**. This reduces the resting membrane potential, i.e. makes it less negative **(Figure 3.7)**. The partial depolarization locks a fraction of the voltage-gated Na^+ channels in the inactivated phase of their cycle **(Figure 3.12)**. As a result, the amplitude and rate of rise of the action potential decrease **(Figure 3.7)**.

d. **F** – The T wave has an exaggerated, peaked or tent-like appearance. This is probably because the outward repolarizing K^+ current is increased, due to the activation of K^+ channels by hyperkalaemia.

e. **F** – Acidosis weakens the heart beat. This is probably because the H^+ ions reduce the amount of Ca^{2+} binding to troponin C, by competition for the binding site.

4.12 a. **T** – Beta-blockers reduce the effect of the tonic sympathetic activity on heart rate and stroke volume. Beta-blockers therefore reduce cardiac work and O_2 demand.

b. **F** – Verapamil and diltiazem are Ca^{2+}-channel inhibitors, so they have a *negative* inotropic (weakening) effect. They are sometimes used to treat hypertension or angina.

c. **T** – Lignocaine is a Na^+ channel inhibitor.

d. **T** – Intravenously, adenosine is used to terminate supraventricular tachycardia.

e. **F** – Ivabradine *slows* the heart rate (the clue is in the name!), by inhibiting the pacemaker 'funny' current i_f. Ivabradine can be used to treat angina.

CHAPTER 5

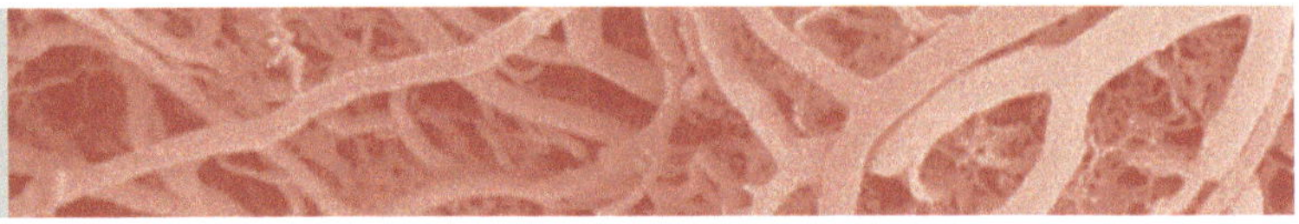

Electrocardiography and arrhythmias

T F

5.1 In the electrocardiogram (ECG) of a healthy human,

a. the P wave is generated by the pacemaker current.
b. the P–R interval is normally 0.3 seconds.
c. the QRS complex coincides with ventricular depolarization.
d. atrial repolarization generates the T wave.
e. exercise shortens the ST interval.

5.2 In the typical lead II electrocardiogram of a resting human,

a. the height of the QRS complex is approximately 100 mV.
b. the P–P interval is typically about 100 milliseconds.
c. the ST segment duration indicates, approximately, the duration of ventricular systole.
d. the T wave is upright because subendocardial action potentials last longer than subepicardial action potentials.
e. the T wave shortly precedes the second heart sound.

5.3 The cardiac dipole,

a. is a vector representing the negative and positive external charges on the heart during ventricular depolarization.
b. rotates clockwise in the frontal plane, viewed from the front.
c. at its maximum size, points along the electrical axis of the heart.
d. is recorded in the horizontal plane by limb lead III.
e. points in roughly the same direction during repolarization and depolarization.

5.4 In an ECG recording,

a. lead aVR usually resembles a lead II recording turned upside down.
b. shortening of the R–R interval during inspiration indicates sinus arrhythmia.
c. a broad, slurred QRS complex is typical of a ventricular extrasystole.
d. an R wave that is larger in lead II than leads I or III indicates left axis deviation.
e. regular P waves and regular QRS complexes can occur in complete heart block.
f. an R–R interval of about 2 seconds is associated with Stokes–Adams attacks.

5.5 In patients with a cardiac arrhythmia,

a. delayed after-depolarization can trigger a ventricular ectopic beat (extrasystole).
b. a ventricular ectopic beat is accompanied by an unusually large pulse.

T F

c. pathological ventricular tachycardia or fibrillation can be maintained by a circus pathway. ☐ ☐
d. the PR interval is the 'vulnerable period' when a ventricular ectopic is most likely to trigger ventricular fibrillation. ☐ ☐
e. atrial fibrillation causes loss of P waves and an irregularly irregular pulse. ☐ ☐

5.6 In ischaemic heart disease,

a. ST segment displacement is usually caused by injury current. ☐ ☐
b. a reversible elevation of the ST segment during exercise is typical of angina. ☐ ☐
c. reduced Q waves are typical of a full thickness (transmural) myocardial infarct. ☐ ☐
d. inverted T waves develop following a transmural infarct. ☐ ☐
e. the ECG changes caused by a heart attack (coronary artery thrombosis) alter over the course of the first week. ☐ ☐

For a change, here is a numerical problem, which will test your understanding of the cardiac dipole. You will need a calculator.

5.7 The electrical axis of a patient's heart.

An ECG recording showed an R wave 10.4 mm high in lead I and 6 mm high in lead aVF.

a. Is the size difference indicative of cardiac disease?
b. What angle in the frontal plane does a lead I recording represent?
c. What angle in the frontal plane does a lead aVF recording represent?
d. What angle is the patient's cardiac electrical axis? (Hint: review **Figure 5.3**, and remember Pythagorus from your schooldays!)
e. Is this electrical axis typical of left ventricular hypertrophy?

Answers

5.1 a. **F** – The pacemaker current is too small to register. The P wave is generated by atrial muscle depolarization **(Figure 5.1)**.

b. **F** – The interval is due chiefly to slow transmission through the AV node, and should not exceed 0.2 s **(Figure 5.1)**. An interval of 0.3 s indicates heart block **(Figure 4.3c)**.

c. **T** – The ventricles represent a large mass of muscle fibres that depolarize almost synchronously. The depolarization current generates the large QRS complex **(Figure 5.1)**.

d. **F** – The T wave is due to *ventricular* repolarization **(Figure 5.1)**. Atrial repolarization does not produce a significant deflection of the ECG, as becomes obvious during complete heart block **(Figure 4.3e)**.

e. **T** – The QT interval depends on the duration of the ventricular action potential. The latter is shortened by sympathetic stimulation during exercise **(Figure 3.11)**.

5.2 a. **F** – The QRS complex is about 1 mV **(Figure 5.1)**. Its small voltage is due to the attenuation of the signal as it passes from heart to skin. The skin potential difference is ~1% of the 100 mV action potential.

b. **F** – P–P is the time between two heart beats, which is typically ~1 s for a resting adult. At 100 ms (0.1 s) per cardiac cycle, the heart would be beating at 600 beats per minute! This may be OK for a shrew, but it would kill a human.

c. **T** – The ST segment represents the duration of the ventricle action potential. This is roughly the same as the duration of ventricular systole **(Figure 2.2)**.

d. **T** – The difference in duration is shown in **Figure 5.1**. How this gives rise to an upright T wave is explained in **Figure 5.2**.

e. **T** – As the ventricle repolarizes (T wave), it relaxes, closely followed by the closure of the aortic and pulmonary valves (second heart sound) **(Figure 2.2)**.

5.3 a. **T** – The concept of a dipole is illustrated in **Figure 5.3**.

b. **F** – The dipole rotates anticlockwise during ventricular excitation **(Figure 5.4)**.

c. **T** – This is the definition of electrical axis. It is about 40° in **Figure 5.4**.

d. **F** – Limb lead III is left arm to left leg; so it 'looks' at the dipole from an angle of 120° from the horizontal **(Figure 5.5)**.

e. **T** – This is why the T wave is in the same direction as the R wave **(Figure 5.2)**.

5.4 a. **T** – Lead aVR 'looks' at the heart from the opposite direction to lead II **(Figure 5.5)**.

b. **T** – Shortening of the R–R interval means that the heart rate has increased. This is normal during inspiration (sinus arrhythmia, **Figure 4.3a**). It is caused by the withdrawal of cardiac vagal inhibition during inspiration.

c. **T** – The QRS is broad and slurred **(Figure 4.3b)**. This is because ventricular excitation spreads out from an abnormal point in the myocardium, not via the usual fast-conducting His–Purkinje pathway.

d. **F** – Amongst the frontal leads, lead II has the biggest R wave in most normal subjects **(Figure 5.5)**. This is because the electrical axis (direction of largest dipole in frontal plane) is typically ~40–50° below the horizontal and lead II (right arm to left leg) 'looks' at the heart from a similar angle, 60° **(Figure 5.6)**. Left axis deviation would cause a large R wave in lead aVL.

e. **T** – Each is regular but dissociated from the other, i.e. the QRS waves do not follow the P waves **(Figure 4.3e)**. This is because atrial excitation is not transmitted to the ventricles. A slow, emergent pacemaker in the ventricle maintains the regular, independent ventricular beat.

f. **T** – A Stokes–Adams attack is a sudden loss of consciousness due to the very low cardiac output caused by complete heart block. The ventricular rate is 30–40 min^{-1}, driven by an emergent ventricular pacemaker **(Figure 4.3e)**.

5.5 a. **T** – If the DAD reaches threshold, it triggers a premature action potential and contraction, i.e. a ventricular extrasystole **(Figure 3.16)**.

b. **F** – The pulse is weak or undetectable, because the ventricle has not had time to fill properly (**Figure 4.3b**, upper trace).

c. **T** – The circular (circus) pathway causes the re-entry of excitation **(Figure 5.7)**.

d. **F** – The vulnerable period is the late part of the T wave **(Figure 4.3g)**. Repolarization is heterogeneous at this time point (some myocytes have repolarized, some not), creating favourable conditions for a circus pathway.

e. **T** – The transmission of excitation from a fibrillating atrium to the ventricles is very erratic, so the timing and volume of the pulse are wildly irregular **(Figure 4.3f)**.

5.6 a. **T** – The myocyte membrane potential is reduced in the affected, ischaemic region. The potential difference between these myocytes and those in healthier regions creates injury currents, which displace the ST segment **(Figure 5.8A)**.

b. **F** – The ST segment is *depressed* by the transient myocardial ischaemia as increased myocardial O_2 consumption exceeds supply **(Figure 5.8A)**. The depression disappears on terminating the exercise.

c. **F** – Deep pathological Q waves appear a few days after a full thickness infarct, due to the 'electrical window' created by cell death **(Figure 5.8B)**.

d. **T** – T wave inversion is caused by the electrical window effect **(Figure 5.8B)**.

e. **T** – In the first few hours, the infarcted cells remain electrically active, leading to ST segment elevation **(Figure 5.8B)**. Pathological Q waves and T wave inversion appear later as cells become electrically quiescent.

5.7 a. No, this is normal **(Figure 5.5)**. Each lead detects the cardiac dipole from a different angle, and accordingly 'sees' more or less of the dipole **(Figure 5.6)**.

b. Lead I is aligned horizontally, which by convention is taken to be zero degrees **(Figure 5.5)**.

c. Lead aVF is orientated 90° below the horizontal. The 'F' refers to Foot **(Figure 5.5)**.

d. Thirty degrees. Here's how. Draw a horizontal arrowed line, pointing right, 10.4 mm long (direction and size of the lead I record). Draw a second arrowed line from the same starting point, 6 mm long and pointing vertically down, i.e. at 90° to horizontal, to represent the signal recorded by lead aVF. Complete the rectangle as in **Figure 5.3**. The dipole that created these two R waves must be the diagonal *d*. The angle between the dipole and the horizontal is the electrical axis (θ in **Figure 5.3**). You could measure this with a protractor or calculate it from the length of the sides. The dipole is the hypotenuse of a right angle triangle. Pythagorus' famous theorem tells us that the square of the hypotenuse equals the sum of the squares of the other two sides; so the dipole must be 12 mm long ($12^2 = 10.4^2 + 6^2$). The sine of angle θ is, by definition, opposite/hypotenuse, or 6/12. The angle whose sine is 0.5 is 30°.

e. The electrical axis is perfectly normal here. If he/she had left ventricular hypertrophy, the angle would be less than zero, i.e. negative.

CHAPTER 6

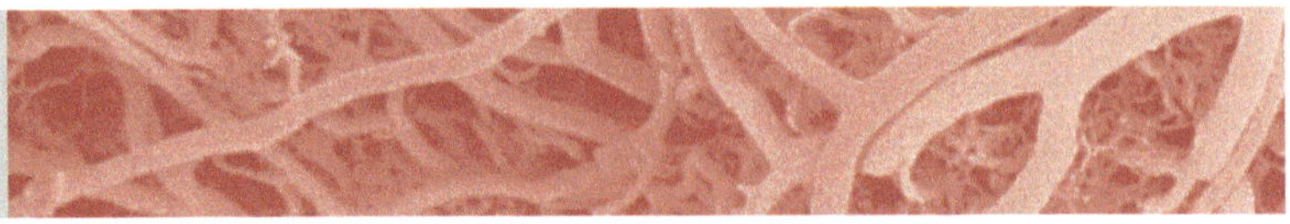

Control of stroke volume and cardiac output

T F

6.1 Cardiac output is

a. typically 4–6 l/min in a resting adult.
b. increased by a rise in central venous pressure.
c. increased by a rise in arterial blood pressure.
d. increased when circulating catecholamine concentration falls.
e. regulated by both sympathetic and parasympathetic autonomic nerves.

6.2 When a myocardial muscle strip is stimulated to contract,

a. its contractile force is increased if the muscle is first stretched by a 'preload'.
b. the contraction force has a similar sensitivity to resting sarcomere length as in skeletal muscle.
c. the development of tension without shortening is called 'isotonic contraction'.
d. stretch prior to stimulation reduces the actin–myosin sensitivity to sarcoplasmic Ca^{2+}.
e. the degree of shortening declines if the afterload is raised.

6.3 Concerning the load experienced by ventricular muscle before and during a contraction,

a. preload is the force per unit cross-sectional area of muscle during diastole.
b. preload is increased by a rise in end-diastolic pressure.
c. afterload is the ventricular wall stress after the aortic valve closes.
d. afterload is influenced by the arterial blood pressure.
e. preload and afterload are reduced by an increase in chamber radius.

6.4 The Frank–Starling mechanism

a. is an increase in cardiac contractility brought about by an increase in heart rate.
b. is mediated by the autonomic nerve fibres innervating the heart.
c. is triggered by stretch receptors in the aorta wall and carotid sinus.
d. causes stroke volume to increase when the heart is distended.
e. accounts for a reduction in arterial blood pressure following a haemorrhage.

6.5 Starling's law of the heart

a. helps equalize the outputs of the left and right ventricles.
b. brings about a fall in cardiac output when a supine person stands up.
c. accounts for most of the increase in cardiac output during exercise.
d. mediates a rise in left ventricular stroke volume during inspiration.
e. underlies the rise in arterial pressure that follows a blood transfusion.

T F

6.6 If stroke work is plotted as a function of end-diastolic pressure,

a. the vertical axis (stroke work) equals stroke volume × heart rate.
b. the horizontal axis (end-diastolic pressure) is an index of ventricular stretch at the onset of systole.
c. the ventricle is shifted up the curve by a rapid intravenous saline infusion.
d. the curve is depressed by activation of cardiac β_1 receptors.
e. movement from a low point on the curve to a higher point on the curve is called an increase in contractility.

6.7 In a plot of left ventricle pressure (vertical axis) versus left ventricle blood volume (horizontal axis),

a. the area inside the pressure–volume loop represents left ventricle stroke work.
b. the incisura of the arterial pulse coincides with the top right corner of the plot.
c. increasing the end-diastolic volume of the ventricle increases the width of the loop.
d. raising the arterial blood pressure reduces the height of the loop.
e. sympathetic stimulation increases loop area, but shifts the loop leftwards, to a smaller end-systolic and end-diastolic volume.

6.8 Cardiac filling pressure in humans

a. can be reduced by contracting the calf muscles.
b. can be raised by sympathetic vasomotor fibre activity.
c. is higher when upright than supine.
d. is reduced by a substantial haemorrhage.
e. in the upright position is increased during exercise.

6.9 Laplace's law

a. states that the pressure inside a sphere equals the wall tension × radius.
b. predicts a fall in mechanical efficiency when the heart is dilated.
c. underpins the use of diuretics to treat heart failure.
d. predicts that ventricular ejection gets easier as it proceeds.
e. like Starling's law, predicts an increase in systolic pressure generation following diastolic distension.

6.10 A rise in arterial blood pressure

a. tends to reduce left ventricular stroke volume.
b. triggers a baroreflex increase in the sympathetic drive to the heart.
c. can affect stroke volume via Starling's law of the heart.
d. lowers myocardial contractility over 5–10 min.
e. can evoke concentric left ventricular hypertrophy in the long term.

6.11 The following raise cardiac contractility:

a. noradrenaline.
b. the Frank–Starling mechanism.
c. atenolol.
d. phosphodiesterase inhibitors.
e. verapamil.
f. local ischaemia.

T F

6.12 Increased sympathetic drive to the heart

a. reduces the cardiac ejection fraction.
b. increases the rate of pressure increase during ejection.
c. increases the systolic ejection time.
d. reduces the rate of ventricular relaxation.
e. reduces ventricular volume in diastole and systole.
f. leads to a fall in coronary blood flow.

6.13 Sympathetic drive to the human heart

a. is absent at rest.
b. is high during exercise.
c. increases in response to a rise in arterial blood pressure.
d. decreases when angiotensin II levels increase.
e. increases during a mental stress test.

6.14 Propanolol

a. is a non-selective α-adrenoceptor blocker.
b. reduces myocardial oxygen demand.
c. attenuates exercise-induced tachycardia.
d. increases the stroke volume.

6.15 Acute myocardial ischaemia

a. causes intracellular alkalosis.
b. impairs ventricular contractility.
c. can cause arrhythmia through intracellular Ca^{2+} depletion.
d. increases the action potential duration and size.
e. may be followed by cell injury on reperfusion.

6.16 During upright exercise,

a. ejection pressure increases in both the right and left ventricles.
b. human left ventricular end-diastolic volume increases.
c. left ventricular end-systolic volume increases.
d. diastolic filling time increases.
e. peripheral resistance increases.

6.17 Myocardial metabolism

a. maintains a virtually constant intracellular ATP level, even at raised cardiac outputs.
b. requires so much O_2 that greater than two-thirds of coronary blood O_2 is extracted even in a resting subject.
c. and coronary blood flow increase in linear proportion during exercise.
d. uses free fatty acids as the major energy source in diabetics but not healthy subjects.
e. can utilize circulating lactate, because myocytes express lactic dehydrogenase.

Answers

6.1 a. **T** – Human cardiac output in health and ischaemic heart disease is summarized in **Table 6.1**.
b. **T** – A rise in central venous pressure (CVP) increases contractile force and therefore stroke volume (Starling's law) **(Figures 6.1 and 6.2)**.
c. **F** – Arterial pressure opposes the opening of the aortic valve, so a rise in arterial pressure reduces stroke volume **(Figures 6.1 and 6.3)**.
d. **F** – The catecholamines noradrenaline and adrenaline stimulate both heart rate **(Figure 4.6)** and contractility **(Figures 3.11)**.
e. **T** – Both branches of the autonomic system innervate the pacemaker to control heart rate; and sympathetic fibres innervate ventricular muscle to regulate contractility and stroke volume **(Figure 4.1)**.

6.2 a. **T** – This is called the 'length–tension relation' **(Figure 6.4a)**. It is the basis of Starling's law of the heart.
b. **F** – Myocardium is much more responsive to stretch than skeletal muscle **(Figure 6.5)**.
c. **F** – Tension without shortening is called 'isometric' contraction (*iso-*, same; *-metric*, length). An isotonic contraction is shortening under a constant tension (*iso-*, same, *-tonic*, tension).
d. **F** – Resting stretch *increases* the sensitivity of the contractive filaments to Ca^{2+}. Consequently, contractile force increases without requiring an increase in the sarcoplasmic free Ca^{2+} transient **(Figure 6.6)**.
e. **T** – Afterload reduces contraction velocity and degree of shortening **(Figure 6.4b,c)**. This is why a high arterial blood pressure impairs the stroke volume.

6.3 a. **T** – The term arose from experiments where weights (loads) were used to set the initial length of an isolated strip of resting muscle **(Figure 6.4, left)**. A given weight represents a bigger load for a thin muscle than a thick muscle, so the load is expressed as the force per unit cross-sectional area of muscle (stress).
b. **T** – The passive stress (tension) in the relaxed ventricle wall increases if the pressure distending the ventricle increases, i.e. end-diastolic pressure.
c. **F** – Afterload is the wall stress during systole. The term arose from studies in which an additional weight (afterload) is picked up by a muscle as it begins to contract **(Figure 6.4, left)**.
d. **T** – The higher the arterial pressure, the higher the intraventricular pressure during ejection, and therefore the higher the wall stress (afterload) during ejection.
e. **F** – From Laplace's law, wall stress = pressure × radius / $2w$, where w is wall thickness. So an increase in radius *increases* preload and afterload **(Figure 6.7)**.

6.4 a. **F** – The effect of pacing rate on contractility is called the interval–tension relation or Bowditch effect. It is of relatively little physiological importance. The Frank–Starling mechanism is an increase in contractile force in response to diastolic distension **(Figure 6.2)**.
b. **F** – The Frank–Starling mechanism (increased contractile energy in response to diastolic stretch) is an *intrinsic* property of cardiac muscle, stemming from the length–tension relation. It is present in an isolated, denervated heart **(Figure 6.2a)**.
c. **F** – The Frank–Starling mechanism is driven by increases in resting sarcomere length **(Figure 6.4a)**.
d. **T** – Starling's experiments with isolated, canine hearts showed that diastolic distension increases stroke volume. This occurs in humans too **(Figure 6.2)**.
e. **T** – Following a haemorrhage, the reduced blood volume lowers central venous pressure and cardiac distension. This reduces contractile force and stroke volume (Frank–Starling

mechanism), as in the points labelled 'phlebotomy' in **Figure 6.2b**. The fall in stroke volume reduces the arterial blood pressure.

6.5 a. **T** – Output equalization is the single most important role of Starling's law. The process is explained in **Figure 6.8**. Imagine that CVP increases or falls, then work through the sequence to see how the right and left ventricles will respond.

b. **T** – On standing up, gravity causes venous pooling in the legs, which reduces the venous filling pressure at heart level **(Figure 6.9)**. This reduces diastolic ventricular distension and, through Starling's law, stroke volume.

c. **F** – There is indeed diastolic distension during dynamic upright exercise, which triggers the Frank–Starling mechanism and contributes to a moderate increase in stroke volume **(Figure 6.10)**. However, most of the increase in cardiac output is due to the tachycardia **(Table 6.2)**.

d. **F** – Starling's law brings about a *fall* in left ventricle stroke volume and arterial blood pressure during inspiration. The lung blood vessels expand during inspiration, reducing the return of blood to the left ventricle. With less ventricular distension, the left ventricular stroke volume falls.

e. **T** – A hypovolaemic patient has a low CVP. Blood transfusion raises the CVP, which increases stroke volume by the Frank–Starling mechanism **(Figure 6.2b)**. This helps restore arterial pressure to normal.

6.6 a. **F** – Stroke volume × heart rate is cardiac output. Stroke work is stroke volume × rise in blood pressure. Stroke work equals the area inside the ventricle pressure volume loop of **Figure 2.7**.

b. **T** – The pressure filling the ventricle at the end of diastole (start of systole) governs the stretch of the muscle fibres and hence the degree of activation of the length–tension mechanism.

c. **T** – **Figure 6.11** shows a plot of stroke work versus filling pressure. An increase in blood volume increases the filling pressure of the heart – as in the points labelled 'reinfusion' and 'dextran 400 ml' in **Figure 6.2b**.

d. **F** – Sympathetic stimulation and circulating adrenaline shift the curve upwards **(Figure 6.11, arrows)**. This shift is called an increase in contractility.

e. **F** – Movement along a given curve, as in the points on **Figure 6.2**, is simply an increase in force of contraction due to stretch, i.e. the Frank–Starling (length–tension) mechanism. An increase in contractility is an increase in force of contraction at a given degree of stretch, e.g. the upward displaced ventricular function curves as in **Figure 6.11**.

6.7 a. **T** – Work is force × distance moved. For a fluid, this equates to change in pressure × change in volume. Therefore, work is the sum of all the little strips labelled $\Delta P \cdot dV$ in **Figure 6.12a**, top, i.e. the total loop area.

b. **F** – The incisura marks aortic valve closure **(Figure 2.2)**. This occurs at the top left corner of the pressure–volume loop **(Figure 6.12, point D)**.

c. **T** – The loop width is the stroke volume. An increase in end-diastolic stretch increases contractile energy (Starling's law) and hence stroke volume **(Figure 6.12b, loop 2)**.

d. **F** – The upper line of the loop represents aortic blood pressure as well as ventricular pressure, since the aortic valve is open **(Figure 2.7)**. So raising arterial pressure *increases* the loop height **(Figure 6.12b, loops 3 and 4)**.

e. **T** – Loop area (stroke work) increases, because β_1-adrenoceptor activation increases contractility **(Figure 6.13a, loop 2)**. End-systolic volumes (L side of loop) shifts to the left, because the ejection fraction has increased. The end-diastolic volume (R side of loop) shifts too, because more blood is being pumped out of the central veins, reducing central venous pressure and volume **(Figure 6.14)**. During exercise, a fall in central venous pressure is prevented by the calf muscle pump and peripheral venoconstriction **(Figure 6.13b, loop 3)**.

6.8 a. **F** – The calf muscle pump shifts venous blood into the thorax, raising central filling pressure.
b. **T** – Sympathetic venoconstriction in the renal, splanchnic and cutaneous circulations **(Figure 6.15)** reduces peripheral venous blood volume. The displaced blood moves into the central veins and thorax, raising cardiac filling pressure.
c. **F** – In the upright position, gravity distends the veins in the lower body, thereby shifting blood out of the thorax and lowering CVP **(Figure 6.9)**.
d. **T** – Blood volume is a major determinant of central venous pressure, because two-thirds of the blood is in the venous system. A fall in blood volume therefore reduces central venous pressure.
e. **T** – The calf muscle pump and peripheral venoconstriction together increase the central blood volume, which increases the diastolic filling of the heart **(Figure 6.10)**.

6.9 a. **F** – Pressure P is proportional to tension T, but *inversely* proportional to radius R. Laplace's law is $P = 2T/R$.
b. **T** – The greater the radius, the less the pressure generated by a given wall tension. This is because the angle of the tensile force become increasingly flat as radius increases **(Figure 6.7)**.
c. **T** – Failing hearts are very dilated, due to a raised filling pressure **(Figure 6.16)**. Diuretics reduce the plasma volume, which reduces the filling pressure and cardiac radius. This improves the conversion of contractile tension into systolic pressure (Laplace's law).
d. **T** – The radius of the ventricle falls as ejection proceeds, so a given systolic wall tension generates more systolic pressure, facilitating the late phase of ejection.
e. **F** – Laplace's biophysical law predicts a fall in systolic pressure as radius increases. Starling's biological law describes a rise in systolic pressure as radius increases (e.g. **Figure 6.12b, loop 2**). In normal hearts the Starling effect is bigger and 'wins'. In dilated failing hearts, the Laplace effect is bigger.

6.10 a. **T** – More of the contractile energy goes into raising the intraventricular pressure high enough to open the aortic valve, leaving less energy for ejection. This is a fundamental property of any pump, as depicted by the pump function curve **(Figure 6.3)**.
b. **F** – A rise in arterial pressure triggers a baroreflex-mediated *reduction* in cardiac sympathetic nerve activity. This reduces cardiac output, so as to bring the arterial pressure back down to normal **(Figure 6.17)**.
c. **T** – Stroke volume falls initially due to the rise in arterial pressure; but ventricular distension then increases, due to the returning blood. This increases contractile force (Starling's law) and partly restores the reduced stroke volume **(Figure 6.17)**.
d. **F** – The immediate Starling effect is followed by a *rise* in contractility over 5–10 min – the Anrep effect **(Figure 6.17)**. The Anrep effect is due to the 'slow force response' to stretch **(Figure 6.6)**.
e. **T** – Concentric hypertrophy, leading eventually to failure, is one of the complications of clinical hypertension.

6.11 a. **T** – $Beta_1$ adrenoceptor stimulation by noradrenaline, the sympathetic transmitter, increases the sarcoplasmic Ca^{2+} transient **(Figure 3.11)**.
b. **F** – An increase in contractility is defined as an increase in contractile force that is *independent of length*. It is thus a shift in the entire Starling curve **(Figure 6.11)**. Movement along a

given Starling curve alters contractile force, but not contractility. Changes in contractility require changes in the systolic Ca^{2+} transient, the Starling effect does not.

c. **F** – Atenolol is a β_1-blocker. Beta-blockers reduce the stimulatory effect of tonic sympathetic activity on contractility, so they are negative inotropes **(Figure 3.14)**.

d. **T** – Caffeine and milrinone inhibit the phosphodiesterase that breaks down cAMP, so they raise intracellular cAMP **(Figure 3.14)**. Consequently, they have a similar effect to β_1 adrenoceptor stimulation. The cAMP boosts contractility by activating protein kinase A.

e. **F** – Verapamil and diltiazem are L-type Ca^{2+} channel inhibitors, so they reduce the plateau inward Ca^{2+} current **(Figure 3.14)**. This leads to a reduced sarcoplasmic Ca^{2+} transient and reduced contractility.

f. **F** – Ischaemia causes intracellular acidosis and eventually ATP rundown, with negative inotropic effects **(Figure 6.18)**.

6.12 a. **F** – Ejection fraction is stroke volume divided by end-diastolic volume. Sympathetic stimulation *increases* the ejection fraction (normal 67%, maximum ~90%) **(Figures 6.13a loop 2, Figure 6.10)**.

b. **T** – The raised ventricular contractility increases dP/dt_{max}, which is one of several indices of contractility used by cardiologists **(Figure 6.19a)**.

c. **F** – Ejection is *faster* during sympathetic stimulation **(Figure 6.19a)**, so systole is *shorter* **(Figure 2.4)**.

d. **F** – Sympathetic stimulation *increases* the rate of relaxation **(Figure 6.19a)**. This is due to stimulation of the SR Ca^{2+} uptake pump **(Figure 3.14)**.

e. **T** – Diastolic and systolic volumes decrease **(Figure 6.19b; Figure 6.13a loop 2)**. The fall in diastolic volume is caused by a fall in CVP, brought about by the increased rate of transfer of blood out of the venous system **(Figure 6.14)**. The increased ejection fraction contributes further to the fall in end-systolic volume.

f. **F** – Coronary vessels do indeed have a sympathetic vasoconstrictor fibre innervation, yet coronary blood flow increases upon sympathetic stimulation. This is because cardiac work increases, eliciting a powerful metabolic vasodilatation of the coronary vessel **(Figures 6.20)**. The metabolic vasodilatation overwhelms the sympathetic vasoconstrictor effect.

6.13 a. **F** – Sympathetic activity is tonic and present even at rest. It partially offsets the tonic vagal (parasympathetic) drive to the pacemaker. It also contributes to coronary resistance vessel tone.

b. **T** – Increased cardiac sympathetic activity accounts for much of the increase in heart rate and stroke volume during exercise.

c. **F** – A rise in arterial pressure activates the baroreflex, which elicits a reflex *fall* in cardiac sympathetic activity **(Figure 6.21)**. The ensuing fall in heart rate and stroke volume help return the arterial pressure to normal **(Figure 6.17)**.

d. **F** – Angiotensin II *increases* sympathetic drive through multiple actions. It acts on the brainstem, the postganglionic sympathetic neurons and the sympathetic terminal varicosities to boost sympathetic activity and facilitate noradrenaline release.

e. **T** – The resulting increases in cardiac work can trigger angina in some patients with coronary artery disease.

6.14 a. **F** – Propanolol is a non-selective β-adrenoceptor blocker **(Figure 3.14)**.

b. **T** – Beta-blockers reduce the effect of sympathetic noradrenaline on the pacemaker and myocardium. They therefore reduce cardiac output and oxygen demand. Beta-blockers are therefore used to prevent attacks of angina.

c. **T** – Beta-blockers reduce the effect of sympathetic noradrenaline and circulating adrenaline on the pacemaker, so they reduce exercise-induced tachycardia.
d. **F** – Beta-blockers *decrease* stroke volume, by blocking the inotropic effect of the tonic sympathetic activity.

6.15 a. **F** – The switch to anaerobic metabolism leads to metabolic acidosis **(Figure 6.18)**.
b. **T** – Intracellular acidosis strongly impairs contractility – probably because H^+ ions interfere with the activation of the troponin–tropomyosin complex by Ca^{2+}.
c. **F** – Ischaemia triggers increased sympathetic activity. This increases the plateau inward Ca^{2+} current **(Figure 3.14)** and reduces Na^+–K^+-ATPase pumping, leading to a fall in Ca^{2+} expulsion by the Na–Ca exchanger. These changes leads to Ca^{2+} store *overload* **(Figure 6.18)**. Discharge of the overloaded store creates a delayed after-depolarization (DAD), which can trigger arrhythmia **(Figure 3.16)**.
d. **F** – The resting potential and the size of the action potential are both reduced by ischaemia **(Figure 5.8)**. So too is action potential duration **(Figure 3.13)**. The heterogeneous changes in myocyte potential create suitable conditions for re-entry circuits to develop. Re-entry circuits maintain arrhythmias, such as fibrillation.
e. **T** – Ischaemia-reperfusion injury is caused by myocyte contracture and free oxygen radical damage.

6.16 a. **T** – A more rapid, forceful ventricular systole raises systolic pressure in both the systemic circulation **(Figures 6.22)** and pulmonary circulation **(Figure 6.23)**.
b. **T** – Human end-diastolic volume increases by ~20 ml **(Table 6.2)**, as shown by echocardiography **(Figure 6.10)**. This expansion is due to increased venous filling pressure, brought about by peripheral venoconstriction and the calf muscle pump.
c. **F** – End-systolic volume is reduced **(Table 6.2)**. This is because the ejection fraction is raised by the increased cardiac sympathetic activity.
d. **F** – The duration of diastole falls markedly, due to the shortened cycle duration **(Figure 2.4)**.
e. **F** – Total peripheral resistance falls, due to the dilatation of resistance vessels in the active muscles **(Figure 6.22)**. This helps prevent an excessive rise in arterial pressure (afterload) as cardiac output rises. The responses of the heart and peripheral circulation are thus coordinated during exercise.

6.17 a. **T** – The rate of mitochondrial oxidative phosphorylation closely matches the rate of ATP consumption by myosin ATPase. This is called the 'metabolic stability paradox'.
b. **T** – Coronary O_2 extraction is higher than in most other tissue **(Figure 6.24)**. The blood supply is only just adequate – perhaps surprisingly for such a vital organ.
c. **T** – Increased myocardial performance requires increased ATP production and therefore increased O_2 supply. To meet this requirement, coronary blood flow increases in direct proportion to myocardial metabolic rate over most of the range **(Figure 6.20)**.
d. **F** – Free fatty acids are the normal heart's favourite food and account for 50–65% of energy production.
e. **T** – Exercising skeletal muscle releases lactate into the circulation. The lactate is used as an energy source by the myocardium. Release of myocyte lactic dehydrogenase into the circulation from damaged myocardium serves as a biochemical test for a heart attack.

CHAPTER 7

Assessment of cardiac output and peripheral pulse

T F

7.1 Human cardiac output

a. can be calculated from a subject's O_2 consumption and the O_2 concentrations in the radial artery and antecubital vein.
b. can be assessed by echocardiography.
c. can be estimated using pulsed Doppler ultrasound directed at the aorta.
d. can be calculated from blood temperature in the pulmonary artery following a cold saline injection into the left ventricle.
e. can be assessed from the pulse pressure and heart rate.

7.2 When cardiac output is measured using the Fick principle,

a. pulmonary blood flow is equated with cardiac output.
b. cardiac output is calculated as pulmonary O_2 uptake (U) multiplied by the difference between the O_2 content of arterial blood (A) and the mixed venous blood entering the lungs (V); $CO = U(A - V)$.
c. cardiac catheterization is necessary.
d. a six-fold increase in oxygen uptake indicates a six-fold increase in cardiac output.
e. the subject must be in a steady state.

7.3 When cardiac output is measured by the indicator dilution method,

a. the measured flow is the combined outputs of the right and left ventricles.
b. the key relation is that indicator concentration = cardiac output × blood volume.
c. it is essential to know the mass of indicator injected.
d. the indicator recirculates via the coronary circulation in about 20 seconds.
e. the indicator should ideally be confined to the circulation.

7.4 When cardiac output is estimated from the peripheral arterial pulse,

a. the pulse pressure is calculated as diastolic pressure plus one-third of systolic pressure.
b. the pulse pressure serves as an index of the left ventricle stroke volume.
c. the pulse pressure increases in direct proportion to arterial compliance.
d. it is necessary to measure the heart rate too.
e. the output may be underestimated, due to flow out of the arterial system during ventricular ejection.

For a change, here is a different type of question.

7.5 The different cardiac outputs of three subjects

In three subjects (two healthy, one with a cardiac disorder), O_2 consumption was measured by collecting expired air in a Douglas bag. Arterial blood oxygen concentration was measured in a sample drawn from the femoral artery. Mixed venous oxygen concentration was measured in a sample obtained from the right ventricle outflow tract by cardiac catheterization. The results were as follows.

	Subject A	Subject B	Subject C
Pulse rate (min^{-1})	75	150	75
Mean arterial blood pressure (mmHg)	90	100	95
Arterial pulse pressure (mmHg)	40	50	100
Mean right atrial pressure (mmHg)	1	1	5
O_2 uptake from lungs (ml O_2 min^{-1})	250	1250	260
Femoral arterial O_2 content (ml O_2/litre)	195	195	195
Mixed venous O_2 content (ml O_2/litre)	145	95	145
Arterial compliance (ml/mmHg)	1.67	1.67	1.67

Insert the most appropriate answer from the list below into the following passage.

Cardiac output can be estimated in two different ways from the data table, namely by the __________ or more approximately by the __________. Based on the oxygen data, the cardiac output of subject A was __________, while that of subject B was __________ and subject C was __________. The total peripheral resistance of subject B, namely __________ differed markedly from that of subject A, namely __________. Based on the above cardiac output values, and the fact that stroke volume is related to cardiac output by the relation stroke volume = __________, the stroke volumes of the subjects were approximately __________ for subject A, __________ for subject B and __________ for subject C. There is an alternative way, however, to estimate the stroke volume from the data, namely using the relation stroke volume equals (approximately) __________. When applied to subjects A and B, this second method gave similar results to the first method, but when applied to subject C the stroke volume works out to be __________. Based on these results, it is likely that subject A fits the description __________, subject B fits the description __________ and subject C fits the description __________.

5 litre min^{-1}	15.2 litre min^{-1}	5.2 litre min^{-1}	12.5 litre min^{-1}
Doppler flow	Pulse pressure method	Echocardiography	Fick principle
17.8 mmHg/(litre/min)	7.9 mmHg/(litre/min)	pulse pressure × arterial compliance	cardiac output/heart rate
167 ml	83 ml	69 ml	67 ml
aortic valve stenosis	aortic valve incompetence	normal, exercising	normal, resting

Answers

7.1 a. **F** – A mixed venous sample must be taken from the right ventricle to calculate cardiac output by the Fick method. The antecubital venous O_2 concentration does not represent the average venous O_2 concentration for the whole body, i.e. pulmonary artery O_2 concentration.

b. **T** – Echocardiography records the separation of the ventricle walls in diastole and systole **(Figure 6.10)**. This is converted into stroke volume, using assumptions about chamber shape. Then stroke volume × heart rate = cardiac output.

c. **T** – The altered frequency of ultrasound reflected by red cells in the aorta is used to calculate aortic blood velocity **(Figure 7.1)**. Aortic diameter too can be measured by ultrasound. Proximal aorta flow ($cm^3\ s^{-1}$) = velocity ($cm\ s^{-1}$) × cross-sectional area (cm^2) = cardiac output − coronary blood flow. Coronary blood is drawn from the root of the aorta, at the sinuses of Valsalva **(Figure 2.1)**.

d. **F** – In the thermal dilution method cold saline is injected into the right ventricle or base of the pulmonary trunk.

e. **T** – The pulse pressure depends on stroke volume **(Figure 7.2)**. This is the basis of automated cardiac output monitoring in intensive care units.

7.2 a. **T** – The entire output of the right ventricle passes through the lungs.

b. **F** – The Fick principle states that U = CO (A − V). So CO = U/(A − V) **(Figure 7.3)**.

c. **T** – The right ventricle has to be catheterized to obtain a sample of mixed venous blood.

d. **F** – During exercise the O_2 uptake increases much more than the cardiac output, because the venous O_2 concentration (V) decreases **(Figure 6.22)**.

e. **T** – It takes several minutes to measure O_2 consumption, so the cardiac output has to remain steady over this time.

7.3 a. **F** – Cardiac output is *always* the output of a single ventricle.

b. **F** – The key relation is that the arterial concentration of indicator, C, equals the mass of indicator injected, m, divided by the volume of blood in which it is distributed V_D. $C = m/V_D$. The time that the indicator volume takes to flow past a given point is recorded **(Figure 7.4a)**.

c. **T** – The cardiac output (CO) is calculated as injected mass m divided by area in under the arterial concentration versus time plot, Ct. $CO = m/Ct$ **(Figure 7.4b)**.

d. **T** – This causes a hump in the arterial concentration time course beyond 20 s **(Figure 7.4c)**. This limitation of the dye dilution method is circumvented in the thermal dilution method, due to thermal equilibration of the blood in the tissues.

e. **T** – If the indicator escapes from the bloodstream between the injection point and the sampling point, the true intravascular mass of indicator is smaller than the known, injected mass, m.

7.4 a. **F** – Pulse pressure is systolic pressure minus diastolic pressure **(Figure 7.2a)**.

b. **T** – The rise in arterial pressure is caused by the temporary accommodation of most of the stroke volume in the elastic arteries **(Figure 7.2b)**.

c. **F** – The bigger the arterial compliance (distensibility), the smaller the pulse pressure generated by a given stroke volume. Pulse pressure is *inversely* proportional to compliance. Compliance is change in volume per unit change in pressure.

d. **T** – Cardiac output = heart rate × stroke volume.

e. **T** – A volume of blood equal to 20–30% of the stroke volume flows out of the distal arteries during the time taken for ventricular ejection.

7.5 Cardiac output can be estimated in two different ways from the data table, namely by the **Fick principle** or more approximately by the **pulse pressure method**. Based on the oxygen data, the cardiac output of subject A was **5 litre min^{-1}**, while that of subject B was **12.5 litre min^{-1}** and subject C was **5.2 litre min^{-1}**. The total peripheral resistance of subject B, namely **7.9 mmHg/(litre/min)**, differed markedly from that of subject A, namely **17.8 mmHg/(litre/min)**. Based on the above cardiac output values, and the fact that stroke volume is related to cardiac output by the relation stroke volume = **cardiac output/heart rate**, the stroke volumes of the subjects were approximately **67 ml** for subject A, **83 ml** for subject B and **69 ml** for subject C. There is an alternative way, however, to estimate the stroke volume from the data, namely using the relation stroke volume equals (approximately) **pulse pressure × arterial compliance**. When applied to subjects A and B, this second method gave similar results to the first method; but when applied to subject C the stroke volume works out to be **167 ml**. Based on these results, it is likely that subject A fits the description **normal, resting**, subject B fits the description **normal, exercising** and subject C fits the description **aortic valve incompetence**.

CHAPTER 8

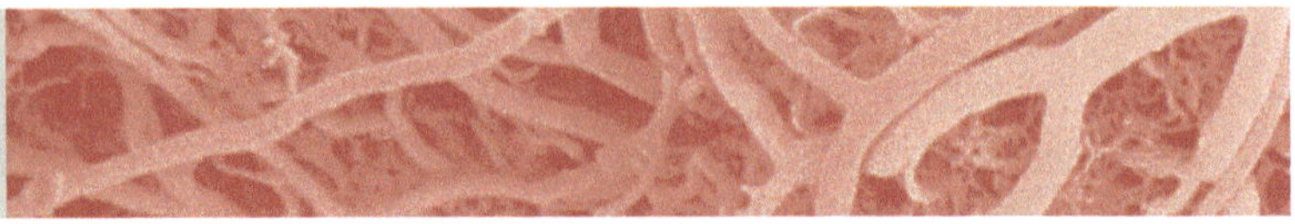

Haemodynamics: flow, pressure and resistance

T F

8.1 For a liquid flowing through a set of tubes,

a. Darcy's law states that the flow equals the pressure drop across the tubes divided by resistance.
b. Darcy's law applies to laminar and turbulent flow.
c. the total resistance of tubes linked in series is the sum of their individual resistances.
d. the total resistance of tubes arranged in parallel is one minus the sum of the resistances.

8.2 The relations between cardiac output (CO), total peripheral resistance (TPR), mean arterial blood pressure (BP), stroke volume (SV), heart rate (HR) and venous return (VR) are approximately as follows, if right atrial pressure is at atmospheric pressure.

a. CO = SV/HR
b. BP = CO × TPR
c. VR = BP/TPR
d. TPR = BP/(HR × SV)
e. SV = HR/TPR

8.3 During walking, blood flows from the proximal aorta to the dorsalis pedis artery of the foot because

a. arterial blood pressure is higher in the aorta than in the foot.
b. the calf muscle pump propels the blood through the legs.
c. the leg arteries have a lower resistance than the aorta.
d. the sum of pressure and gravitational energy in the aorta exceeds that in the foot.
e. the kinetic energy of blood in the foot is greater than in the aorta.

Next comes a little problem that tests your understanding of how circulations operate in parallel.

8.4 Concerning circulations arranged in parallel.

The skin and muscle of the arm are supplied from the same artery, the axillary artery (blood pressure, P_A). Both tissues drain into the same vein, the axillary vein (pressure, P_V). Assume that pressures P_A and P_V are *constant*. Skin blood flow is Fs, muscle blood flow Fm, skin vascular resistance Rs and muscle vascular resistance Rm.

T F

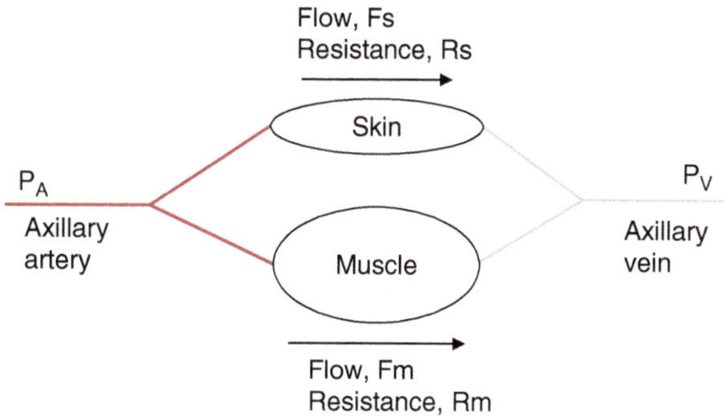

Are the following statements true or false?

a. Blood flow through the skin (Fs) equals $(P_A - P_V)/Rs$.
b. Total blood flow through the arm (skin and muscle) equals $(P_A - P_V)/(Rs + Rm)$.
c. If muscle vascular resistance Rm decreases, muscle blood flow Fm will increase.
d. If skin resistance Rs increases in cold weather, muscle blood flow will increase.
e. The net resistance to flow through the arm (skin and muscle) is $1/Rs + 1/Rm$.
f. If muscle blood flow is $2\,ml\,min^{-1}\,100\,g^{-1}$ and $P_A - P_V$ is 80 mmHg, muscle vascular resistance Rm is $0.025\,ml\,min^{-1}\,100\,g^{-1}\,mmHg^{-1}$.

8.5 Blood flow

a. in most blood vessels exhibits a parabolic velocity profile.
b. in the venae cavae is turbulent.
c. through capillaries depends on red cell deformability.
d. creates the highest shear rate near the vessel wall.
e. generates a marginal, red cell-enriched layer.

8.6 The tendency for blood flow to develop turbulence is greater

a. during peak cardiac ejection, when blood velocity is highest.
b. in a narrow artery than a wide artery.
c. when the haematocrit is reduced by anaemia.
d. when the vessel lumen is irregular, due to atheroma.
e. across a normal heart valve than a stenosed valve.

8.7 The arterial pulse pressure

a. equals the sphygmomanometer cuff pressure that just obliterates the radial pulse.
b. is about 30–40 mmHg in the pulmonary artery.
c. increases when stroke volume increases.
d. is raised by arteriosclerosis.
e. falls when a human stands up.

8.8 Increased stiffness of the walls of elastic arteries

a. raises systolic arterial pressure.
b. raises diastolic arterial pressure.
c. increases the total peripheral resistance.
d. can be measured using the pulse velocity.
e. lowers the oxygen consumption of the heart.

T F

8.9 Arterial compliance

a. is the increase in blood pressure required to distend the arterial system by 1 ml. ☐ ☐
b. decreases as arterial blood pressure is raised. ☐ ☐
c. increases with advancing age. ☐ ☐
d. is reduced when the rate of ventricular ejection increases. ☐ ☐
e. is reduced in patients with hypertension. ☐ ☐

8.10 Arterial pulse pressure can be increased by

a. a moderate haemorrhage. ☐ ☐
b. sympathetic stimulation of the heart. ☐ ☐
c. clinical hypertension. ☐ ☐
d. exercise. ☐ ☐
e. clinical shock. ☐ ☐

8.11 The aortic pressure wave in a resting human

a. rises quickly in systole, but falls only slowly in diastole. ☐ ☐
b. has a notch, the incisura, that marks opening of the aortic valve. ☐ ☐
c. is transmitted to the periphery faster than the stroke volume. ☐ ☐
d. is conducted more quickly in the young than the elderly. ☐ ☐
e. may show a late diastolic wave in young humans or during hypotension. ☐ ☐
f. may show an inflexion on the systolic upstroke in elderly humans or hypertensives. ☐ ☐

8.12 A systemic arterial pulse

a. that gets palpably weaker during each inspiration is called pulsus alternans. ☐ ☐
b. that fluctuates greatly from beat to beat is typical of atrial fibrillation. ☐ ☐
c. with an abnormally large pulse pressure occurs in mitral valve stenosis. ☐ ☐
d. with a slowly rising systolic phase is associated with aortic valve stenosis. ☐ ☐

8.13 In the measurement of blood pressure by the auscultatory method,

a. the first Korotkov sound as cuff pressure is lowered indicates systolic pressure. ☐ ☐
b. the complete disappearance of sound is commonly taken to be diastolic pressure. ☐ ☐
c. the estimate of systolic pressure tends to be lower than the true value. ☐ ☐
d. a wider-than-normal cuff is required for an obese arm. ☐ ☐
e. the upper arm should be raised above heart level. ☐ ☐

8.14 Mean arterial blood pressure

a. in the brachial artery is diastolic pressure plus systolic pressure divided by 2. ☐ ☐
b. is regulated by both peripheral resistance *and* cardiac output. ☐ ☐
c. is the sole determinant of the blood flow through an organ. ☐ ☐
d. can be increased by raising the blood volume. ☐ ☐
e. can be reduced by raising the blood haematocrit. ☐ ☐
f. when chronically raised, increases the risk of strokes. ☐ ☐

8.15 Systolic blood pressure in the brachial artery

a. is typically ~120–125 mmHg in a healthy, resting 20-year-old man. ☐ ☐
b. is typically ~105–110 mmHg in a 10-year-old child. ☐ ☐

T F

c. is reduced by exercise.
d. can be raised by a visit to the doctor.
e. is typically ~200 mmHg at 70 years of age.

8.16 Mean systemic arterial blood pressure usually increases in response to

a. stimulation of the carotid sinus baroreceptors.
b. stimulation of peripheral chemoreceptors.
c. brainstem compression/asphyxia.
d. atropine.
e. ganglionic blocking drugs.
f. sleep.
g. pregnancy.

8.17 The velocity of blood

a. in the ascending aorta falls to nearly zero at the onset of diastole.
b. becomes non-pulsatile in arterioles.
c. is slower in capillaries than arteries.
d. is slower in veins than capillaries.

8.18 According to Poiseuille's law for flow along a cylindrical tube,

a. flow is linearly proportion to the transmural pressure difference.
b. resistance to flow is proportional to vessel length.
c. flow increases two-fold if the vessel radius is doubled.
d. polycythaemia increases the vascular resistance to flow.
e. local vasoconstriction will reduce local blood flow.
f. generalized systemic vasoconstriction will raise the blood pressure if the cardiac output is held constant.

8.19 The effective viscosity of blood

a. is raised in patients with iron deficiency.
b. is lower in arterioles than in arteries.
c. is lowered by cooling.
d. is raised in climbers acclimatised to high altitudes.
e. is increased by a raised plasma protein concentration in multiple myeloma.

8.20 Laplace's law for tubes predicts that

a. the wall tension is proportional to the transmural pressure difference.
b. the wall tension is bigger in a small artery than a large artery.
c. the wall stress increases as wall thickness increases.
d. tension is increased in the wall of an abdominal aortic aneurysm.
e. in capillaries the wall tension is low and wall stress is high.

8.21 After a healthy subject has changed position from supine to standing,

a. the jugular veins become visible in the neck.
b. arterial pressure is increased in the lower limbs.
c. venous pressure is increased in the lower limbs.
d. the drag of gravity slows the venous drainage from the legs.
e. the volume of blood in the thorax decreases.

T F

8.22 In the human jugular veins,

a. the venous pulsation can be palpated in the neck when supine. ☐ ☐
b. the pressure is raised in right ventricular failure. ☐ ☐
c. the pulsation is exaggerated in atrial fibrillation. ☐ ☐
d. the pressure is reduced in patients with tricuspid valve incompetence. ☐ ☐
e. the pulse is exaggerated when the P wave of the ECG occurs during the S–T interval in a patient with complete heart block. ☐ ☐

8.23 The volume of blood in peripheral veins

a. is very sensitive to venous pressure, because veins can collapse. ☐ ☐
b. can be increased by activation of their sympathetic innervation. ☐ ☐
c. can be increased by the muscle pump. ☐ ☐
d. is about the same as the volume of blood in the arteries. ☐ ☐

8.24 Venous blood pressure

a. inside the thoracic cavity increases during inspiration. ☐ ☐
b. is about 20 mmHg in the venae cavae at heart level. ☐ ☐
c. is subatmospheric in the venous sinuses of the skull when standing. ☐ ☐
d. in the foot during standing is roughly equal to blood pressure in the ascending aorta. ☐ ☐
e. in the foot is increased by walking. ☐ ☐
f. in the antecubital vein at heart level is ~8–10 mmHg. ☐ ☐
g. in the hepatic portal vein is lower than in the inferior vena cava. ☐ ☐

Answers

8.1 a. **T** – Flow = pressure drop × conductance = pressure drop/resistance **(Figure1.5)**.
b. **F** – Darcy's law applies only to laminar flow. When turbulence sets in, much of the increased pressure energy is dissipated in cross-currents; further increases in flow are proportional to the square root of the pressure difference **(Figure 8.1)**.
c. **T** – If one tube has a resistance of 1 unit and the next in series has a resistance of 3 units (e.g. a terminal artery feeding an arteriole), the total resistance to flow is 4 units **(Figure 8.2)**.
d. **F** – When tubes are connected in parallel (e.g. capillaries), their *conductances* add up **(Figure 8.2)**. Conductance is 1/resistance.

8.2 a. **F** – Cardiac output equals stroke volume *multiplied* by heart rate. CO = SV × HR.
b. **T** – This is Darcy's law applied to the whole systemic circulation, for which the flow is the cardiac output. Flow = pressure drop/resistance, so CO = BP/TPR, taking central venous pressure as zero mmHg above atmospheric pressure. Rearranging this, BP = CO × TPR.
c. **T** – Venous return equals cardiac output in the steady state. So this is again Darcy's law applied to the whole systemic circulation. From (b), VR = CO = BP/TPR.
d. **T** – This again follows from the Darcy equation in (b), with HR × SV substituted for cardiac output; CO = HR × SV = BP/TPR. Rearranging, TPR = BP/(HR × SV).
e. **F** – Stroke volumes equal cardiac output divided by heart rate; SV = CO/HR.

8.3 a. **F** – Arterial pressure is actually higher in the foot in the upright position, due to the drag of gravity **(Figure 8.3)**.
b. **F** – The calf muscle pump propels blood up the venous system, not down the arterial system, because limb veins have valves, unlike arteries **(Figure 8.4)**.
c. **F** – The aorta is the widest of all arteries, so it has the lowest resistance.
d. **T** – Bernoulli's theory states that total *energy* gradient drives flow, not pressure alone. Aortic blood has more potential energy (gravitational energy) than blood in the foot, due to its height above the foot.
e. **F** – Kinetic energy is mass × velocity^2. The mass and velocity of blood in the dorsalis pedis are smaller than in the aorta.

8.4 a. **T** – This is Darcy's law of flow **(Figure 1.5)**.
b. **F** – Resistances in parallel do not summate. For the muscle, Fm = $(P_A - P_V)$/Rm. Total flow in skin and muscle is Fs + Fm = $(P_A - P_V)$/Rs + $(P_A - P_V)$/Rm = $(P_A - P_V)$(1/Rs + 1/Rm). In parallel circuits the conductances 1/Rs and 1/Rm summate **(Figure 8.2)**. Conductance is 1/resistance.
c. **T** – Muscle perfusion = $(P_A - P_V)$/Rm, so if Rm decreases, as happens during exercise, the muscle perfusion increases.
d. **F** – Muscle blood flow is $(P_A - P_V)$/Rm; none of these terms have changed. Students often get this wrong, because they think there is a *fixed* flow going through the arm; they then argue that, since less blood is going through the skin, more must be going through the muscle. But total arm blood flow is *not* fixed – it decreases when skin resistance increases. The driving pressure P_A, on the other hand, is held relatively constant by the baroreflex. This example illustrates the virtue of circulations in parallel, namely that the flow through one tissue (muscle in this case) does not depend on what is happening in a parallel tissue (skin).

e. **F** – The parameter 1/Rs + 1/Rm is the net (combined) conductance of the two tissues. Conductances in parallel summate **(Figure 8.2)**. The net resistance is 1/net conductance, or 1/(1/Rs + 1/Rm).

f. **F** – The stated value is flow per unit pressure gradient, so it is *conductance*. From Darcy's law, resistance = pressure drop/flow, so its units are mmHg per unit flow. Here, it is 40 mmHg min 100 g ml^{-1}.

8.5 a. **T** – Blood moves fastest in the vessel centre and has zero velocity at the vessel wall during laminar flow **(Figure 8.5a, top right)**.

b. **F** – Flow is laminar in healthy veins and arteries.

c. **T** – Capillaries are narrower than red cells, so red cells have to deform to file through them **(bolus flow, Figure 8.5b)**. In sickle cell anaemia, stiffening of the red cells can impair capillary perfusion, causing an ischaemic crisis.

d. **T** – Due to the parabolic velocity profile, the rate at which one layer slides (shears) over the next is greatest at the wall **(Figure 8.5a)**. This stimulates endothelium to secrete NO. If the wall is weak, the high shear stress can trigger a dissecting aortic aneurysm.

e. **F** – Laminar flow creates a marginal plasma stream that is deficient in red cells, and consequently is of low viscosity **(Figure 8.5a, right)**. This helps blood flow in narrow tubes, such as the arterioles **(the Farheus–Lindquist effect, Figure 8.6)**.

8.6 a. **T** – When a high velocity raises the Reynold's number above ~2000, turbulence develops **(Figure 8.1)**. The Reynold's number is velocity × diameter × density/viscosity. Turbulence during peak ejection can cause an innocent systolic murmur.

b. **F** – The Reynold's number tells us that turbulence is promoted by a wide diameter.

c. **T** – Anaemia reduces viscosity, which raises the Reynold's number. For this reason, an innocent systolic ejection murmur is not uncommon during pregnancy.

d. **T** – An atheromatous plaque can cause local turbulence. This may be audible through a stethoscope (a 'bruit'), and is sometimes even palpable (a 'thrill').

e. **F** – The abrupt change in velocity and diameter across a stenosed valve creates turbulence, producing a cardiac murmur **(Figure 2.6 top)**.

8.7 a. **F** – Pulse pressure is the difference between systolic and diastolic pressure **(Figure 8.7)**. The cuff pressure that just obliterates the pulse is systolic pressure **(Figure 8.8)**.

b. **F** – Pulse pressure is only ~13–16 mmHg in the low pressure pulmonary circulation **(Figure 1.6)**.

c. **T** – The addition of a bigger stroke volume to the elastic arteries raises the arterial blood pressure more **(Figures 7.2 and 8.9, top)**.

d. **T** – Arteriosclerosis is a stiffening of the tunica media of elastic arteries (reduced compliance). Therefore, a greater rise in pressure is needed to stretch the walls sufficiently to accommodate the stroke volume **(Figure 8.9, bottom)**.

e. **T** – Standing up causes venous pooling in the lower limbs, which reduces central venous pressure **(Figure 6.9)**. The fall in central venous pressure reduces stroke volume (Starling's law of the heart) and therefore pulse pressure.

8.8 a. **T** – Stiffness (elastance) is 1/compliance (distensibility). In order to distend a stiff artery sufficiently to accommodate the stroke volume, a greater increase in pressure is required – so systolic pressure is raised **(Figure 8.9, bottom)**.

b. **F** – If mean blood pressure is unchanged (because it is determined by peripheral resistance and cardiac output), a rise in elastic artery stiffness would actually *reduce* diastolic pressure.

This is because pressure falls more sharply as blood drains out of a stiff vessel. Arterial stiffness determines the size of the oscillation in pressure (systolic–diastolic) around the mean.

c. **F** – Elastic arteries make no significant contribution to peripheral resistance, as shown by the pressure profile of the circulation **(Figure 1.6)**.

d. **T** – The speed with which the pulse spreads along the arterial tree depends on wall stiffness. The stiffer the vessels, the faster the pulse is transmitted from aorta to radial artery.

e. **F** – Stiffening of the aorta, which occurs with ageing and clinical hypertension, raises the systolic pressure, which is the afterload on the left ventricle. This increases cardiac work and thus *raises* oxygen consumption.

8.9 a. **F** – Arterial compliance (distensibility) is the increase in arterial blood volume produced by 1 mmHg increase in blood pressure. Its reciprocal, the increase in pressure per ml distension, is called elastance (stiffness) **(Figure 8.9, bottom)**.

b. **T** – The pressure–volume relation is a steepening curve, not a straight line. Its slope is the elastance (stiffness). This increases with stretch, as with a bicycle tyre. Compliance (1/elastance) therefore falls when pressure is raised **(Figure 8.9, middle)**.

c. **F** – Elastic arteries get stiffer with age due to arteriosclerosis; so their compliance (distensibility) decreases. The stiff, ageing aorta is similar to the stiff, hypertensive aorta **(Figure 8.10)**.

d. **T** – The artery wall is viscoelastic – meaning that its passive tension relaxes over time. If ejection is rapid, relaxation time is reduced and the wall becomes effectively stiffer; compliance is reduced.

e. **T** – The pressure–volume curve of the hypertensive aorta is steeper than normal, i.e. compliance is reduced **(Figure 8.10)**.

8.10 a. **F** – A fall in blood volume reduces central venous pressure (CVP), which reduces stroke volume (Starling's law) **(Figure 6.2b, phlebotomy points)**. This reduces the pulse pressure **(Figure 8.11)**.

b. **T** – The rise in stroke volume and the increased rate of ejection both raise the pulse pressure **(Figures 6.13a, loop 2 and 6.19, left)**.

c. **T** – Pulse pressure (as opposed to mean pressure) increases in clinical hypertension for two reasons. (1) Large artery compliance is reduced **(stiffness increases, Figure 8.10)**. (2) Early return of the faster travelling reflected pressure wave augments the systolic pressure **(Figure 8.12c)**.

d. **T** – Stroke volume and ejection rate increase during exercise, raising the pulse pressure.

e. **F** – Clinical shock is a state of reduced stroke volume, so pulse pressure falls.

8.11 a. **T** – The pressure pulse is *not* a sine wave – contrary to drawings by some students! Systole is shorter than diastole in a resting human **(Figure 8.7)**.

b. **F** – The incisura is caused by aortic valve *closure* **(Figures 2.2)**.

c. **T** – The stroke volume advances ~20 cm along the aorta in 1 s, whereas the pulse travels at 4–15 m/s; it reaches the periphery in a fraction of a second **(Figure 1.7)**.

d. **F** – The elderly have stiffer arteries, due to arteriosclerosis, and conduction velocity increases with wall stiffness.

e. **T** – The low stiffness of the artery wall in young people slows the conduction velocity. The slow reflected wave arrives back in the proximal aorta during diastole, creating a diastolic wave **(Figure 8.12a)**. The same effect occurs during hypotension, because the artery wall is slacker at the lower pressure.

f. **T** – The systolic inflection is caused by the rapid return of the reflected wave, due to fast conduction by the stiff arterial system **(Figure 8.12c)**.

8.12 a. **F** – This phenomenon is called pulsus paradoxus – a sign of cardiac tamponade. Pulsus alternans is alternating strong and weak beats – a sign of severe cardiac failure.

b. **T** – When the atria are fibrillating, the filling time for the ventricle is irregular, so stroke volume is erratic **(Figure 4.3f, radial pulse trace)**.

c. **F** – A large pulse pressure is the characteristic feature of aortic valve incompetence **(Figure 8.7, top right inset)**. It can cause a crossed leg to bob markedly in time with pulse.

d. **T** – Blood is ejected slowly through the narrow valve **(Figures 8.7, top left inset and 2.6)**.

8.13 a. **T** – Blood first starts to spurt under the cuff when cuff pressure is lowered just below systolic blood pressure, causing the onset of the Korotkov sounds **(Figure 8.8)**.

b. **T** – When cuff pressure is less than diastolic pressure, flow through the brachial artery is continuous and laminar, so it is silent **(Figure 8.8)**. (Nevertheless, the point of silences often underestimates true diastolic pressure by several mmHg.)

c. **T** – The estimate is actually about 10 mmHg below the true value.

d. **T** – In a big arm, a wider cuff is needed to compress the deep brachial artery adequately.

e. **F** – Arterial blood pressure falls in arteries raised above heart level, due to the drag of gravity **(Figure 8.3)**.

8.14 a. **F** – The time-averaged pressure of blood in the brachial artery is diastolic + one-third pulse pressure **(Figures 8.7)**. This is due to the shape of the pressure wave, which is tall but thin in the brachial artery. In the aorta, mean pressure is indeed close to (diastolic + systolic)/2.

b. **T** – Mean BP = cardiac output × peripheral resistance. Both components are regulated, via the baroreflex control of sympathetic nerve activity to the heart and blood vessels.

c. **F** – Blood flow through an organ is regulated chiefly by changes in the local resistance vessels, in accordance with Darcy's law; flow = pressure gradient/resistance. Blood flow through an exercising skeletal muscle can increase by 2000% (20×) yet blood pressure during exercise increases by only ~10%.

d. **T** – This is how saline or blood transfusions produce therapeutic benefit in hypovolaemic patients. An increase in blood volume raises central venous pressure, which increases stroke volume via Starling's law of the heart **(Figure 6.2b, point labelled 'reinfusion')**.

e. **F** – Raising the haematocrit (e.g. polycythaemia) increases the blood viscosity **(Figure 8.13)**, and therefore the resistance to flow. Peripheral resistance depends on fluid viscosity, as well as vessel radius (Poiseuille's law).

f. **T** – Strokes correlate particularly with systolic pressure elevation (systolic hypertension). This is a major reason for treating asymptomatic clinical hypertension.

8.15 a. **T** – See **Figure 8.7**. The pressure is slightly lower in a woman **(Figure 8.14)**.

b. **T** – Blood pressure is low in children and increases with age **(Figures 8.14)**.

c. **F** – The increase in stroke volume and ejection velocity during exercise raise the systolic pressure, even if diastolic pressure falls **(Figure 8.15)**.

d. **T** – The effects of stress (adrenaline and increased sympathetic activity, raised cardiac output, peripheral vasoconstriction) cause 'white coat hypertension'.

e. **F** – Systolic pressure does indeed increase with age, but not this much (severe hypertension). The average systolic pressure at 70 in the English population is ~140 mmHg **(Figure 8.14)**.

8.16 a. **F** – The baroreflex is a negative feedback loop that lowers blood pressure **(Figure 8.16)**.
b. **T** – Peripheral chemoreceptor activation activates sympathetic activity to support blood pressure during a severe haemorrhage, and to increase cerebral blood flow during asphyxia.
c. **T** – Cushing's reflex is a reflex rise in blood pressure evoked by brainstem compression and asphyxia **(Figure 8.17)**. This helps preserve local cerebral blood flow and oxygen supply.
d. **T** – Atropine blocks muscarinic M_2 receptors for parasympathetic acetylcholine on the pacemaker **(Figure 3.14)**. This raises the heart rate, and therefore cardiac output and blood pressure.
e. **F** – Blockers of the sympathetic ganglia inhibit postganglionic sympathetic activity. The fall in sympathetic vasoconstrictor fibre activity causes peripheral vasodilatation, lowering peripheral resistance and therefore blood pressure.
f. **F** – Pressure falls during sleep.
g. **F** – Blood pressure falls during mid-pregnancy, because the fall in total peripheral resistance (TPR) outweighs the concurrent increase in cardiac output.

8.17 a. **T** – Flow actually goes into reverse during closure of the aortic valve **(Figure 8.18, bottom)**.
b. **F** – Flow is still pulsatile, even down to the level of arterial capillaries **(Figure 1.6)**.
c. **T** – The huge increase in the total cross-sectional area of the vascular bed at the level of capillaries slows the velocity of the blood **(Figure 1.6)**. Velocity (cm s^{-1}) is the flow (i.e. the cardiac output, $cm^3\ s^{-1}$) divided by total cross-sectional area (cm^2).
d. **F** – As microvessels unite to form venules and then veins, the total cross-sectional area of the circulation falls, so the blood velocity increases **(Figure 1.6)**.

8.18 a. **F** – 'Transmural' ('across-wall') means the difference in pressure between the inside and outside of the tube, whereas it is the *internal* pressure difference between the entry and exit of the tube that drives flow **(Figure 8.19)**. Transmural pressure only affects flow if it alters the tube width.
b. **T** – This is part of Poiseuille's law **(Figure 8.19)**. The shortness of the capillaries contributes to their low resistance to flow.
c. **F** – A key feature of Poiseuille's law is that radius to the fourth power governs flow **(Figure 8.19)**. If the radius increases 2-fold, conductance and flow increase $2^4 = 16$-fold.
d. **T** – Polycythaemia raises blood viscosity **(Figure 8.13)**. Viscosity is one of the three factors determining resistance to flow through a tube **(Figure 8.19)**. A comparison of the flow curves for saline and blood through an organ highlights the effect of viscosity on flow **(Figure 8.20)**.
e. **T** – Vasoconstriction reduces vessel radius, so flow falls markedly, due to the Poiseuille r^4 effect; see **Figure 8.20**, curve labelled 'Blood + noradrenaline'.
f. **T** – Widespread vasoconstriction raises TPR and therefore arterial blood pressure **(Figure 8.21)**, BP = CO × TPR. An everyday example is the response to stress.

8.19 a. **F** – Iron deficiency causes anaemia, which reduces viscosity. Blood viscosity depends chiefly on haematocrit **(Figure 18.13)**.
b. **T** – Effective blood viscosity varies with tube radius – the Fahreus–Lindqvist effect **(Figure 8.6)**. The Fahreus–Lindqvist effect reduces the resistance of the microcirculation **(Figure 8.13)**.

c. **F** – Blood viscosity is raised by cooling. This increases the resistance to flow through the skin in cold hands.
d. **T** – An adaptive polycythaemia raises blood viscosity.
e. **T** – In multiple myeloma, which is a cancerous overproduction of plasma cells, excessive globulin production increases the blood viscosity.

8.20 a. **T** – Laplace's law states that wall tension = ($P_{inside} - P_{outside}$) × radius **(Figure 8.22)**.
b. **F** – The bigger the radius, the bigger the tension produced by a given pressure **(Figure 8.23)**. So the aorta has the highest wall tension.
c. **F** – Stress is tension per unit cross-sectional area of wall. The thicker the wall, the less the stress on each element in the wall. Thus, in clinical hypertension, increases in wall thickness in the resistance vessels and left ventricle help normalize wall stress.
d. **T** – An aneurysm has a bigger radius than the normal vessel, so a bigger wall tension.
e. **T** – Wall tension is low in capillaries due to the tiny radius, but stress is high due to the extreme thinness of the wall **(Figure 8.23)**. This contributes to capillary fragility.

8.21 a. **F** – The jugular veins are normally visible only when recumbent or during forced expiration **(Figure 8.24)**. This is because central venous pressure is only a few cmH_2O.
b. **T** – The drag of gravity on the vertical column of arterial blood raises arterial pressure is the legs **(Figure 8.3)**.
c. **T** – The venous valves are open when standing still, since blood is flowing continuously up the veins. The pull of gravity on the vertical column of venous blood raises venous pressure is the legs **(Figures 8.3 and 6.9)**.
d. **F** – Gravity does not affect flow through a U tube (leg artery to leg vein). This is the siphon principle **(Figure 8.25)**. Flow does in fact decrease, but for a different reason, namely postural vasoconstriction of the resistance vessels in the legs.
e. **T** – The rise in lower limb venous pressure distends the veins, which results in a transfer of blood from thorax to the lower limbs **(Figure 6.9)**. This reduces the central venous pressure and therefore stroke volume (Starling's law).

8.22 a. **F** – The magnitude of the venous pulse in only a few mmHg. This is too small to feel. Only the arterial pulse is palpable.
b. **T** – The jugular veins are connected via the superior vena cava to the right atrium, with no intervening valves. Right atrial and central venous pressure are raised during right ventricular failure. A raised jugular venous pressure (JVP) is an important clinical sign of right heart failure.
c. **F** – When the atria do not contract in a co-ordinated manner, the 'a' wave of the jugular venous pulse disappears. The normal jugular venous waveform is similar to that shown for the atrium in **Figure 2.2**.
d. **F** – The 'v' wave of the jugular pulse becomes exaggerated, due to regurgitation from the right ventricle through the leaking valve during systole.
e. **T** – The first labelled P wave in **Figure 4.3e** shows a P-on-ST situation. The atria contract just after the P wave. If the tricuspid valve is closed at this point, as it is during the S–T interval, an exaggerated 'a' wave occurs and is transmitted into the jugular veins.

8.23 a. **T** – Unsupported veins change from a circular cross-section to an elliptical and then figure-of-eight cross-section (i.e. they collapse), as pressure is lowered from ~15 cmH_2O to a few cmH_2O below atmospheric **(Figure 8.26)**.

b. **F** – Venous sympathetic fibres release noradrenaline and cause venoconstriction, reducing peripheral blood volume **(Figures 8.26 and 6.15)**.
c. **F** – The intermittent squeezing of local veins by rhythmically contracting muscle groups (e.g. calf during walking) *reduces* local venous volume, which boosts central venous pressure **(Figure 8.4)**.
d. **F** – The veins are the capacitance vessels and contain about two-thirds of the blood volume.

8.24 a. **F** – Inspiration lowers all intrathoracic pressures.
b. **F** – Vena cava pressure is ~3 mmHg, being close to that in the right atrium **(Tables 2.1)**. 20 mmHg would indicate severe heart failure.
c. **T** – The drag of gravity reduces pressures within the skull **(Figure 8.3)**. A traumatic or surgical breach in the venous sinuses in the upright position therefore carries the risk of air embolism.
d. **T** – Gravity greatly increases venous pressure in the foot during standing **(Figures 8.3 and 8.27)**. A breached dependent vein will therefore bleed profusely, unless raised to heart level.
e. **F** – The calf muscle pump *reduces* distal venous pressure **(Figure 8.4)**. This increases the local arterio-venous pressure difference driving the blood flow **(Figure 8.27)**. It also reduces capillary filtration pressure.
f. **T** – This is the most common site for venepuncture. Pressures are shown in **Figure 1.6**.
g. **F** – Blood flows from the portal vein through the liver into the vena cava **(Figure 1.4)**. The pressure must, therefore, be higher in the portal vein than the vena cava.

CHAPTER 9

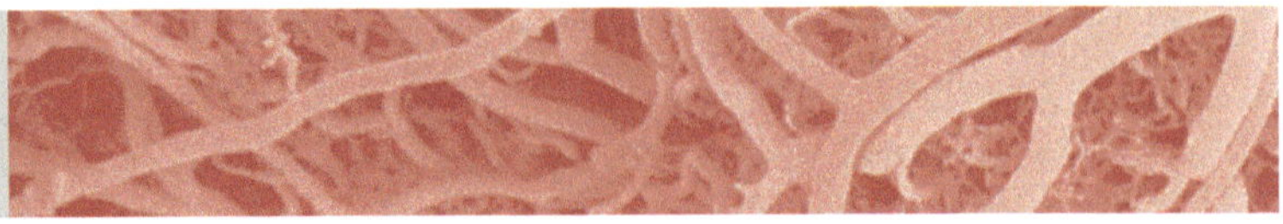

The endothelial cell

T F

9.1 Endothelial cells

a. line the entire cardiovascular system, except the cardiac chambers.
b. are usually joined together by continuous, unbroken junctional strands of protein.
c. can communicate through electrically conductive gap junctions.
d. have a semipermeable coat of biopolymers on the luminal surface.
e. resist the shearing force of blood through β_1 integrin-collagen bonds.

9.2 Endothelial cells express

a. K^+ channels that contribute to a negative intracellular membrane potential.
b. Ca^{2+}-conducting channels that close in response to inflammatory mediators.
c. Ca^{2+}-conducting channels activated by Ca^{2+} store depletion.
d. Ca^{2+}-activated potassium channels that depolarize the cell.
e. an enzyme that is activated via a rise in cytosolic Ca^{2+} and catalyses the production of a vasodilator agent.

9.3 Endothelium-generated nitric oxide (NO)

a. is produced continuously from citrulline.
b. is a circulating hormone that induces widespread vasodilatation.
c. induces vasodilatation by raising intracellular cAMP in vascular smooth muscle.
d. is produced tonically in response to the shear stress of flowing blood.
e. contributes to the characteristic heat and redness of inflammation.

For a change, here is a different style of question.

9.4 Factors produced by endothelium.

Endothelial cells produce many biologically active agents. The well known vasodilator gas __________ is also an inhibitor of __________ and __________, so it has an __________ action. The identity of another endothelium-dependent vasodilator, called __________, is controversial. Endothelium also secretes a derivative of arachidonic acid, __________, which inhibits __________ and __________. In addition, endothelium secretes a peptide related to snake venom, called __________, that causes long-lasting __________. Lung endothelium possess a surface peptide-degrading enzyme that generates the circulating hormone __________, another agent that causes __________. Not all endothelial secretions are vasoactive, however. For example, a glycoprotein involved in the clotting cascade, called __________, is secreted continuously, and is also stored inside endothelium in a structure called a __________.

Choose the right word from the list below, using a word/phrase as often as required or not at all, as appropriate.

caveolae	endothelin	nitrous oxide	initiates platelet activation
vesicles	Factor VIII	nitric oxide	vasoconstriction
Weibel–Palade body	adrenaline	von Willebrand factor	vasodilatation
cadherin	prostacyclin	platelet aggregation	stimulates vascular myocyte growth
histamine	anti-atheroma	pro-atheroma	vascular myocyte proliferation
bradykinin	angiotensin II	endothelium-derived hyperpolarizing factor	natriuretic peptide

T F

9.5 In most tissues the permeability of capillary endothelium

a. to glucose depends on the transporter GLUT-1 in the endothelial cell membrane. ☐ ☐
b. to respiratory gases is determined primarily by their water solubility. ☐ ☐
c. to plasma proteins is attributed partly to transport by vesicles. ☐ ☐
d. to albumin is greatly restricted by a negatively charged glycocalyx. ☐ ☐
e. can be increased by β_2-adrenoceptor agonists. ☐ ☐
f. is increased by vascular endothelial growth factor (VEGF). ☐ ☐
g. can be reduced by atrial natriuretic peptide. ☐ ☐

9.6 In the inflammatory response,

a. endothelial nitric oxide production is stimulated by inflammatory mediators. ☐ ☐
b. gaps formed in arterial capillaries are responsible for plasma protein leakage. ☐ ☐
c. endothelial P-selectin initiates the rolling capture of circulating leukocytes. ☐ ☐
d. leukocyte arrest is brought about by β_1 integrin insertion into the endothelial surface. ☐ ☐
e. lack of β_2 integrin expression by leukocytes can prevent leukocyte emigration. ☐ ☐

9.7 Regarding angiogenesis,

a. the primary event is often a lateral sprouting of capillary endothelium. ☐ ☐
b. VEGF is expressed abundantly by the placenta and other growing tissues. ☐ ☐
c. new capillaries are of abnormally low permeability. ☐ ☐
d. thrombospondin and angiostatin normally hold angiogenesis in check. ☐ ☐
e. tumour growth is critically dependent on new vessel formation. ☐ ☐

9.8 In atheromatous arteries,

a. cholesterol accumulates in the tunica media. ☐ ☐
b. acetylcholine may cause vasoconstriction rather than vasodilatation. ☐ ☐
c. superoxide production is impaired. ☐ ☐
d. nitric oxide availability is reduced. ☐ ☐
e. endothelial dysfunction promotes plaque formation. ☐ ☐

Answers

9.1 a. **F** – Endothelium lines the *entire* cardiovascular system, including the cardiac chambers.

b. **F** – The junctional strands have breaks that allow water and small lipid-insoluble solutes (glucose, etc.) to pass from blood to tissue **(Figure 9.1)**. The blood–brain barrier is an exception to this rule.

c. **T** – Homocellular gap junctions are common in arterial endothelium **(Figure 9.2)**. They are part of the mechanism underlying conducted vasodilatation. Heterocellular (myoendothelial) gap junctions are common in small vessels **(Figure 1.8)**. They often account for endothelium-dependent hyperpolarization of vascular smooth muscle (EDHF).

d. **T** – A thin polymer coating, the glycocalyx, renders endothelium semipermeable, i.e. permeable to water and small solutes but relatively impermeable to plasma proteins **(Figure 9.3)**.

e. **T** – The integrins link up internally with the actin stress fibres and externally with the type IV collagen of the basal lamina at focal contact points **(Figure 9.3)**.

9.2 a. **T** – Inward rectifier K_{ir} channels conduct an outward K^+ current that generates a negative intracellular potential **(Figure 9.2)**. The negative potential contributes to the electrochemical force driving Ca^{2+} entry, e.g. during inflammation.

b. **F** – Inflammatory agents *activate* receptor-operated Ca^{2+} channels **(Figure 9.2)**.

c. **T** – Store-operated channels are an important route for Ca^{2+} entry in endothelium **(Figure 9.2)**.

d. **F** – Endothelial cells express K_{Ca} channels that conduct an outward K^+ current that *hyperpolarizes* the cell. This increases the electrochemical gradient driving Ca^{2+} entry.

e. **T** – Endothelial nitric oxide synthase (eNOS) is activated by Ca^{2+}–calmodulin complex and generates the vasodilator nitric oxide **(Figure 9.4)**.

9.3 a. **F** – NO is produced by cleavage of the nitro-group from the amino acid *arginine* by eNOS (endothelial nitric oxide synthase), leaving behind citrulline **(Figure 9.4)**.

b. **F** – The half-life of NO is only seconds, so it only acts locally; it is not a circulating hormone, such as adrenaline.

c. **F** – NO activates smooth muscle guanylate cyclase, which catalyses cGMP production **(Figure 9.4)**. cAMP, by contrast, mediates the vasodilator effect of adrenaline-activated β_2 receptors.

d. **T** – Shear stress is thought to be the main tonic stimulus to basal NO production. It activates eNOS via PI3 kinase **(Figure 9.4)**.

e. **T** – Inflammatory mediators, such as bradykinin and histamine, and other agonists such as parasympathetic acetylcholine, activate eNOS through a rise in Ca^{2+}–calmodulin complex **(Figure 9.4)**. The resulting vasodilatation increases local blood flow, which causes the characteristic heat and redness of inflammation.

9.4 Endothelial cells produce many biologically active agents. The well known vasodilator gas **nitric oxide** also inhibits **platelet aggregation/vascular myocyte proliferation**, and **platelet aggregation/vascular myocyte proliferation**, so it has an **anti-atheroma** action. The identity of another endothelium-dependent vasodilator, called **endothelial derived hyperpolarizing factor**, is controversial. Endothelium also secretes a derivative of arachidonic acid, **prostacyclin**, which inhibits **platelet aggregation/vasoconstriction** and **platelet aggregation/vasoconstriction**. In addition, endothelium secretes a peptide related to snake venom, called **endothelin**, that causes long lasting **vasoconstriction**. Lung endothelium possess a surface peptide-degrading enzyme that generates the circulating hormone **angiotensin II**, another agent that causes **vasoconstriction**. Not all endothelial secretions are vasoactive, however. For example, a glycoprotein involved in the clotting cascade, called **von Willebrand factor**, is secreted continuously, as well as being stored inside endothelium in a structure called a **Weibel–Palade body**.

9.5 a. **F** – Glucose diffuses through the intercellular clefts, via breaks in the junctional strands **(Figure 9.5)**. GLUT-1 carrier-based transport is only necessary in blood–brain barrier capillaries.
b. **F** – Gas permeation depends primarily on lipid solubility. Oxygen and carbon dioxide, being lipid-soluble (lipophilic), diffuse directly through the endothelial plasma membrane **(Figure 9.6)**.
c. **T** – Plasma proteins can cross the wall via vesicles **(Figure 9.6)**, although this may not be the sole or even major route (controversial).
d. **T** – The glycocalyx is the semipermeable layer; it is permeable to water but largely impermeable to albumin and most other plasma proteins **(Figure 9.6)**.
e. **F** – Beta$_2$-adrenoceptor agonists raise endothelial cAMP, which increases the number of junctional strands and thereby *reduces* permeability.
f. **T** – VEGF was originally called vascular permeability factor. Newly grown capillaries are therefore abnormally leaky.
g. **F** – Atrial natriuretic peptide is a hormone that reduces plasma volume, partly by actions on the kidney and partly by increasing capillary permeability to water.

9.6 a. **T** – Bradykinin, histamine, etc., increase eNOS activity by raising cytosolic [Ca^{2+}] **(Figure 9.4)**.
b. **F** – Gaps form in *venular* endothelium during inflammation, increasing immunoglobulin permeation.
c. **T** – P selectin is translocated to the luminal membrane from a store in the Weibel–Palade body **(Figure 9.7)**.
d. **F** – Leukocytes are arrested by the insertion of vascular cell adhesion molecules (VCAM) and intercellular adhesion molecules (ICAM) into the luminal membrane **(Figure 9.7)**. Abluminal endothelial β_1 integrin attaches endothelium to its basement membrane **(Figure 9.3)**.
e. **T** – Leukocyte β_2 integrin is the ligand for the VCAM and ICAM **(Figure 9.7)**. Rare individuals lacking β_2 integrin have difficulty dealing with bacterial infections.

9.7 a. **T** – New vessels often form from endothelial outgrowths, called sprouts **(Figure 9.5)**.
b. **T** – Vascular endothelial growth factor stimulates endothelial sprouting.
c. **F** – They are hyperpermeable, e.g. to fibrinogen, creating a loose, hydrated matrix called granulation tissue that is suitable for further angiogenesis. VEGF used to be called vascular permeability factor.
d. **T** – These agents counter the angiogenic action of VEGF.
e. **T** – Tumours bigger than ~1 mm need a capillary blood supply. Drugs that block angiogenesis are now being used clinically to inhibit tumour growth.

9.8 a. **F** – Cholesterol, the major constituent of low density lipoprotein, accumulates in the *subendothelial* space, not the tunica media. Atheroma (atherosclerosis) is primarily a disease of the tunica intima.
b. **T** – Acetylcholine normally causes vasodilatation, by stimulating endothelium to produce extra nitric oxide. NO availability is reduced, however, in atheromatous arteries. The direct vasoconstrictor action of acetylcholine on vascular smooth muscle is then revealed **(Figure 9.8, bottom left)**.
c. **F** – Hypercholesterolaemia, smoking and diabetes *increase* superoxide production.
d. **T** – The NO reacts with superoxide to form harmful peroxynitrite **(Figure 9.8)**.
e. **T** – Endothelial NO normally exerts multiple anti-atheroma actions. A fall in endothelial NO thus contributes to atheroma formation.

CHAPTER 10

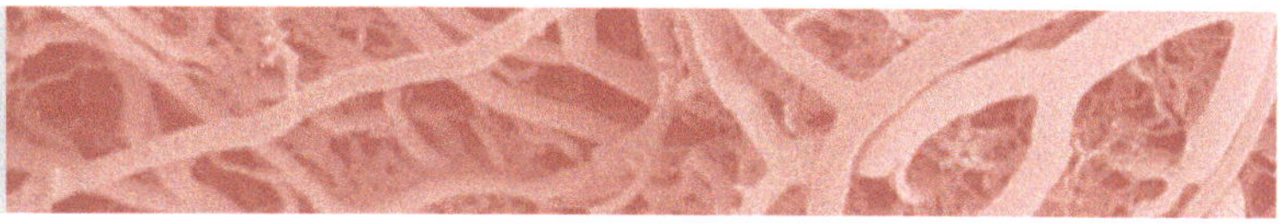

The microcirculation and solute exchange

T F

10.1 Of the three main types of capillary,

a. continuous capillaries predominate in the liver.
b. fenestrated capillaries are abundant in exocrine glands.
c. discontinuous capillaries are found in the bone marrow.
d. fenestrated capillaries are less permeable to water than continuous capillaries.
e. discontinuous capillaries are more permeable to plasma proteins than continuous capillaries.

10.2 Regarding the permeation of different solutes across the wall of a continuous capillary,

a. general anaesthetics permeate rapidly, because they are lipid soluble.
b. glucose is generally carried across the wall chiefly by plasma ultrafiltration.
c. urea enters the capillary chiefly by diffusion down a concentration gradient.
d. oxygen permeation is more than 1000 times faster than glucose permeation.
e. net water transport depends on diffusion down the water concentration gradient.
f. plasma proteins do not cross the capillary wall.

10.3 When a solute diffuses from the capillary bloodstream into a tissue,

a. the mass transported per unit time is proportional to the fourth power of the concentration gradient.
b. doubling the endothelial surface area will double the mass transported per unit time, for a given concentration gradient.
c. the diffusion rate is inversely proportional to the solute diffusion coefficient.
d. the diffusion coefficient of a solute increases in proportion to its molecular mass.
e. the mean oxygen concentration along the capillary increases with blood flow.

10.4 The permeability of a continuous capillary

a. equals the concentration gradient needed to drive 1 unit of solute across unit wall area per second.
b. to small lipid-insoluble solutes is mediated by small pores of radius ~3–5 nm.
c. to small lipid-insoluble solutes depends on the extent of the breaks in the interendothelial junctional strands.
d. is raised by steric exclusion of solute at the pore entrance and restricted diffusion inside the pore.
e. is much greater to small solutes than large solutes.

T F

10.5 The specialized capillaries of the brain

a. are impermeable to many small, lipophobic molecules, such as L-glucose, that readily permeate capillaries in other tissues.
b. lack breaks in the intercellular junctional strands.
c. have an abundant caveola–vesicle system to transport amino acids into the brain.
d. express the endothelial carrier protein GLUT-1 for glucose transport.
e. depend on facilitated diffusion for oxygen transport into the brain.

10.6 When a metabolic substrate or drug diffuses from the bloodstream into the tissue,

a. the mass leaving the blood per minute is called the 'extraction'.
b. the fraction of the substance removed per minute is called the 'clearance'.
c. the quantity removed per minute equals the blood flow × arterio-venous concentration difference.
d. the quantity removed per minute is given by the Fick principle.
e. the mean capillary concentration of a drug is 6 mM if the arterial concentration is 8 mM and local venous concentration is 4 mM.

10.7 Vasodilatation of the arterioles in skeletal muscle is likely to

a. increase the number of capillaries perfused with blood at any one moment.
b. increase the arterio-venous difference in oxygen content.
c. reduce the partial pressure of CO_2 in the local venous blood.
d. lower muscle capillary blood pressure.
e. neither increase nor decrease muscle lymph flow.

10.8 Regarding the effect of blood flow on transcapillary solute flux,

a. the solute exchange is flow-limited if plasma and interstitial concentrations equilibrate before the end of the capillary.
b. O_2 uptake by pulmonary capillaries is an example of diffusion-limited exchange.
c. doubling the blood flow doubles the transcapillary solute exchange when exchange is flow-limited, if concentration outside the capillary is constant.
d. exchange is diffusion-limited when the capillary plasma and interstitial concentrations fail to equilibrate by the end of the capillary.
e. raising the blood flow greatly enhances solute exchange if the latter is diffusion-limited.

10.9 The diffusive transfer of glucose from blood to skeletal muscle is increased many fold during exercise by

a. an increase in endothelial exchange area due to capillary recruitment
b. a decrease in the average diffusion distance.
c. a rise in interstitial glucose concentration.
d. an increase in capillary permeability to glucose.
e. a fall in the glucose concentration gradient.

Lastly, here is a numerical problem, to enhance your familiarity with permeability and diffusion. The questions are of the single best answer (SBA) type.

10.10 Regarding the delivery of glucose to muscle by the bloodstream,

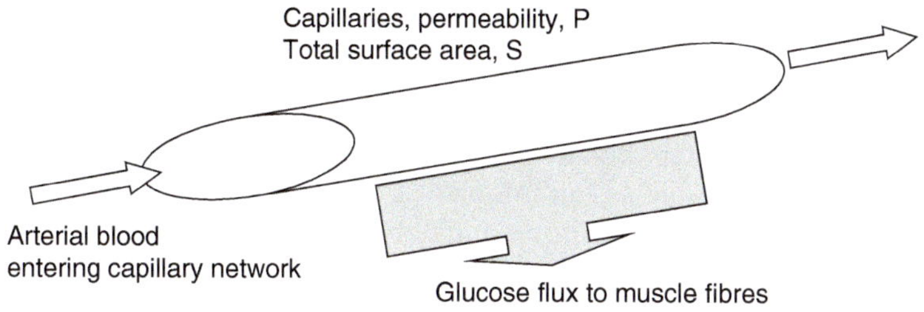

A) A resting skeletal muscle consumes 2.8 μmol glucose per minute. The glucose permeability (*P*) × surface area (*S*) product, *PS*, for the muscle capillary network is 5 cm^3 min^{-1}. The glucose concentration difference across the capillary wall is

a. 10.4 micromoles per ml.
b. 14.0 micromoles per ml.
c. 0.56 micromoles per litre.
d. 0.56 millimoles per litre.

☐

B) The subject then undertakes sustained exercise, raising the muscle glucose consumption to 30 μmol min^{-1}. The glucose concentration difference between capillary plasma and tissue increases to 1.5 mM. The capillary permeability × surface area *PS* is now approximately

a. 5 cm^3 min^{-1}.
b. 7.5 cm^3 min^{-1}.
c. 15 cm^3 min^{-1}.
d. 20 cm^3 min^{-1}.
e. 54 cm^3 min^{-1}.

☐

Answers

10.1 a. **F** – Liver capillaries are discontinuous or 'sinusoidal' **(Figure 10.1)**. Continuous capillaries are found in skin, muscle, connective tissue and the nervous system.

b. **T** – Fenestrated capillaries are found in tissues specialized for water exchange, including all the exocrine glands, e.g. salivary glands, pancreas **(Figure 10.1b)**.

c. **T** – The wide gaps in the wall allow red cells to enter the circulation **(Figure 10.1c)**.

d. **F** – The extremely thin fenestral membrane confers a very high permeability to water and to small lipophobic solutes, but not plasma proteins.

e. **T** – The gaps in the endothelial lining of discontinuous capillaries are wider than plasma protein molecules, which therefore escape readily.

10.2 a. **T** – The vast surface area of the capillary network, comprising the entire lipid endothelial membrane, is available for the diffusive permeation of lipid-soluble solutes **(Figure 9.6)**. Consequently, general anaesthetics act on the brain extremely rapidly.

b. **F** – Transcapillary fluid filtration is too slow to carry much glucose across the wall, except in the renal glomeruli (where the capillaries are fenestrated, not continuous). Transcapillary glucose transport in skeletal muscle (continuous capillaries) is by diffusion down the glucose concentration gradient.

c. **T** – If a concentration gradient is present, the transport of any small solute across the capillary wall is chiefly by diffusion, via the intercellular cleft **(Figure 10.2)**.

d. **T** – The permeability to lipid-soluble O_2 is huge **(Figure 10.3)**. This is because O_2 can access the entire (lipid) capillary surface **(Figure 9.6)**. The diffusion of lipid-insoluble solutes such as glucose is limited to the narrow, water-filled intercellular clefts **(Figure 10.2)**.

e. **F** – This is a common 'red herring'. The net transfer of water across capillaries is a process of hydraulic flow, not diffusion, being proportional to the net driving pressure (hydraulic pressure gradient minus osmotic pressure gradient).

f. **F** – The capillary reflection coefficient to plasma proteins, though high, is generally less than 100%, so interstitial fluid has a substantial plasma protein concentration – contrary to the impression given in some textbooks.

10.3 a. **F** – Fick's first law of diffusion states that diffusive transport (mass/time) is directly proportional to the concentration gradient dC/dx **(Figure 10.4)** (cf. Poiseuille's law of hydraulic flow – flow is proportional to radius^4, **Figure 8.19**).

b. **T** – Diffusive transport (J_s, mass/time) is directly proportional to surface area A. Fick's first law of diffusion states: $J_s = -DA(dC/dx)$, where D is the diffusion coefficient. So the massive capillary surface area A in the lungs allows a correspondingly massive rate of O_2 uptake.

c. **F** – Fick's first law states that diffusive transport (mass/time) is directly proportional to the diffusion coefficient D. D represents the speed at which the solute molecule slips through the solvent molecules.

d. **F** – The bigger the solute (e.g. plasma protein compared with glucose), the more friction it encounters with the solvent, so the slower it diffuses. Diffusivity D is approximately inversely proportional to the square root of molecular mass (**Figure 10.3**, dashed line 'Free diffusion').

e. **T** – The rate of O_2 diffusion out of the capillaries (J_s) normally equals the tissue O_2 consumption, e.g. myocardial O_2 consumption, so increasing the O_2 delivery to the capillary leaves more residual O_2 in the venous capillary (concentration, C_V), if tissue consumption has not increased. This follows from the Fick principle; $C_A - C_V = J_s$/blood flow **(Figure 10.5)**. The rise in C_V increases the mean O_2 concentration along the capillary **(Figure 10.6)**.

10.4 a. **F** – Permeability P is the solute transfer rate J_s (mass/time) per unit concentration difference ΔC across unit surface area A of membrane, $P = J_s/C \cdot A$. It has units of velocity, cm s^{-1}.

b. **T** – The fall-off in permeability as solute molecules approach 3–5 nm in radius reveals the pore size **(Figure 10.3)**. The small pores are the spaces in the network of biopolymer molecules making up the glycocalyx, which covers the entrance to the intercellular cleft **(Figure 9.3)**.

c. **T** – The more abundant the breaks, the greater the fraction of the intercellular junction that is available for solute and water permeation **(Figures 9.1, 9.3 top and 10.2)**. Agents that increase the number of junctional strands (cAMP-raising agents) reduce the open fraction of the cleft, and thus reduce capillary permeability.

d. **F** – When the ratio of solute radius to pore radius is >1:10, the solute experiences difficulty in entering the pore (steric exclusion) and diffusing inside it (restricted diffusion). These biophysical effects *reduce* permeability.

e. **T** – Small solutes experience less steric exclusion and restriction to diffusion **(Figure 10.3)**.

10.5 a. **T** – The endothelial cells create a blood–brain barrier. L-glucose, the stereoisomer of natural D-glucose (dextrose) and other small molecules, such as mannitol and catecholamines, cannot penetrate this barrier.

b. **T** – The continuous junctional strands create the barrier.

c. **F** – There are few caveolae or vesicles, so little protein is transported across the barrier. Amino acids are transported across the barrier by specialized carrier proteins in the endothelial cell membrane.

d. **T** – This is how natural glucose, D-glucose, the brain's primary energy source, is transported across the barrier. The process is a facilitated, carrier-mediated diffusion.

e. **F** – The respiratory gases are lipid soluble, so they diffuse through the cerebral capillary wall without hindrance **(Figure 9.6)**.

10.6 a. **F** – Extraction is the *fraction* of the solute removed **(Figure 10.5)**. For example, if the arterial concentration is 8 mM and the local venous concentration is 4 mM, half the solute has been extracted; the extraction is 50%.

b. **F** – Clearance is the volume of plasma that would be cleared of the substance per minute, so its units are millilitres/minute – as in renal clearance. The clearance equals the mass of substance removed per minute (J_s) divided by arterial plasma concentration (C_A). For example, if J_s is 2 millimoles/min and the arterial concentration is 8 millimoles/litre, the clearance is 2/8 = 0.25 litre/min = 250 ml/min.

c. **T** – This is the Fick principle **(Figures 7.3 and 10.5)**. Example: if the arterial concentration is 8 mM and local venous concentration is 4 mM, the A–V difference is 4 millimoles/litre. If the blood flow is, say, 0.5 litre/min, the solute flux J_s is $(8 - 4) \times 0.5 = 2$ millimoles/min.

d. **T** – The statement in 'c' was in fact the Fick principle; solute flux J_s = blood flow $\times (C_A - C_V)$ **(Figure 7.3)**.

e. **F** – Concentration does not fall linearly along a capillary, because outward diffusion is fastest in the early part of the capillary, where the concentration is highest **(Figure 10.5)**. The true mean is lower than the arithmetical average.

10.7 a. **T** – This is called capillary recruitment **(Figure 10.7)**. Recruitment facilitates gas exchange in exercising muscle.

b. **F** – Vasodilatation increases the blood flow. If the metabolic demand of the tissue has not increased, less O_2 needs to be extracted from each ml of blood when flow is increased.

The venous O_2 therefore rises and the A–V difference declines. This follows from the Fick principle, $(A - V)_{O_2} = O_2$ consumption/blood flow **(Figure 10.5)**.

c. **T** – Applying the Fick principle, we see that $(V - A)_{CO_2} = CO_2$ production/blood flow. A rise in blood flow will therefore reduce venous CO_2 concentration (and thus P_{CO_2}), provided that muscle metabolic rate has not increased.

d. **F** – Vasodilatation reduces the arteriolar resistance guarding the capillaries. Blood loses less pressure energy in traversing the dilated arteriole and capillary pressure rises **(Figure 11.7)**.

e. **F** – The rise in capillary pressure increases the capillary filtration rate, which increases the rate of lymph production.

10.8 a. **T** – The flow $\dot{Q}$ is delivering solute less rapidly than solute diffuses across the wall, due to the high diffusion capacity of the wall (permeability–surface area product, *PS*). Flow-limited exchange occurs when the ratio $PS/\dot{Q}$ is $\geqslant 5$ (**Figure 10.6a**, curves 1–2).

b. **F** – Raising the blood flow through the lungs (cardiac output) during exercise increases the O_2 uptake. This, then, is an example of flow-limited exchange.

c. **T** – Applying the Fick principle, solute flux J_s = blood flow$\times(C_A - C_V)$. Doubling the blood flow doubles the solute exchange, if venous concentration C_V (which has equilibrated with the surrounding concentration) is unchanged on raising flow, e.g. in the lungs (**Figure 10.6a** curves 1–3; **Figure 10.6b** points 1 and 2).

d. **T** – The flow $\dot{Q}$ is delivering material faster than it can escape, due to the limited diffusion capacity of the wall (*PS*) (**Figure 10.6a** curves 5–7). The ratio $PS/\dot{Q}$ is $\leqslant 1$. An example is glucose in exercising muscle.

e. **F** – Raising blood flow has little effect on diffusion-limited exchange (**Figure 10.6b**, points 5–7). This is because diffusion capacity *PS*, not blood flow, is limiting the exchange rate. In the Fick formula, flux J_s = flow $\times$ $(C_A - C_V)$, the effect of the increase in flow is almost cancelled out by a rise in venous concentration C_V. C_V rises because each unit of blood has less time in the capillary to exchange its contents.

10.9 a. **T** – Metabolic vasodilatation of the muscle arterioles recruits capillaries that had little flow at a given instant during rest. This increases the homogeneity of perfusion and the endothelial surface area available for exchange **(Figure 10.7)**.

b. **T** – Capillary recruitment reduces the radius of the Krogh cylinder, i.e. the cylinder of muscle fibres that a given capillary has to supply **(Figure 10.7)**.

c. **F** – The increased glucose consumption of the muscle lowers the interstitial glucose concentration. This is reflected in the fall in venous glucose concentration **(Figure 10.8, middle)**.

d. **T** – Capillary permeability to a range of small lipophobic solutes is increased by flow.

e. **F** – The concentration gradient from plasma to tissue, $\Delta C/\Delta x$, increases, due partly to the fall in tissue glucose concentration (which raises the concentration difference ΔC) and partly to capillary recruitment (which reduces the diffusion distance Δx).

10.10 Part A. The single correct answer is (d). Permeability *P* is by definition solute flux J_s per unit surface area *S* per unit concentration drop ΔC. Re-arranging this definition, $\Delta C = J_s/PS = 2.8\,\mu\text{mol min}^{-1}/5\,\text{cm}^3\text{ min}^{-1} = 0.56\,\mu\text{mol/cm}^3 = 0.56$ millimoles/litre.

Part B. The single correct answer is again (d). From the definition of permeability, $PS = J_s/\Delta C = 30\,\mu\text{mol min}^{-1}/1.5\,\mu\text{mol cm}^{-3} = 20\,\text{cm}^3\text{ min}^{-1}$. *PS* is four times bigger than in resting muscle, due to capillary recruitment, and probably also an increase in permeability stimulated by the increased blood flow.

CHAPTER 11

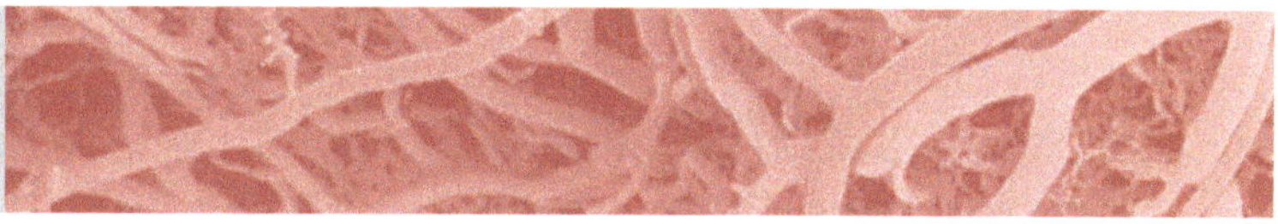

Circulation of fluid between plasma, interstitium and lymph

T F

11.1 The transfer of fluid across the capillary wall contributes importantly to

a. the regulation of interstitial fluid volume.
b. antigen transport to lymph nodes.
c. the transport of glucose into the tissues.
d. the formation of urine.
e. the enhancement of plasma volume after a haemorrhage.

11.2 The capillary

a. wall is normally a perfect semipermeable membrane.
b. reflection coefficient for plasma protein is closer to 0.9 than 0.5.
c. filtration rate is governed by just two forces, blood pressure and plasma colloid osmotic pressure.
d. glycocalyx is responsible for the semipermeability of capillaries.
e. wall hydraulic conductance is lower in fenestrated capillaries than in continuous capillaries.

11.3 Regarding the forces that influence transcapillary fluid movement in a healthy human,

a. mid-capillary pressure at heart level is ~25–30 mmHg.
b. globulins contribute more than albumin to plasma colloid osmotic pressure.
c. interstitial colloid osmotic pressure is typically one-third or more of plasma colloid osmotic pressure.
d. plasma colloid osmotic pressure is ~15 mmHg.
e. interstitial fluid pressure is subatmospheric in the subcutis.

11.4 Capillary blood pressure

a. in the foot of a standing man is about the same as aortic blood pressure.
b. can be regulated by sympathetic vasomotor fibres.
c. declines in the tissues upstream of a deep venous thrombosis.
d. is reduced after a haemorrhage.
e. is about 25 mmHg in the lungs of a resting human.

11.5 The net microvascular filtration rate

a. is typically ~20% of the plasma flow in most tissues.
b. is reduced by venous congestion.
c. is increased by hypoproteinaemia.
d. is reduced in exercising skeletal muscle.
e. is increased in the skin in hot weather.
f. is increased in inflamed tissues.
g. is increased in all forms of oedema.

T F

11.6 The concentration of plasma proteins in the interstitial fluid

a. of a given tissue is a fixed quantity. ☐ ☐
b. of the lungs is higher than in the legs. ☐ ☐
c. is increased when capillary filtration rate increases. ☐ ☐
d. falls when interstitial fluid is absorbed by capillaries. ☐ ☐
e. acts as a buffer against sustained fluid absorption. ☐ ☐

11.7 Regarding the 'balance' of Starling pressures along a capillary,

a. the sum of the Starling pressures is greater in arterial than venous capillaries. ☐ ☐
b. the Starling pressures add up to a sustained absorption force in most venous capillaries. ☐ ☐
c. plasma colloid osmotic pressure exceeds the sum of the other Starling pressures during a severe haemorrhage. ☐ ☐
d. the sum of the Starling pressures results in an increase in plasma volume during standing. ☐ ☐
e. the sum of the Starling pressures leads to a fall in plasma volume during exercise. ☐ ☐

Here is a numerical problem that highlights the importance of interstitial factors for filtration versus absorption.

11.8 A tissue in stable fluid balance exhibited the following Starling parameters,

Mean capillary pressure, P_c	9 mmHg
Plasma colloid osmotic pressure, π_p	26 mmHg
Interstitial fluid pressure, P_i	−2 mmHg
Interstitial colloid osmotic pressure, π_i	15 mmHg
Endothelial reflection coefficient for plasma proteins, σ	0.8
Capillary filtration capacity (hydraulic permeability, Lp × total surface area, A)	0.3 ml min^{-1} $mmHg^{-1}$ per kg tissue

a. Does the difference between capillary pressure and plasma colloid osmotic pressure favour plasma filtration or interstitial fluid absorption?
b. Was there net filtration or absorption between the plasma and interstitial compartment?
c. What tissue might this be?
d. What was the rate of lymph production?

T F

11.9 Interstitial fluid

a. volume is ~20–28 l in a human adult. ☐ ☐
b. mobility is high due to the interstitial glycosaminoglycan chains. ☐ ☐
c. in the oedematous subcutis is readily displaced by finger pressure. ☐ ☐
d. pressure is very sensitive to acute changes in interstitial fluid volume in the physiological range. ☐ ☐
e. pressure is very sensitive to changes in interstitial fluid volume in the oedema range. ☐ ☐
f. pressure is around +2 mmHg in oedematous subcutis. ☐ ☐

T F

11.10 The lymphatic system

a. is essential for the tissue volume homeostasis. ☐ ☐
b. is the chief means of clearing escaped plasma proteins from the interstitium. ☐ ☐
c. is vital for the immunosurveillance of tissue antigens. ☐ ☐
d. transports fatty products of digestion from the intestine to the bloodstream. ☐ ☐
e. commences peripherally as endothelial tubes with tight intercellular junctions. ☐ ☐
f. empties centrally into the pulmonary veins. ☐ ☐

11.11 Lymph nodes

a. contain a network of blood capillaries that can absorb afferent lymph. ☐ ☐
b. phagocytose particulate materials washed into them in the lymph. ☐ ☐
c. release activated lymphocytes into the nodal bloodstream. ☐ ☐
d. possess specialized blood vessel called low-endothelial arterioles. ☐ ☐
e. take up circulating lymphocytes from nodal blood vessels. ☐ ☐

11.12 The flow of lymph

a. increases when capillary pressure increases. ☐ ☐
b. is reduced by tissue movement. ☐ ☐
c. is promoted by active contraction in large lymphatic vessels. ☐ ☐
d. is unidirectional, due to semilunar valves in many lymphatics. ☐ ☐
e. is increased in filariasis. ☐ ☐
f. is increased by lymph node excision as part of cancer treatment. ☐ ☐

11.13 The contractile activity of lymphatic vessels

a. is initiated by depolarization-triggered action potentials. ☐ ☐
b. can generate pressures as high as 40 mmHg, if obstructed. ☐ ☐
c. depends on L-type Ca^{2+} channels in the smooth muscle membrane. ☐ ☐
d. is preceded by a diastolic filling phase, with the downstream (central) valve open and upstream (distal) valve closed. ☐ ☐
e. is stimulated by moderate distension. ☐ ☐
f. is inhibited by sympathetic noradrenergic fibres. ☐ ☐

11.14 Oedema often develops when

a. arterial blood pressure is high (essential hypertension). ☐ ☐
b. venous blood pressure is raised by chronic cardiac failure. ☐ ☐
c. arterioles are dilated by Ca^{2+} channel blocking drugs. ☐ ☐
d. plasma colloid osmotic pressure is increased in multiple myeloma. ☐ ☐
e. axillary lymph nodes are resected during breast cancer treatment. ☐ ☐

11.15 Factors that prevent or mitigate dependent oedema (oedema of the feet) include

a. a locally low extravascular colloid osmotic pressure. ☐ ☐
b. a locally reduced interstitial fluid pressure. ☐ ☐
c. reduced leg lymph flow. ☐ ☐
d. a rise in local peripheral vascular resistance. ☐ ☐
e. the calf muscle pump. ☐ ☐

T F

11.16 During acute inflammation,

a. the oedema fluid has an unusually low fibrinogen content.
b. wide gaps appear in venular endothelium.
c. vasoconstriction lowers the capillary filtration pressure.
d. the endothelial osmotic reflection coefficient for plasma proteins decreases.
e. the hydraulic conductance of the venular wall decreases.
f. histamine is a common, early mediator.

11.17 The hyperpermeability of inflammation can be mediated by

a. a rise in endothelial cytoplasmic Ca^{2+}.
b. a fall in endothelial nitric oxide production.
c. a rise in endothelial cAMP.
d. the redistribution of junctional cadherin.
e. increased vascular endothelial growth factor (VEGF) in rheumatoid joints.

Here is a quantitative problem, designed to enhance familiarity with the classic Starling principle. Assume, as a first approximation, that subglycocalyx osmotic pressure equals that in the interstitial compartment.

11.18 The effect of a haemorrhage on fluid exchange.

In a patient prior to haemorrhage, mean capillary blood pressure P_c in the leg muscles (supine) was 25 mmHg; plasma colloid osmotic pressure π_p was 25 mmHg; interstitial fluid pressure P_i was −1 mmHg; interstitial fluid colloid osmotic pressure π_i was 6 mmHg; the protein reflection coefficient σ was 0.96; and the capillary filtration capacity K was 0.003 ml min^{-1} mmHg^{-1} per 100 g muscle.

a. What was the rate of fluid filtration per 100 g muscle?
b. If the muscle blood flow was 6 ml/min per 100 g, and the haematocrit was 0.45, what was the filtration fraction?
c. If the muscle mass in the leg was 10 kg, what was the leg lymph flow?

The patient then suffered a severe, acute haemorrhage. This reduced the capillary blood pressure to 10 mmHg. Assume that the other pressure terms have not yet changed.

d. In which direction was net fluid transfer after the haemorrhage?
e. How much fluid was transferred between the muscle interstitial compartment and plasma compartment per minute in the muscle of the whole leg (10 kg)?
f. If fluid exchange occurred at a similar average rate in the entire body, of mass 70 kg, how much fluid was transferred over 30 min? Could this affect the patient's survival?
g. Had the haematocrit increased, decreased or not changed at 30 min?

Answers

11.1 a. **T** – Interstitial fluid is continuously replenished by capillary filtrate **(Figure 11.1)**. Excessive filtration causes oedema.

b. **T** – Capillary filtrate forms interstitial fluid, which drains into lymphatics, carrying antigens from the tissue to the lymph nodes for immunosurveillance **(Figure 11.2)**.

c. **F** – Glucose diffuses down its concentration gradient much faster than it is washed into the tissue by the relatively slow stream of capillary filtrate.

d. **T** – Glomerular capillary filtration is the first stage in urine formation.

e. **T** – Capillaries absorb interstitial fluid after a haemorrhage, thus boosting the depleted plasma volume – the 'internal transfusion'.

11.2 a. **F** – The wall is an *imperfect* semipermeable membrane; it allows some plasma protein permeation (reflection coefficient $\sigma < 1.0$). A perfect semipermeable membrane totally excludes the osmotically active solute ($\sigma = 1.0$).

b. **T** – About 90% of the plasma protein osmotic pressure is exerted in practice; the osmotic reflection coefficient σ is 0.9 (90%). Sigma falls below 0.5 during inflammation, due to gap formation.

c. **F** – Four forces must always be considered, not just two. Filtration rate is proportional to the *difference in* hydraulic pressure across the membrane minus the *difference* in the effective colloid osmotic pressure across the membrane (Starling's principle of fluid exchange, **Figure 11.3**).

d. **T** – The glycocalyx comprises a biopolymer network **(Figure 9.3)**. The small pores between the polymer fibres impede plasma protein passage, relative to water and small solutes **(Figure 11.3b)**.

e. **F** – The extremely thin membranes of the fenestrations are highly permeable to water and small solutes, though not to plasma proteins **(Figure 10.1)**.

11.3 a. **T** – These are typical values in human skin at heart level, as measured through a micropipette **(Figures 11.3, top and 11.4, left)**.

b. **F** – Albumin comprises only approximately half of the plasma protein mass, but accounts for approximately two-thirds of the plasma colloid osmotic pressure (COP). This is because fixed negative charges on the albumin molecule attract Na^+ ions, which contribute to the osmotic pressure (Gibbs–Donnan effect).

c. **T** – The value depends on the tissue and on capillary filtration rate, but typically ranges from 23% (leg) to 70% (lung) of plasma COP **(Figures 11.3, top and 11.4, left)**. There is a widespread misconception that interstitial COP is negligible.

d. **F** – Human plasma COP averages ~25 mmHg (range, 21–29 mmHg) **(Figure 11.3, top)**. A general rule across different species is that mid-capillary pressure and plasma COP are approximately equal.

e. **T** – Measurements using the wick-in-needle and servo-null micropipettes indicate that interstitial fluid pressure is −1 to −3 mmHg in skin and subcutis **(Figures 11.3, top and 11.5)**.

11.4 a. **T** – Direct micropuncture studies show that capillary pressure in the human foot during standing is about 90 mmHg (120 cmH_2O) **(Figure 11.6)**.

b. **T** – Capillary pressure depends partly on the pre- to postcapillary resistance ratio **(Figure 11.7)**, and the precapillary resistance vessel diameter is controlled by sympathetic vasoconstrictor fibres. Sympathetic activity raises the precapillary resistance, causing blood to lose more pressure before it reaches the capillary; capillary pressure thus falls.

c. **F** – A deep vein thrombosis (DVT) raises the *post*-capillary resistance, and thus raises capillary pressure. A DVT therefore causes acute limb oedema.
d. **T** – Haemorrhage triggers a reflex, sympathetic-mediated vasoconstriction. This raises the pre- to postcapillary resistance ratio **(Figure 11.7)**; also arterial and venous pressures may fall. The resulting fall in capillary pressure allows the plasma colloid osmotic pressure to absorb interstitial fluid – the 'internal transfusion' **(Figure 11.4, middle)**.
e. **F** – Pressures are much lower in the pulmonary circulation than the systemic circulation. Pulmonary capillary pressure is ~9–13 mmHg at rest.

11.5 a. **F** – The filtration fraction is only 0.2–0.3% in most tissues. It reaches 20% in the specialized, highly fenestrated capillaries of the renal glomerulus.
b. **F** – A rise in venous pressure increased the capillary pressure and therefore filtration rate. This is a common cause of oedema **(Figure 11.8)**.
c. **T** – Hypoproteinaemia reduces plasma colloid osmotic pressure, the force retaining water in the circulation. The increased capillary filtration rate can lead to oedema.
d. **F** – A rise in interstitial osmolarity in the exercising muscle increase filtration rate. This is compounded by metabolic vasodilatation of the arterioles, which raises capillary pressure **(Figure 11.7)**.
e. **T** – Heat causes cutaneous arterioles to dilate. This reduces precapillary resistance and thus raise capillary pressure **(Figure 11.7)**. The resulting increase in interstitial fluid volume explains why a ring on the finger becomes much tighter in hot weather.
f. **T** – Inflammation causes gaps to form in the post-capillary venule wall. Gaps increase the wall's hydraulic conductance and reduce its osmotic reflection coefficient, raising the filtration rate **(Figure 11.9)**. This leads to the rapid, severe tissue swelling that is a major feature of inflammation.
g. **F** – Although most forms of oedema are indeed caused by increased capillary filtration rate, lymphoedema is caused by reduced lymphatic drainage.

11.6 a. **F** – Interstitial protein concentration is set by the ratio of protein leakage rate to water filtration rate. Since the latter is a dynamic variable, dependent on capillary pressure, so too is interstitial protein concentration and COP **(Figure 11.10)**.
b. **T** – Since capillary pressure is low in the pulmonary circulation, filtration rate and lymph flow are low, so interstitial protein concentration and COP are high **(Figure 11.10)**. Due to the high interstitial COP, lung capillaries filter fluid despite their low capillary pressure. This illustrates the need to take account of the interstitial forces when considering fluid exchange.
c. **F** – Raising the filtration rate reduces interstitial protein concentration **(Figure 11.10)**.
d. **F** – Extravascular plasma protein concentration increases as interstitial fluid is absorbed, due to the reflection of the extravascular proteins by the capillary wall.
e. **T** – The process described in (d) raises extravascular colloid osmotic pressure. This progressively slows and eventually halts the absorption process **(Figure 11.4, right)**.

11.7 a. **T** – Capillary blood pressure falls along the length of the capillary, so the net filtration force is low in venous capillaries and venules **(Figure 11.4, left)**.
b. **F** – This fallacy has been perpetuated for over half a century, based usually on inappropriate values for the interstitial forces. When all four Starling pressures are measured in the same tissue, they add up to a slight net filtration force in most venous capillaries and venules **(Figures 11.4 and 11.11)**. Fluid absorption is not sustained at venous capillary pressure in most tissues (**Figure 11.12**, steady-state curve).

c. **T** – Capillary pressure falls during a severe haemorrhage. Transient fluid absorption ensues **(Figure 11.4, middle panel)**.

d. **F** – During orthostasis the capillary pressure increases in the tissues below heart level. Consequently, the filtration rate increases over much of the body, reducing the plasma volume by 6% or more.

e. **T** – In exercising muscle the arteriolar vasodilatation raises capillary blood pressure. Also, interstitial osmolarity is raised by crystalloids (lactate, K^+) released by the contracting muscle fibres. The resulting increase in local capillary filtration rate reduces plasma volume by as much as 20%.

11.8 a. Since the osmotic suction pressure of the plasma proteins π_p (26 mmHg) exceeds capillary filtration pressure P_c (9 mmHg), this difference strongly favours fluid absorption.

b. Despite the answer to (a), there is actually net filtration in this tissue – because fluid movement depends on interstitial, as well as intravascular forces. Starling's principle states that the net force driving fluid movement is $(P_c - P_i) - \sigma(\pi_p - \pi_i)$ (neglecting differences between interstitium and subglycocalyx). This is $(9 - (-2)) - 0.8(26 - 15) = 2.2$ mmHg. There is thus a net filtration gradient from plasma to interstitium.

c. The lung. The very low mean capillary pressure is typical of the low-pressure pulmonary circulation (lowest, left point, **Figure 11.11**). So too are the high interstitial colloid osmotic pressure and high capillary filtration capacity (CFC).

d. According to the classic Starling principle (neglecting differences between interstitium and subglycocalyx), the filtration rate $J_v = L_pA\{(P_c - P_i) - \sigma(\pi_p - \pi_i)\} = 0.3\{2.2\} = 0.66$ ml min^{-1} kg^{-1}. Over a day, therefore, the human lungs (which weigh ~1 kg) should produce ~950 ml of prenodal lymph.

11.9 a. **F** – Interstitial fluid volume is ~10–12 l **(Figure 11.1)**. *Intracellular* fluid volume is double this, ~20 l (female) to 28 l (male).

b. **F** – Interstitial glycosaminoglycan chains fill in the spaces between the collagen fibrils, thus creating a high resistance to flow **(Figure 11.13)**. Consequently, interstitial fluid mobility is normally low and normal tissue does not pit readily to external pressure.

c. **T** – Dilution of the interstitial glycosaminoglycans by oedema fluid raises the fluid mobility. Consequently, an oedematous tissue 'pits' readily – the clinical 'pitting test' for oedema **(Figure 11.14)**.

d. **T** – The sigmoidal pressure–volume relation is steep at normal hydrations **(Figure 11.5)**. This is because the suction effect of the glycosaminoglycans (their osmotic pressure or 'swelling pressure'), which contributes to the subatmospheric pressure, depends on their concentration – which is altered by acute changes in volume.

e. **F** – The pressure–volume relation is very flat in the oedema range **(Figure 11.5)**. The glycosaminoglycan osmotic pressure has been reduced to zero by dilution. Due to the flatness of the relation, oedema fluid can accumulate with little increase in opposing force.

f. **T** – This is a typical value, e.g. in human limb lymphoedema.

11.10 a. **T** – The lymphatics are the normal route by which the capillary filtrate is returned to the bloodstream **(Figures 11.1 and 11.2)**.

b. **T** – The hydraulic and diffusive gradients across the capillary wall prevent net reuptake of escaped plasma proteins into the microcirculation.

c. **T** – Lymph carries viral and other antigens to the lymph nodes. Although all vertebrates have a lymphatic system, only mammals and certain birds have lymph nodes.

d. **T** – Intestinal lacteals transport chylomicra to the cisterna chyli **(Figure 11.2)**. The observation of these milky vessels led to the discovery of the lymphatic system.

e. **F** – The initial lymphatics are indeed endothelial tubes, but the intercellular junctions are very loose. They act as flap valves that allow interstitial fluid entry **(Figure 11.15)**.

f. **F** – The main lymphatic vessel, the thoracic duct, drains into the left subclavian vein in the root of the neck **(Figure 11.2)**.

11.11 a. **T** – Lymph node capillaries absorb up to half the water and electrolytes in the incoming afferent lymph **(Figures 11.1 and 11.2)**. Efferent lymph thus has a smaller volume and higher protein concentration than afferent lymph.

b. **T** – The sinuses of a lymph node are lined by phagocytic cells that take up particles; carbon particles blacken the hilar nodes in the lungs of smokers.

c. **F** – Nodes release lymphocytes into the *efferent lymph*, which therefore has a higher lymphocyte count than afferent lymph **(Figure 11.2)**.

d. **F** – Nodes contain specialized blood vessels called *high-endothelial venules* **(Figure 11.2)**. These vessels express a receptor for L-selectin on circulating lymphocytes.

e. **T** – Lymphocytes adhere to the high endothelial venules and migrate into the node through the high endothelium, completing their own 'circulation' between lymph and blood.

11.12 a. **T** – Increased capillary pressure raises capillary filtration rate. In the steady state, interstitial fluid drainage (lymph flow) must equal interstitial fluid formation (capillary filtration) **(Figure 11.1)**.

b. **F** – Tissue movement causes cyclic squeezing of the small lymphatics, which promotes lymph flow.

c. **T** – Large lymphatics have smooth muscle in the wall and contract rhythmically. The lymphatic pressure–volume loop is comparable with that of the ventricle **(Figure 11.16)**.

d. **T** – The larger lymphatic vessels have semilunar valves **(Figures 11.2 and 11.15a)**.

e. **F** – Filariasis, a nematode worm infection, blocks lymphatics. It is the most common cause of lymphoedema worldwide.

f. **F** – Nodal excision obstructs lymphatic drainage. It is the most common cause of lymphoedema in the West.

11.13 a. **T** – A slow depolarization triggers a burst of action potentials, which in turn trigger contraction **(Figure 11.16a)**.

b. **T** – Human arm and leg lymphatics can pump to these pressures if obstructed. Therefore, the tourniquet pressure applied to cases of snake or spider envenomation has to be >40–50 mmHg – otherwise venom-laden lymph can be pumped centrally.

c. **T** – Lymphatic smooth muscle action potentials are generated partly by activated Ca^{2+} channels.

d. **F** – In the diastolic filling phase, the distal, upstream valve is open and the proximal, downstream valve is closed – similar to the cardiac ventricular filling phase. **(Figure 11.16b; compare to Figure 2.7)**.

e. **T** – Moderate lymphatic distension boosts both contractile force and frequency **(Figure 11.16b)**. Excessive distension reduces contractile force.

f. **F** – Large lymphatics have a sympathetic noradrenergic innervation that *increases* contractility and ejection fraction, e.g. after a haemorrhage **(Figure 11.16b, dashed loop)**.

11.14 a. **F** – Oedema is not a feature of clinical hypertension, unless heart failure supervenes. Hypertension is due to increased precapillary resistance; so the pressure drop across the precapillary resistance vessels is bigger than usual. This protects the capillary from any substantial rise in pressure.

b. **T** – A rise in venous pressure increases the capillary pressure and filtration rate **(Figure 11.8)**, leading to peripheral and pulmonary oedema. Deep vein thrombosis has a similar effect in the drainage territory of the obstructed vein.

c. **T** – A fall in the precapillary resistance raises capillary pressure **(Figure 11.7)**. This can lead to oedema, a recognized complication of Ca^{2+} blockers. These drugs may also inhibit lymphatic contractility.

d. **F** – Multiple myeloma is a cancer of globulin-secreting cells that causes hyperproteinaemia. But it is *hypo*proteinaemia that causes oedema, by reducing plasma colloid osmotic pressure, the force retaining water in the circulation.

e. **T** – Up to a quarter of women treated in this way for breast cancer develop lymphoedema of the arm.

11.15 a. **T** – The extravascular plasma protein concentration is low due to capillary filtration. This reduces the extravascular colloid osmotic pressure, which in turn attenuates the filtration rate **(Figure 11.17a)**.

b. **F** – Interstitial fluid pressure *rises* as capillary filtration and interstitial fluid volume are increased by dependency **(Figure 11.17b)**. The rise in interstitial pressure reduces the pressure gradient driving capillary filtration.

c. **F** – Lymph flow *increases*, because capillary filtration delivers more fluid to the interstitium, raising interstitial fluid volume **(Figure 11.17c)**.

d. **T** – Precapillary resistance vessel contract in the dependent tissue (postural vasoconstriction) **(Figure 11.6)**. The increased precapillary resistance reduces local capillary pressure to almost the minimum possible, namely venous pressure.

e. **T** – The calf muscle pump lowers the venous pressure in the dependent leg **(Figure 8.4)**. Since capillary pressure is close to venous pressure, it too falls, reducing the filtration rate.

11.16 a. **F** – Inflammation oedema is an 'exudate', i.e. rich in plasma proteins, especially the large ones such as fibrinogen (due to gaps in the endothelium). The high fibrinogen content can cause problems, e.g. fibrin adhesions between loops of bowel following peritonitis.

b. **T** – The gaps between and/or through the venular endothelial cells increase the hydraulic permeability of the wall, leading to rapid, severe tissue swelling **(Figure 11.9a)**.

c. **F** – Inflammation is characterized by vaso*dilatation*, which raises capillary filtration pressure **(Figure 11.7)**. Vasodilatation accounts for two of the classic signs of inflammation – heat and redness.

d. **T** – The venular gaps allow easy passage of the plasma proteins. The resulting fall in the osmotic reflection coefficient contributes to the rapid fluid filtration.

e. **F** – The hydraulic conductance of the venule wall increases sharply, due to the gap formation **(Figure 11.9b, slope of line)**. This promotes rapid tissue swelling.

f. **T** – Histamine is released from mast cells and basophilic leukocytes in inflammatory reactions, such as urticaria, anaphylaxis and asthma. It causes intercellular gap formation.

11.17 a. T – Endothelium expresses receptor-operated and store-operated Ca^{2+}-conducting channels (Figure 9.2). These raise endothelial Ca^{2+} concentration between four- and ten-fold at the onset of acute inflammation (Figure 11.18). If the rise in Ca^{2+} is suppressed, so is the hyperpermeability response.

b. F – The rise in Ca^{2+}-calmodulin *increases* the activity of eNOS and hence the production of NO, a pro-inflammatory agent in venules (Figure 11.19). Deletion of eNOS blocks the inflammatory response.

c. F – Agents that raise intracellular cAMP, such as isoprenaline, *reduce* permeability. One of the downstream effects of NO is to activate a phosphodiesterase that degrades cAMP (Figure 11.19).

d. T – Fragmentation of the peripheral ring of actin, to which the junctional proteins are anchored (Figure 9.3), coupled with phosphorylation of the junctional proteins themselves, loosens the intercellular junction (Figure 11.19).

e. T – Vascular endothelial growth factor causes a chronic increase in endothelial permeability. It is raised at many chronic inflammatory sites, including rheumatoid joints.

11.18 a. From the classic Starling principle, filtration rate $J_v = K\{[P_c - P_i] - \sigma[\pi_p - \pi_i]\} = 0.003\{[25 - (-1)] - 0.96[25 - 6]\} = 0.0233\,\text{ml min}^{-1}$ per 100 g muscle. This highlight the fact that capillary filtration is normally a *very* slow process.

b. Plasma was 55% of the blood volume ($1 - 0.45 = 0.55$). The plasma flow was therefore $6 \times 0.55 = 3.3\,\text{ml min}^{-1}$ per 100 g. The filtration fraction is therefore 0.0233 ml filtrate min^{-1}/3.3 ml plasma min^{-1}, or 0.007. Fluid filtration is thus very slow relative to plasma flow in continuous capillaries.

c. Lymph flow equals capillary filtration rate in the steady state, i.e. $0.0233\,\text{ml min}^{-1}$ per 100 g. This is $2.33\,\text{ml min}^{-1}$ for the whole leg (10 kg muscle). Lymph production is thus very low.

d. After the haemorrhage, the classic Starling principle predicts a net filtration force of $[10 - (-1)] - 0.96[25 - 6] = -7.24$ mmHg. The minus sign means that the net force is now a force directed into the capillary lumen, i.e. an absorption force. Fluid will move from the interstitial compartment into the bloodstream.

e. The rate of fluid absorption predicted by the classic Starling principle is $J_V = K\{[P_C - P_i] - \sigma[\pi_p - \pi_i]\} = 0.003\{-7.24\} = -0.022\,\text{ml min}^{-1}$ per 100 g. For 10 kg muscle this is $2.2\,\text{ml min}^{-1}$.

f. Over 30 min, scaling up to a 70 kg body mass, the volume of fluid transferred from the interstitial compartment to the plasma compartment would be $2.2 \times 30 \times 7 = 462$ ml. This rough calculation ignores differences in K between tissues and the progressive changes in the extravascular forces; but it suffices to indicate a major internal transfusion of interstitial fluid, of ~0.5 l, into the volume-depleted circulation. This improves the patient's chances of survival.

g. The haematocrit would have declined, due to haemodilution by the internally transfused fluid.

CHAPTER 12

Vascular smooth muscle: excitation, contraction and relaxation

T F

12.1 Vascular myocytes

a. are spindle-shaped cells aligned longitudinally along the vessel axis. ☐ ☐
b. form homocellular gap junctions that provide electrical coupling. ☐ ☐
c. are striated due to the presence of myosin and actin. ☐ ☐
d. have actin filaments that are rooted in Z lines. ☐ ☐
e. store Ca^{2+} in the sarcoplasmic reticulum. ☐ ☐

12.2 Vascular contraction differs from cardiac contraction in that

a. vascular contraction does not always depend on depolarization, unlike cardiac contraction. ☐ ☐
b. vascular contraction requires myosin activation, as opposed to actin filament activation in cardiac myocytes. ☐ ☐
c. vascular contraction can be maintained despite a fall in cytosolic free Ca^{2+}. ☐ ☐
d. cardiac contraction lasts much longer than vascular myocyte contraction, in general. ☐ ☐
e. sympathetic fibres can initiate vascular contraction, but not cardiac contraction. ☐ ☐

For a change, here is a 'choose the right phrase' question.

12.3 The ion channels of vascular myocytes

Vascular myocytes typically have a basal membrane potential of around ______. This is generated in part by an ______ current of ______ through the abundant ______. Other channels that can increase the membrane potential (hyperpolarize it) include ______, which help prevent vasospasm, and ______, which contribute to vasodilatation in ischaemic tissue. When the sympathetic fibres to a resistance vessel are activated, a slow depolarization called a slow ______ may arise due to the activation of two currents – an ______ current carried by ______ composed of TRP proteins, and an outward movement of negative charge through ______. In resistance vessels, the slow depolarization activates the abundantly expressed ______. The latter may result in an ______ in some vessels.

Insert the right word or phrase from the list below. A word can be used more than once or not at all.

−94 mV	−80 mV	−55 mV	Ca^{2+} ions
inward	outward	Na^{+} ions	K^{+} ions
ATP-dependent K^{+} channels	inward rectifier K^{+} channels	calcium-dependent K^{+} channels	voltage-dependent Na^{+} channels
receptor-operated cation channels	calcium-activated chloride channels	acetylcholine-activated K^{+} channels	voltage-sensitive Ca^{2+} channels
inhibitory junction potential	excitatory junction potential	repolarization	action potential

T F

12.4 Vascular smooth muscle agonists can raise the cytosolic free Ca^{2+} through

a. inositol trisphosphate (IP_3) mediated release of an intracellular Ca^{2+} store.
b. action potentials mediated by sarcolemmal voltage-sensitive sodium channels.
c. diacylglycerol (DAG)-mediated activation of receptor-operated cation channels.
d. the activation of calmodulin.
e. Beta$_2$-adrenergic receptor stimulation.

12.5 Large artery contraction is mediated by different pathways to resistance vessel contraction, because

a. resistance vessels usually express very few voltage-sensitive Ca^{2+} channels.
b. resistance vessels commonly show depolarization-dependent contraction.
c. large arteries often exhibit depolarization-independent contraction.
d. sympathetic stimulation inhibits contraction in small arterial vessels.

12.6 Calcium sensitization in vascular myocytes

a. is achieved by maintaining a high level of free Ca^{2+} ions in the cytosol.
b. often contributes to the maintenance of vascular tone over long periods.
c. is mediated by the activation of myosin light chain phosphatase.
d. is brought about by receptor-induced activation of rhoA kinase.

12.7 Regarding adrenoceptors on vascular myocytes,

a. the α_1-,α_2-adrenoceptor blocker phentolamine reduces vascular tone.
b. Alpha$_1$-adrenoceptors bind adrenaline more avidly than noradrenaline.
c. the activation of α_1-adrenoceptors inhibits the phospholipase C pathway.
d. Alpha$_2$-adrenoceptors activate the cAMP pathway.
e. Beta$_1$-adrenoceptors are more common than β_2 in most blood vessels.
f. Beta$_2$-adrenoceptors bind adrenaline more avidly than noradrenaline.

12.8 Action potentials in vasomotor sympathetic fibres can trigger

a. the release of vesicles containing noradrenaline and ATP from varicosities.
b. fast excitatory junction potentials on vascular myocytes mediated by α_1-adrenoceptors.
c. a slow depolarization of vascular myocytes mediated by α_1-adrenoceptors.
d. the hydrolysis of phosphoinositol bisphosphate (PIP_2) in the myocyte membrane.
e. the activation of vascular L-type Ca^{2+} channels and/or non-selective cation channels.

12.9 Vascular myocyte relaxation can be brought about by

a. adrenaline via an increase in intracellular cGMP.
b. the dephosphorylation of myosin heads by myosin light chain phosphatase.
c. a fall in the cytosolic free Ca^{2+} concentration.
d. reduced sympathetic fibre activity.
e. vascular myocyte hyperpolarization.

12.10 Pharmacological agents that alter vascular tone include

a. adrenaline, which causes vasoconstriction in many tissues.
b. nitrodilators, such as glyceryl trinitrate, which raise intracellular cAMP.

	T	F
c. sildenafil (Viagra), which raises intracellular cGMP.	☐	☐
d. losartan, which inhibits angiotensin II receptors to evoke vasodilatation.	☐	☐
e. nifedipine, which stimulates the sarcolemmal Ca^{2+} pumps.	☐	☐

Here is a short quantitative problem that should help clarify the role of chloride ions.

12.11 Regarding the role of chloride-conducting channels in vascular smooth muscle (VSM), the concentration of chloride ions in extracellular fluid (Cl_o) is 120 mM, while the intracellular concentration (Cl_i) is 50 mM – considerably higher than in central neurons (7 mM).

a. What is the equilibrium potential for chloride in VSM?
b. What effect does sympathetic activity have on chloride channels in the VSM membrane?
c. If the membrane potential of VSM is −60 mV, in which direction would the potential change if the chloride conductance of the membrane were increased.
c. If the membrane potential of a central neuron is −70 mV, in which direction would neuron potential change if the chloride conductance of the membrane increased?

Answers

12.1 a. **F** – Vascular myocytes are wrapped around the circumference of the vessel, so that their tension can regulate the vessel diameter **(Figures 1.8 and 10.7)**.

b. **T** – Homocellular gap junctions, formed of connexin, connect the cytoplasm one myocyte to the next **(Figure 12.1)**. Heterocellular, myoendothelial gap junctions also link the innermost myocytes electrically to endothelial cells **(Figures 1.8 and 9.5)**.

c. **F** – The myosin and actin are not aligned in register across the cell **(Figure 12.1)**, unlike skeletal and cardiac muscle **Figure 3.3**). Consequently, vascular smooth muscle is not striated.

d. **F** – Vascular myocyte actin filaments are rooted in non-aligned dark bodies composed of α-actinin, and in the dense bands of the sarcolemma **(Figure 12.1)**.

e. **T** – The release of the sarcolemmal Ca^{2+} store by IP_3 is an important factor in vascular contraction **(Figure 12.2)**.

12.2 a. **T** – Depolarization-independent contraction is common in large arteries **(Figure 12.3c)**. It is triggered by biochemical signals **(Figure 12.4b)**. Any associated change in membrane potential is secondary, and not the cause of contraction **(Figure 12.5a)**. Action potentials are essential for cardiac contraction, and for contraction in some blood vessels (resistance vessels, portal vein) **(Figures 12.3a and 12.4a)**.

b. **T** – A rise in vascular Ca^{2+}–calmodulin complex activates myosin light chain kinase (MLCK). MLCK phosphorylates the myosin heads to initiate crossbridge formation **(Figure 12.6)**. By contrast, cardiac contraction is brought about by Ca^{2+} binding to troponin, which exposes binding sites on the actin filament **(Figure 3.4)**.

c. **T** – Vascular agonists, e.g. noradrenaline, can maintain contractile tension during the tonic, sustained phase by increasing the sensitivity of the myocyte to Ca^{2+} **(Figure 12.7)**. This is achieved by inhibiting the 'relaxing enzyme', myosin light chain phosphatase **(Figure 12.6)**; and also through caldesmon, a protein that regulates actin binding site availability.

d. **F** – A cardiac contraction lasts ~300 ms. Vascular contraction can be sustained almost indefinitely.

e. **T** – Sympathetic activity is a major mediator of vascular myocyte contraction **(Figures 12.5 and 12.8)**. The pathways involved are shown in **Figure 12.4**. In the heart, sympathetic activity does not *initiate* cardiac contraction, though it can *modify* contractile strength.

12.3 Vascular myocytes typically have a basal membrane potential of around **−55mV**. This is generated in part by an **outward** current of **K^+ ions** through the abundant **inward rectifier K^+ channels**. Other channels that can increase the membrane potential **hyperpolarize it** include **calcium-dependent K^+ channels**, which help prevent vasospasm, and **ATP-dependent K^+ channels**, which contribute to vasodilatation in ischaemic tissue. When the sympathetic fibres to a resistance vessel are activated, a slow depolarization called a slow **excitatory junction potential** may arise due to the activation of two currents – an **inward** current carried by **receptor-operated cation channels** composed of TRP proteins, and an outward movement of negative charge through **calcium-activated chloride channels**. In resistance vessels, the slow depolarization activates the abundantly expressed **voltage-sensitive Ca^{2+} channels**. The latter may result in an **action potential** in some vessels.

12.4 a. **T** – G_q-coupled receptors, such as α_1-adrenoceptors, activate phospholipase Cβ, which cleaves IP_3 from the membrane phospholipid PIP_2. IP_3 receptors on the sarcoplasmic reticulum trigger the release of its stored Ca^{2+} **(Figure 12.4b)**.

b. **F** – Membrane depolarization opens voltage-gated *calcium* channels **(Figure 12.4a)**. The ensuing rise in intracellular Ca^{2+} triggers depolarization-dependent contraction. Vascular myocytes lack the voltage-sensitive Na^+ channels that carry the action potential current in cardiac myocytes and nerve fibres.

c. **T** – The activation of a G_q-coupled receptor (e.g. α_1-adrenoceptor) triggers the cleavage of PIP_2 by phospholipase Cβ, forming soluble IP_3 and membrane-bound DAG. The DAG binds to certain TRP channels, activating their conductivity to cations **(Figure 12.4b)**.

d. **F** – Calmodulin *binds* Ca^{2+}, forming a complex that activates myosin light chain kinase, leading to contraction **(Figure 12.6)**.

e. **F** – $Beta_2$-adrenergic receptors are activated by circulating adrenaline and trigger a fall in cytosol-free Ca^{2+}, leading to vasorelaxation **(Figure 12.9)**.

12.5 a. **F** – Resistance vessel myocytes have abundant voltage-sensitive Ca^{2+} channels. This enables them to generate action potentials **(Figures 12.4a and 12.8)**.

b. **T** – Depolarization activates the voltage-sensitive Ca^{2+} channels, leading to a rise in cytosolic free $[Ca^{2+}]$ and contraction **(Figure 12.4a and 12.5b)**.

c. **T** – Contraction in some arteries is mediated by receptor-operated, Ca^{2+}-conducting TRP channels. These are activated via DAG generation **(Figure 12.4b)**. Consequently, contraction is independent of any concomitant depolarization **(Figures 12.3c and 12.5a)**.

d. **F** – Sympathetic activity is a major *vasoconstrictor* influence on all resistance vessels. The sympathetic vasoconstrictor transmitters are noradrenaline and ATP **(Figures 12.5b and 12.10)**.

12.6 a. **F** – Sensitization is the maintenance of contractile tone despite a *fall* in free Ca^{2+} concentration **(Figure 12.7)**.

b. **T** – Ca^{2+} sensitization contributes to the tonic phase of contraction **(Figure 12.7)**.

c. **F** – Sensitization is brought about by the *inhibition* of MLC phosphatase. The inhibition of this phosphate-removing enzyme tips the balance in favour of MLC kinase, leading to an increase in myosin head phosphorylation **(Figure 12.6)**.

d. **T** – G-protein coupled receptors can initiate, indirectly, the activation of rhoA kinase, which inhibits MLC phosphatase **(Figure 12.6)**.

12.7 a. **T** – Tonically active sympathetic vasomotor fibres release noradrenaline continually, activating α-receptors to help maintain vasoconstrictor tone. Alpha-blockers therefore reduce vascular tone **(Figure 12.5a)**.

b. **F** – $Alpha_1$-adrenoceptor have a greater affinity for noradrenaline than adrenaline.

c. **F** – $Alpha_1$ adrenoceptors are G_q-protein coupled receptors that *activate* PLC-β, leading to the formation of DAG and IP_3 from PIP_2. These agents in turn mediate vasoconstriction **(Figure 12.4a,b)**.

d. **F** – $Alpha_2$ adrenoceptors are coupled to the *inhibitory* G protein, G_i. G_i inhibits adenylate cyclase and therefore *inhibits* the vasodilator cAMP pathway. $Alpha_2$-adrenoceptor activation thus promotes vasoconstriction.

e. **F** – Beta$_1$-adrenoceptors are found mainly on the cardiac pacemaker and myocardial myocytes. They are coupled to the stimulatory G protein, G_s, which stimulates the adenylate cyclase–AMP–PKA pathway **(Figure 3.14)**.

f. **T** – Beta$_2$-adrenoceptors are abundantly expressed by arterial myocytes in the myocardium and skeletal muscle. They are coupled to G_s protein, which stimulates the adenylate cyclase–cAMP–PKA pathway, leading to vasodilatation **(Figure 12.9)**. Adrenaline thus causes vasodilatation in the heart and skeletal muscle, improving blood flow during the alerting response.

12.8 a. **T** – Sympathetic fibres in the tunica adventitia of blood vessels have a string of varicose swellings **(Figure 1.8)**. Each varicosity is packed with vesicles containing the transmitters ATP and noradrenaline **(Figure 12.11)**. Action potentials cause vesicle release.

b. **F** – Sympathetic stimulation does indeed elicit fast EJPs, but they are caused by the release of ATP, which activates purinergic P_{2x1} ionotropic receptors, not adrenoceptors. Ionotropic receptors are part of the same protein as the cation-conducting channel, so there is a fast effect – the fast excitatory junction potential **(Figures 12.5a and 12.10)**.

c. **T** – Alpha$_1$-mediated depolarization is slow **(Figures 12.8)** The reason is that a chain of relatively slow biochemical reactions (Gq $\rightarrow$ PLCβ $\rightarrow$ IP_3/DAG) precedes the ion channel activation that causes the depolarization **(Figure 12.5a)**.

d. **T** – The hydrolysis of the membrane phospholipid PIP_2 by PLCβ generates IP_3 and DAG, which trigger further changes leading to contraction **(Figure 12.6)**.

e. **T** – Depending on the mix of ion channels in a particular vessel and the strength of stimulation, the IP_3 and DAG can lead to depolarization-dependent contraction involving L-type Ca^{2+} channels **(Figure 12.4a)** or depolarization-independent contraction mediated by non-selective cation TRP channels **(Figure 12.4b)**, or both.

12.9 a. **F** – Adrenaline does indeed cause β$_2$-mediated vasodilatation in myocardial and skeletal muscle blood vessels; but it acts by raising intracellular cAMP, not cGMP **(Figure 12.9)**.

b. **T** – Myosin head phosphorylation is essential for vascular myocyte contraction. The degree of phosphorylation depends on a dynamic balance between the phosphorylating enzyme MLC kinase and the dephosphorylating enzyme MLC phosphatase **(Figure 12.6)**. Most pathways mediating relaxation lead, ultimately, to myosin dephosphorylation.

c. **T** – Relaxation is often (but not always) mediated by a fall in the cytosolic free [Ca^{2+}], which reduces the activity of myosin light chain kinase **(Figure 12.9)**. Sensitivity to Ca^{2+} may also be reduced.

d. **T** – Sympathetic vasoconstrictor fibres are normally tonically (continuously) active, contributing to basal vascular tone. A reduction in their firing leads to relaxation, because there is less activation of the vasoconstrictor pathways.

e. **T** – In vessels with abundant L-type Ca^{2+} channels, myocyte hyperpolarization closes the voltage-sensitive Ca^{2+} channels, leading to a fall in cytosolic free Ca^{2+} and vasodilatation **(Figure 12.12)**. Hyperpolarization is brought about by an increase in the open-probability of sarcolemmal K^+ channel, e.g. K_{ATP} channels during ischaemia.

12.10 a. **T** – Adrenaline causes vasoconstriction in all vessels where α-receptors (linked to vasoconstrictor pathways) predominate over β_2-receptors (linked to vasodilator pathways), e.g. skin, gastrointestinal tract, kidneys. Adrenaline causes vasodilatation in myocardium, skeletal muscle and liver.

b. **F** – Nitric oxide-releasing drugs produces vasodilatation by raising intracellular cGMP, not cAMP **(Figure 9.4)**. This effect is used to relieve angina.

c. **T** – Sildenafil inhibits phosphodiesterase-5, the enzyme that degrades intracellular cGMP in the arterial resistance vessels of the penis **(Figure 9.4)**. A rise in cGMP causes vasodilatation, which underlies sexual erection. Sildenafil is therefore prescribed to treat erectile dysfunction.

d. **T** – Angiotensin II receptors cause vasoconstriction in a similar way to α-adrenoceptors. The receptor blocker losartan prevents the tonic stimulation of vascular tone by circulating angiotensin II, so it causes vascular relaxation. Losartan is used in the treatment of heart failure, to reduce the vascular resistance opposing ejection.

e. **F** – Nifedipine cause vasodilatation by inhibiting voltage-sensitive Ca^{2+} channels **(Figure 12.4a)**. Nifedipine and analogous 'calcium blockers' are widely prescribed to treat clinical hypertension.

12.11 a. The Nernst equation tells us that $E_{Cl} = (61.5/\text{valency}) \log (Cl_o/Cl_i) = (61.5/(-1)) \log (120/50)$. This is -23 mV.

b. Activation of α_1-adrenoceptors by the sympathetic transmitter, noradrenaline, leads to a rise in VSM Ca^{2+} concentration. This activates Cl_{Ca} channels (Ca^{2+}-activated chloride channels) in the surface membrane **(Figure 12.4a)**.

c. Cl^- ions will leave the cell as the Cl_{Ca} channels activate, because the membrane potential (-60 mV) is more negative than the chloride equilibrium potential (-23 mV). An increase in Cl^- conductance shifts the membrane potential closer to the Cl^- equilibrium potential. The cell will depolarize to a lower potential. This accounts partly for the slow excitatory junction potential elicited by sympathetic activity.

d. For a central nervous system neuron, such as an α-motorneuron, $E_{Cl} = (61.5/\text{valency}) \times \log (Cl_o/Cl_i) = (61.5/(-1)) \log (120/7)$. This is -76 mV – much more negative than in VSM, due to the lower neuronal Cl^- concentration. This E_{Cl} is more negative than the resting potential, -70 mV. Opening of chloride channels will therefore *hyper*polarize the central neurone – the opposite of the effect in VSM. This is the basis of inhibitory post-synaptic potentials in the central nervous system.

CHAPTER 13

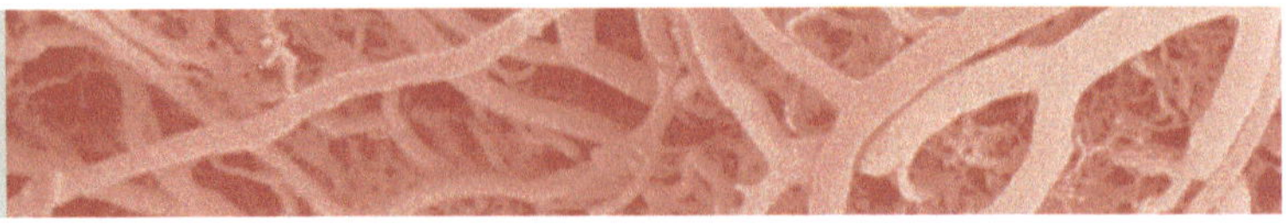

Control of blood vessels: I. Intrinsic control

T F

13.1 Arterioles and the terminal arteries

a. lack basal tone if not stimulated tonically by sympathetic fibres.
b. regulate local blood flow through a tissue.
c. regulate the mean arterial blood pressure.
d. can regulate the number of capillaries perfused with blood at any one moment.
e. increase capillary pressures when they contract.

13.2 Resistance vessel tone is

a. raised by the endothelial secretion of endothelin.
b. reduced by a rise in the pressure of blood in the lumen.
c. raised by the endothelial secretion of nitric oxide.
d. reduced by endothelium-derived hyperpolarization factor (EDHF)
e. raised by vasoactive agents when tissue metabolic rate increases.

13.3 The myogenic response

a. is the dilatation of arterial vessels in response to a rise in blood pressure.
b. is brought about by a fall in sympathetic fibre activity.
c. is mediated by membrane potential changes that alter Ca^{2+} channel activity.
d. helps to maintain a constant glomerular filtration rate.
e. increases cerebral blood flow when arterial pressure rises.

13.4 Nitric oxide

a. dilates large veins and large arteries.
b. is responsible for flow-induced dilatation in conduit arteries during exercise.
c. contributes to the low basal tone of pregnancy.
d. mediates vascular smooth muscle contraction by acetylcholine.
e. mediates erection of the penis.

13.5 The increase in blood flow to human skeletal muscle during moderate, rhythmic exercise

a. is due chiefly to the accompanying rise in arterial blood pressure.
b. is almost linearly proportional to the increase in muscle O_2 consumption.
c. is due partly to the activation of sympathetic vasodilator fibres.
d. is due partly to a fall in interstitial K^+ concentration.
e. may be due partly to local adenosine formation.

T F

13.6 The vascular tone of arteries and resistance vessels

a. is reduced by local hypoxia. ☐ ☐
b. in the brain is increased by hypercapnic acidosis. ☐ ☐
c. is increased by endothelin in heart failure. ☐ ☐
d. is increased by endothelium-derived hyperpolarizing factor (EDHF). ☐ ☐
e. is reduced by bradykinin. ☐ ☐

13.7 Concerning the regulation of blood vessels by autacoids,

a. histamine contributes to the venular hyperpermeability and arteriolar vasodilatation in acute inflammation. ☐ ☐
b. prostaglandin PGI_2 (prostacyclin) contributes to inflammatory vasodilatation. ☐ ☐
c. leukotrienes inhibit venular gap formation and leukocyte migration. ☐ ☐
d. thromboxane release by platelets can contribute to coronary artery vasospasm. ☐ ☐
e. serotonin (5-hydroxytryptamine) release by platelets counteracts haemostasis. ☐ ☐

13.8 The autoregulation of blood flow

a. is an increase in blood flow in response to an increase in demand. ☐ ☐
b. is particularly well developed in the pulmonary circulation. ☐ ☐
c. is often brought about by the myogenic response of resistance vessels. ☐ ☐
d. minimizes the reduction in local tissue perfusion if blood pressure falls. ☐ ☐
e. cannot occur during metabolic hyperaemia. ☐ ☐

13.9 When muscle blood flow increases during exercise,

a. the extra flow is due mainly to the diversion of flow from vasoconstricted, non-exercising tissues. ☐ ☐
b. the increase in blood flow is brought about by capillary dilatation. ☐ ☐
c. the hyperaemia is aided by the dilatation of feed arteries outside the active muscle. ☐ ☐
d. the hyperaemia is aided by the dilatation of the large conduit artery supplying the muscle. ☐ ☐
e. the hyperaemia is due mainly to increased nitric oxide production. ☐ ☐

13.10 In non-emotional, human exercise

a. involving rhythmic muscle contraction, each contraction phase is accompanied by a sharp rise in local muscle blood flow. ☐ ☐
b. the development of muscle hyperaemia lags behind the rise in metabolic rate. ☐ ☐
c. the muscle hyperaemia ceases within a few seconds of terminating the exercise. ☐ ☐
d. muscle blood flow increases less during static (isometric) exercise than dynamic (rhythmic) exercise. ☐ ☐

13.11 If the blood flow to a tissue is cut off for a while,

a. removal of the obstruction after a few minutes results in a higher than normal blood flow. ☐ ☐
b. removal of the obstruction after an hour or so can result in poor reperfusion. ☐ ☐
c. leukocyte adhesion to endothelium can impede microvascular reperfusion. ☐ ☐
d. oxygen free radicals can protect the tissue against reperfusion injury. ☐ ☐
e. intracellular Ca^{2+} depletion can damage myocardium during reperfusion. ☐ ☐

Finally, a quantitative problem relating to the intrinsic control of muscle blood flow:

13.12 Regarding the perfusion of a skeletal muscle, the resting muscle had a blood flow of 9 ml min^{-1} at a mean arterial blood pressure (ABP) of 95 mmHg. When ABP was raised to 140 mmHg, the non-exercised muscle blood flow increased to 10 ml min^{-1}. When the muscle was exercised at the same raised ABP (140 mmHg), the blood flow increased to 135 ml min^{-1}. Venous pressure was 5 mmHg throughout.

a. What was the conductance of the circulation in the resting muscle at ABP 95 mmHg?

b. If the circulation were simply a set of non-expandable plastic tubes, what would the blood flow be at 140 mmHg ABP.

c. What was the conductance of the muscle circulation at 140 mmHg ABP? What caused the change in conductance?

d. What was the conductance of the exercising muscle? What is this phenomenon called?

Answers

13.1 a. **F** – Arterial vessels have basal tone, due to the Bayliss myogenic response and tonic endothelin secretion.

b. **T** – Arterioles and terminal arteries are the main site of vascular resistance **(Figure 1.6)**. Changes in their radius adjust local blood flow over a very wide range **(Figure 13.1)**.

c. **T** – Mean blood pressure = cardiac output × total peripheral resistance (TPR). TPR is determined chiefly by the tone of the resistance vessels.

d. **T** – When resistance vessel tone is high, flow through a fraction of the capillaries is very slow or zero at any one moment. Dilatation of the resistance vessels 'recruits' these capillaries, increasing the transfer capacity of the microcirculation **(Figure 10.7)**.

e. **F** – Contraction of resistance vessel lowers capillary pressure **(Figures 8.21 and 11.7)**. This can tip the balance of Starling forces in favour of interstitial fluid absorption **(Figure 11.4, panel b)**.

13.2 a. **T** – Endothelin has a prolonged vasoconstrictor action.

b. **F** – A rise in transmural pressure elicits *contraction*. This is the Bayliss myogenic response **(Figure 13.2)**.

c. **F** – Nitric oxide causes vasodilatation **(Figure 13.3a)**.

d. **T** – EDHF cause vascular myocyte hyperpolarization and hence vasodilatation **(Figure 13.3b)**.

e. **F** – Increased metabolic activity generates vasodilator agents. This causes metabolic hyperaemia in skeletal muscle **(Figure 13.4)**, myocardium **(Figure 6.20)** and brain **(Figures 15.1 and 15.11)**.

13.3 a. **F** – A rise in transmural pressure causes a transient passive dilatation followed at once by a sustained contraction. The latter is the Bayliss myogenic response **(Figure 13.2)**.

b. **F** – The myogenic response is an intrinsic property of arterial smooth muscle, present in isolated, denervated vessels **(Figure 13.2)**.

c. **T** – Stress-activated channels are thought to induce myocyte depolarization. This activates voltage-sensitive Ca^{2+} channels, leading to myocyte contraction. Ca^{2+} channel inhibitors block the myogenic response **(Figure 13.2)**.

d. **T** – The myogenic response results in the autoregulation of capillary pressure when arterial blood pressure changes **(Figure 13.5b)**. This is particularly important in stabilizing glomerular filtration pressure in the kidneys.

e. **F** – The myogenic stabilizes cerebral flow (prevents it from changing significantly) when arterial flow changes. This is called flow autoregulation **(Figure 13.6)**. Autoregulation helps preserve cerebral blood flow during hypotension, e.g. spinal anaesthesia, moderate haemorrhage.

13.4 a. **T** – Much of the angina-relieving effect of NO donors (e.g. nitroglycerine) is due to venodilatation, which reduce cardiac preload, and large-artery relaxation, which reduces wave reflection and hence afterload.

b. **T** – The shear stress exerted by flow activates the PI3 kinase – eNOS pathway **(Figure 9.4)**. Without the resulting conduit artery dilatation, large-vessel resistance would limit the high blood flow to exercising muscle.

c. **T** – NO counteracts the tone generated by the myogenic response, endothelin and sympathetic nerves. In pregnancy, NO production is raised by high oestrogen levels. Consequently, blood pressure tends to fall during mid-term.
d. **F** – NO mediates the vaso*dilator* effect of acetylcholine **(Figure 13.3a)**.
e. **T** – Dilatation by nitridergic parasympathetic nerves innervating the penis and clitoris produces erection.

13.5 a. **F** – Darcy's law of flow tells us that blood flow = pressure drop/resistance. There is a relatively small increase in blood pressure during dynamic exercise (~1.1–1.2-fold), but a 20-fold or more increase in muscle blood flow **(Figure 13.1)**. The vast majority of the increase, therefore, is due to a fall in muscle vascular resistance (metabolic vasodilatation), not the minor rise in blood pressure.
b. **T** – The major role of metabolic hyperaemia is to ensure that O_2 delivery matches demand as the metabolic rate increases **(Figure 6.20)**.
c. **F** – Metabolic vasodilatation is purely intrinsic in nature, not neural. Moreover, primates (unlike lower species) have no sympathetic cholinergic dilator innervation to muscle blood vessels.
d. **F** – Increased muscle or brain activity *raises* interstitial K^+. This causes hyperpolarization-mediated vasodilatation. The raised K^+ stimulates the electrogenic $3Na^+$–$2K^+$ pump and increases K_{ir} channel activation, shifting the vascular myocyte potential (basal −55 mV) closer to the Nernst equilibrium potential (−94 mV).
e. **T** – Adenosine is a vasodilator agent formed in the interstitial compartment from adenosine monophosphate released by exercising muscle. It is particularly implicated in myocardial vasodilatation.

13.6 a. **T** – Local hypoxia dilates resistance vessels **(Figure 13.7)**.
b. **F** – Acidosis causes vasodilatation. The brain is especially sensitive to CO_2 **(Figure 13.6)**. This helps to maintain cerebral O_2 delivery during partial asphyxia.
c. **T** – Increased levels of this vasoconstrictor peptide contribute to the peripheral vasoconstriction that characterizes patients in heart failure.
d. **F** – Hyperpolarization causes vasodilatation, by reducing the open state probability of depolarization-gated Ca^{2+} channels. EDHF accounts in part for the vasodilatation of small resistance vessels to acetylcholine and bradykinin **(Figure 13.3b)**.
e. **T** – Bradykinin is a nonapeptide that mediates inflammatory vasodilatation. It activates endothelial receptors, which stimulate the endothelium to produce vasodilators (NO, EDHF, prostanoids).

13.7 a. **T** – Histamine is released from mast cells and basophilic leukocytes in allergic reactions (urticaria, anaphylaxis, asthma) and trauma. H_1 receptors on venules are coupled to the G_q–PLC pathway to evoke intercellular gap formation **(Figure 11.19)**. H_2 receptors on arterioles are coupled to the G_s-adenylyl cyclase–cAMP pathway to evoke vasodilatation **(Figure 12.9)**.
b. **T** – Prostacyclin is a vasodilator eicosanoid (arachidonic acid-derived agent) **(Figure 13.8**, lower panels). It contributes to inflammatory vasodilatation and reactive hyperaemia.
c. **F** – Leukotrienes are ecosanoids produced by leukocytes. They powerfully stimulate gap formation and leukocyte migration during inflammation.
d. **T** – Thromboxane is a powerful eicosanoid vasoconstrictor stored in platelets. If platelets become activated by an atheromatous plaque in a coronary artery, downstream vasospasm may ensue, causing angina at rest (variant angina).

e. **F** – Serotonin is a powerful vasoconstrictor agent. When the circulation is breached, platelets encounter collagen, which triggers the release of serotonin. This causes vasospasm and thus helps arrest the bleeding.

13.8 a. **F** – Autoregulation is the maintenance of an almost *constant* blood flow when arterial pressure changes in the physiological range **(Figures 8.20, 13.5a and 13.6)**. Autoregulation also stabilizes capillary pressure **(Figure 13.5b)**. Autoregulation is well developed in skeletal muscle **(Figure 13.5a)**, brain **(Figure 13.6)**, myocardium **(Figure 13.9)** and kidneys. An increase in flow in response to demand is an entirely different phenomenon, called metabolic or active hyperaemia.

b. **F** – This would be self-defeating – pulmonary blood flow has to be allowed to increase when pulmonary pressure rises during exercise! Autoregulation does not occur in the pulmonary circulation, which has an almost linear pressure–flow relation **(Figure 15.14)**.

c. **T** – The myogenic response increases resistance to flow, thus counteracting the effect of the rise in pressure **(Figure 13.2)**, which would otherwise raise the flow.

d. **T** – The myogenic response operates in both directions; it reduces resistance to flow when arterial pressure falls, thereby preserving local blood flow **(Figure 13.5a)**.

e. **F** – When blood flow is increased by metabolic vasodilatation, autoregulation still occurs at the new level of flow, i.e. changes in blood pressure have little effect on the new, raised flow **(Figure 13.9)**.

13.9 a. **F** – Although there is indeed sympathetic-induced vasoconstriction of the inactive tissues, the amount of blood flow 'diverted' is small. When muscle blood flow increases by ~4 l/min during leg exercise, the flow 'diverted' from inactive muscle is only 0.1 l/min **(Figure 13.10)**. So where does all the extra flow come from? The increase in cardiac output, of course.

b. **F** – Capillaries lack smooth muscle and have surprisingly stiff walls at systemic, physiological pressures.

c. **T** – This is called ascending or conducted vasodilatation **(Figure 13.11)**. It is distinct from the flow-mediated dilatation of conduit arteries. Conducted vasodilatation is mediated by endothelial hyperpolarization, which spreads upstream from endothelial cell to endothelial cell and reaches myocytes through myoepithelial gap junctions.

d. **T** – To produce a co-ordinated response, dilatation occurs in not only the intramuscle resistance vessel (metabolic vasodilatation) and small feeding arteries (ascending vasodilatation), but also the large conduit arteries that supply the feed arteries **(Figure 13.11)**. Otherwise, the resistance of the conduit artery, though low, would become a significant part of the total vascular resistance once the other vessels have dilated.

e. **F** – Nitric oxide contributes to the flow-induced vasodilatation of the conduit artery, but it accounts for only one-fifth to one-third of the increase in blood flow. Metabolic vasodilators account for most of the fall in vascular resistance.

13.10 a. **F** – The contracted skeletal muscle compresses the blood vessels within it, reducing blood flow during each contraction **(Figure 13.4)**. Flow occurs mainly during the relaxation phase.

b. **T** – It takes a while for the metabolic vasodilators to accumulate, so the steady-state vasodilatation lags behind ATP consumption. As a result, an O_2 'debt' builds up at the start of exercise **(Figure 13.4)**.

c. **F** – Post-exercise hyperaemia lasts several minutes, as the metabolic debt is repaid and vasodilator metabolites, lactate, etc., are cleared from the muscle **(Figures 13.4 and 13.12)**.

d. **T** – The sustained intramuscle tension during an isometric contraction compresses the blood vessels within the muscle. Consequently, lactate accumulates quickly and the static compression cannot be maintained for a very long period.

13.11 a. **T** – This is called reactive or post-ischaemic hyperaemia **(Figure 13.12)**. It is caused by the myogenic response and the accumulation of vasodilator metabolites in the tissue during the period without blood flow.

b. **T** – Clamping an artery for a long period during surgery can lead to poor reperfusion.

c. **T** – After a prolonged obstruction of flow, the ischaemic endothelium expresses leukocyte-binding selectins **(Figure 9.7)**. Leukocytes are stiff and, when bound to the wall of small vessels, they act as obstacles to flow.

d. **F** – Oxygen radicals are highly toxic. They are generated from the reperfused O_2 by leukocyte NADPH oxidase and, in some tissues, xanthine oxidase.

e. **F** – Cardiac myocytes become *overloaded* with Ca^{2+} during ischaemia. This is due to reduced Na^+–K^+–ATPase pumping, and hence reduced Ca^{2+} extrusion by the Na^+–Ca^{2+} exchanger **(Figure 6.18)**. The rise in Ca^{2+} can lead to cardiac myocyte contracture and cell damage during reperfusion.

13.12 a. From Darcy's law, flow = arterio-venous pressure difference/resistance = pressure difference × conductance. Therefore conductance is flow/pressure difference, namely 9 ml min^{-1}/(95 − 5) mmHg. The answer is 0.1 ml min^{-1} $mmHg^{-1}$.

b. If the circulation consisted of non-expandable plastic tubes, flow would increase linearly with pressure, moving up the line of fixed conductance in **Figure 1.5**. A 50% increase in pressure difference would raise flow by 50% to 13.5 ml min^{-1}. From Darcy's law, flow = pressure difference × conductance = (140 − 5) mmHg × 0.1 ml min^{-1} $mmHg^{-1}$ = 13.5 ml min^{-1}.

c. From Darcy's law, the actual conductance of the resting muscle at 140 mmHg ABP was flow/pressure difference = 10 ml min^{-1}/(140 − 5) mmHg = 0.074 ml min^{-1} $mmHg^{-1}$. The conductance (slope of line in **Figure 13.5a**) has fallen substantially, greatly limiting the rise in flow. The reduced slope of the dashed lines in **Figure 13.9** are an example of this. The fall in conductance is caused by the myogenic response of resistance vessels to a rise in ABP, resulting in autoregulation (stabilization) of blood flow.

d. In the exercising muscle, conductance = flow/pressure difference = 135 ml min^{-1}/(140 − 5) mmHg = 1.0 ml min^{-1} $mmHg^{-1}$. Flow has increased because resistance vessel vasodilatation has raised the vascular conductance. This phenomenon is called metabolic hyperaemia (exercise hyperaemia, active hyperaemia).

CHAPTER 14

Control of blood vessels: II. Extrinsic control by nerves and hormones

T F

14.1 The sympathetic vasoconstrictor system

a. has short preganglionic fibres that release acetylcholine. ☐ ☐
b. has long postganglionic fibres that release adrenaline. ☐ ☐
c. has preganglionic neurons located chiefly in the cervical spinal cord. ☐ ☐
d. is tonically excited by bulbospinal fibres originating in the ventrolateral medulla. ☐ ☐
e. innervates the inner tunica media of arterial blood vessels. ☐ ☐

14.2 Sympathetic postganglionic vasomotor fibres

a. terminate in motor-end plates, similar to those in skeletal muscle. ☐ ☐
b. are normally quiescent in a resting subject. ☐ ☐
c. activate α-adrenoceptors on blood vessels. ☐ ☐
d. activate P_{2x} purinergic receptors on some blood vessels. ☐ ☐
e. 'spill' some noradrenaline into the circulation. ☐ ☐

14.3 A rise in human sympathetic vasomotor fibre activity

a. can raise arterial blood pressure. ☐ ☐
b. enhances local blood flow through a tissue. ☐ ☐
c. increases the capillary filtration rate. ☐ ☐
d. reduces the splanchnic venous blood volume. ☐ ☐
e. in skin can occur at the same time as sympathetic activity falls in skeletal muscle. ☐ ☐

14.4 Neurally mediated vasodilatation

a. can be achieved by reducing sympathetic vasomotor activity. ☐ ☐
b. in skin may be brought about by increased sympathetic cholinergic activity. ☐ ☐
c. in skin may be brought about by a C-fibre axon reflex. ☐ ☐
d. in salivary glands is associated with parasympathetic activity and secretion. ☐ ☐
e. by parasympathetic fibres contributes to vasodilatation in exercising muscle. ☐ ☐
f. by parasympathetic fibres can cause penile erection. ☐ ☐

14.5 An intravenous infusion of adrenaline

a. causes active constriction of resistance vessels in skeletal muscle. ☐ ☐
b. causes active constriction of resistance vessels in the skin. ☐ ☐
c. raises total peripheral resistance. ☐ ☐
d. raises systolic blood pressure more than diastolic pressure. ☐ ☐
e. elicits tachycardia, whereas intravenous noradrenaline causes bradycardia. ☐ ☐
f. reduces plasma glucose concentration. ☐ ☐

T F

14.6 Noradrenaline

a. is stored in the vesicles of sympathetic varicosities.
b. is formed from adrenaline by methyltransferase.
c. raises mean blood pressure.
d. increases cutaneous blood flow.
e. has a greater affinity for α- than β-adrenoceptors.

14.7 Vasopressin

a. is a peptide synthesized by the posterior pituitary gland.
b. is mainly a stimulus for water excretion.
c. release is triggered by a rise in plasma osmolarity.
d. release is reduced following a haemorrhage.
e. secretion during nausea contributes to the grey pallor of skin.

14.8 The renin–angiotensin system

a. is activated by angiotensinogen secreted by juxtaglomerular cells.
b. is stimulated following a loss of blood.
c. depends on endothelium to generate angiotensin II.
d. can induce vasoconstriction.
e. generally shows reduced activity in patients with hypertension.

14.9 Aldosterone secretion

a. promotes NaCl reabsorption in the distal renal tubule.
b. is stimulated by a fall in plasma angiotensin II concentration.
c. is increased following a major haemorrhage.
d. falls in response to a low salt diet.
e. rises during pregnancy.

14.10 The natriuretic peptide

a. ANP (atrial natriuretic peptide) is secreted by atrial myocytes when cardiac filling pressure falls.
b. ANP lowers blood pressure by both natriuresis *and* resistance vessel dilatation.
c. ANP increases plasma volume by reducing capillary and venular filtration rates.
d. BNP (brain natriuretic peptide) is produced in the brain, but not the heart.
e. BNP can increase 200-fold in the circulation during heart failure.

14.11 Regarding the control of veins,

a. peripheral venoconstriction can enhance cardiac filling pressure.
b. splanchnic veins are poorly innerved by sympathetic vasoconstrictor fibres.
c. skeletal muscle veins are well innervated by sympathetic vasoconstrictor fibres.
d. cutaneous veins are reflexly constricted during moderate exercise.
e. veins dilate markedly in response to glyceryl trinitrate.

Here, for a change, is a data interpretation problem. The question is based on a true experiment.

14.12 Regarding the human alerting response, a resting student had a heart rate of 70 min^{-1}, brachial artery blood pressure 125/80 mmHg, forearm blood flow 8 ml min^{-1} (100 g)$^{-1}$ and hand blood flow 10 ml min^{-1} (100 g)$^{-1}$. The sly experimenter then deliberately frightened the student. Within 120 seconds the parameters had changed to 140 min^{-1}, 150/90 mmHg, forearm 48 ml min^{-1} (100 g)$^{-1}$ and hand 7 ml min^{-1} (100 g)$^{-1}$.

a. How might forearm blood flow have been measured, and what tissue does the flow mainly represent?
b. What were the mean arterial blood pressures at rest and when the student was alarmed?
c. How do you explain the failure of blood pressure to increase as much as the heart rate, which doubled?
d. What mechanism is most likely to account for the 6-fold increase in forearm blood flow?
e. How do you account for the fall in hand blood flow at a time when arterial pressure and forearm flow were increasing?

Answers

14.1 a. **T** – Preganglionic spinal neurons activate nicotinic receptors on the postganglionic fibres in the sympathetic ganglia **(Figure 14.1)**.

b. **F** – Postganglionic fibres are long, but they release the neuroeffector noradrenaline. Adrenaline is produced by chromaffin cells in the adrenal medulla **(Figure 14.1)**.

c. **F** – The sympathetic preganglionic neurons are found in the thoracico-lumbar cord, T1-L3 **(Figure 14.1)**.

d. **T** – This is why spinal cord transection causes a sudden fall in sympathetic-mediated vascular tone, causing hypotension.

e. **F** – The axons terminate in the adventitia; they do not penetrate the media **(Figure 1.8)**.

14.2 a. **F** – Sympathetic fibres end in a string of varicosities containing noradrenaline-filled vesicles **(Figures 1.8 and 12.11)**.

b. **F** – Tonic sympathetic vasoconstrictor activity helps maintain vessel tone and blood pressure. Consequently, vasodilatation can be induced by *reducing* sympathetic vasoconstrictor activity.

c. **T** – The sympathetic neuroeffector noradrenaline has a high affinity for α-adrenoceptors, which are highly expressed by most vascular myocytes **(Table 14.1)**.

d. **T** – Some sympathetic varicosities release vesicles containing ATP as well as noradrenaline. The ATP activates the ionotropic P_{2x} purinergic receptors on vascular myocytes **(Figure 12.11)**. The activated channels produce fast excitatory junction potentials, leading to contraction **(Figure 12.10)**.

e. **T** – Much of the circulating noradrenaline derives from spillover from active sympathetic fibres **(Figure 12.11)**. The rest is secreted by the adrenal medulla, along with its major product, adrenaline.

14.3 a. **T** – Mean arterial blood pressure = total peripheral resistance (TPR) × cardiac output. A widespread increase in sympathetic activity raises TPR, which raises arterial pressure (**Figures 8.21 and 14.2**, line labelled 'abdominal aorta'). Sympathetic activity is a major part of our defence against postural and hypovolaemic hypotension.

b. **F** – Alpha-adrenoceptor-mediated vasoconstriction raises local vascular resistance, which reduces local blood flow. Darcy's law tells us that blood flow = pressure gradient/ resistance **(Figure 14.3, marker c)**.

c. **F** – Precapillary resistance vessel constriction lowers capillary pressure **(Figure 11.7)**. This allows a gradual absorption of interstitial fluid, due to the colloid osmotic pressure of the plasma **(Figure 14.3, arrow b)**.

d. **T** – Sympathetic fibres innervate splanchnic veins and cause venoconstriction **(Figure 14.2)**. This displaces peripheral venous blood centrally, raising CVP and stroke volume (Starling's law).

e. **T** – The brainstem control centre is organized organotopically – tissues are represented and controlled separately. During the alerting, fear–flight–fight response, sympathetic activity to skin increases (vasoconstriction – 'white as a sheet' with fear), but sympathetic vasoconstrictor activity to muscle decreases (vasodilatation, preparation for action).

14.4 a. **T** – Sympathetic vasoconstrictor fibres are tonically active, so a *reduction* in activity leads to vasodilatation, e.g. during the regulation of peripheral resistance and hence blood pressure.

b. **T** – Cutaneous vessels are innervated by sympathetic cholinergic vasodilator fibres, as well as sympathetic noradrenergic vasoconstrictor fibres. Cholinergic fibres are involved in core temperature regulation; they elicit cutaneous vasodilatation and sweating.
c. **T** – The nociceptive C-fibre axon reflex mediates the spreading flare around a damaged area. This is part of the Lewis triple response to trauma **(Figure 14.4)**.
d. **T** – The cranial parasympathetic outflow mediates cholinergic vasodilatation in secretory glands. The increased blood flow is needed to supply water for secretion.
e. **F** – Human skeletal muscle has no parasympathetic innervation. Human and primate muscles also lack a sympathetic cholinergic innervation, unlike many species.
f. **T** – The sacral parasympathetic outflow induces erection through nitridergic (NO-producing) fibres.

14.5 a. **F** – The arterial resistance vessels of skeletal muscle, myocardium and liver strongly express β_2-adrenoceptors, which are G_s-coupled to the dilator cAMP system **(Figure 12.9)**. Adrenaline has a high affinity for β_2-adrenoceptors, so it elicits vasodilatation in these tissues **(Table 14.1)**.
b. **T** – Cutaneous vessels express mainly α-adrenoceptors. Their activation by adrenaline causes vasoconstriction in skin and many other tissues **(Table 14.1)**.
c. **F** – Vasodilatation in skeletal muscle (~40% of body mass) outweighs the effect of vasoconstriction in skin, etc., so the total peripheral resistance falls a little **(Figure 14.5)**.
d. **T** – Adrenaline has a positive inotropic action on the heart, raising the ejection fraction, stroke volume and ejection rate. These changes raise the pulse pressure (systolic minus diastolic pressure). Diastolic pressure may even fall slightly, due to the fall in peripheral resistance **(Figure 14.5)**.
e. **T** – Adrenaline stimulates the cardiac pacemaker β_1 receptors to cause tachycardia and increased contractility. Students often expect a rise in circulating noradrenaline to do the same, since noradrenaline activates cardiac pacemaker β_1 receptors. However, circulating noradrenaline, unlike adrenaline, vasoconstricts *all* peripheral tissues. This increases peripheral resistance, raising blood pressure. The resulting baroreceptor reflex slows the heart rate by changing the autonomic outflow to the pacemaker **(Figure 14.5)**.
f. **F** – Adrenaline stimulates liver glycogenolysis, which *raises* plasma glucose.

14.6 a. **T** – An action potential releases just a few hundred vesicles from the thousands of terminal varicosities along a single sympathetic fibre **(Figures 1.8 and 12.11)**.
b. **F** – It is the other way round – adrenaline is formed from noradrenaline by methyltransferase, which add a methyl group (–CH_3) to noradrenaline.
c. **T** – Noradrenaline causes widespread peripheral vasoconstriction, raising total peripheral resistance **(Figure 14.5)**.
d. **F** – Noradrenaline causes vasoconstriction in all tissues, even muscle.
e. **T** – This is why noradrenaline always causes vasoconstriction; the α-adrenoceptor is linked by G_q protein to phospholipase C, which triggers vasoconstrictor pathways **(Figure 12.4)**.

14.7 a. **F** – Vasopressin is *synthesized* by magnocellular neurons in the hypothalamus. It is transported along their axons for *release* in the posterior pituitary gland **(Figure 14.6)**.
b. **F** – Vasopressin *reduces* water excretion, hence its alternative name 'anti-diuretic hormone' (ADH).
c. **T** – Dehydration stimulates osmoreceptors in the hypothalamus, which project to the vasopressin-producing magnocellular neurons **(Figure 14.6)**. The osmoreceptor–vasopressin pathway is a major factor in body fluid homeostasis.

d. **F** – A fall in arterial pressure and blood volume is sensed by cardiovascular receptors that trigger a reflex increase in vasopressin secretion **(Figure 14.6)**.
e. **T** – Nausea powerfully stimulates vasopressin secretion; circulating levels can increase 50-fold.

14.8 a. **F** – The juxtaglomerular cells secrete the enzyme renin. Angiotensinogen is a circulating plasma protein that is the substrate for renin, leading to the production of angiotensin 1.
b. **T** – A fall in blood pressure stimulates the renal arteriolar juxtaglomerular cells to secrete renin. A fall in pressure also reflexly increases renal sympathetic activity, which is another trigger for renin secretion, along with reduced NaCl load at the macula densa **(Figure 14.7)**.
c. **T** – Angiotensin-converting enzyme (ACE) on the surface of pulmonary endothelium convert the decapeptide angiotensin I into the active octapeptide, angiotensin II **(Figure 14.7)**.
d. **T** – Angiotensin II causes resistance vessel constriction, partly by direct action and partly by boosting sympathetic action. This supports the blood pressure after a haemorrhage.
e. **F** – The renin–angiotensin is tonically active in all humans. The hypotensive effect of blocking it (by ACE inhibitors) is particularly marked in patients with hypertension.

14.9 a. **T** – This action retains salt and water in the water **(Figure 14.7)**.
b. **F** – Angiotensin II *stimulates* aldosterone secretion, completing a feedback loop that regulates body salt and water content **(Figure 14.7)**.
c. **T** – The reduced renal artery pressure and increased renal sympathetic activity stimulate the renin–angiotensin system, and angiotensin II stimulates aldosterone secretion **(Figure 14.7)**.
d. **F** – A low salt load at the macula densa of the renal juxtaglomerular apparatus stimulates the renin–angiotensin–aldosterone system. This leads to the conservation of body salt **(Figure 14.7)**.
e. **T** – Aldosterone contributes to the expansion of extracellular fluid and plasma volume during pregnancy.

14.10 a. **F** – ANP secretion is stimulated by a *rise* in cardiac filling pressure, which distends the atria. The actions of ANP then help lower the filling pressure (negative feedback).
b. **T** – ANP evokes renal natriuresis. ANP-evoked dilatation resembles that evoked by nitric oxide, because the intracellular portion of the ANP receptor possesses guanylate cyclase activity.
c. **F** – ANP *reduces* plasma volume by *increasing* capillary pressure (effect of precapillary resistance vessel dilatation) and increasing venular permeability (effect of receptor guanylate cyclase activity).
d. **F** – BNP, despite its name, is also produced by myocardial cells in the ventricles.
e. **T** – BNP may prove a useful biochemical and prognostic index of heart failure.

14.11 a. **T** – Blood displaced from constricted peripheral veins expands the thoracic blood pool, raising cardiac filling pressure and stroke volume **(Figure 14.8)**.
b. **F** – Visceral veins are well innervated by sympathetic constrictor fibres **(Figure 14.8)**. They are reflexly constricted when carotid sinus arterial pressure falls **(Figure 14.2)**.
c. **F** – Muscle veins are poorly innervated by sympathetic constrictor fibres **(Figure 14.8)**.
d. **T** – Cutaneous venoconstriction is graded in proportion to exercise intensity **(Figure 6.15)**.
e. **T** – Nitrodilators relieve angina partly through venodilatation, which reduces cardiac filling pressure (preload), and hence cardiac work and O_2 demand.

14.12 a. Human forearm blood flow is usually measured by venous occlusion plethysmography **(Figure 14.9)**. Plethysmography traces can be seen in **Figure 13.12**. Most of the soft tissue in the forearm is skeletal muscle, so the measured flow is largely muscle perfusion.

b. In the brachial artery, mean pressure = diastolic + one-third pulse pressure **(Figure 8.7)**. So mean blood pressure was 85 mmHg at rest (80 + 45/3) and 110 mmHg when alarmed (90 + 60/3), a 29% increase.

c. Heart rate increased 2-fold but mean pressure increased only 1.29-fold. It is likely that cardiac output, like the heart rate, at least doubled. The explanation for the relatively small increase in blood pressure must therefore be a substantial fall in total peripheral resistance, TPR; mean BP = cardiac output × TPR (so, 1.29 = 2 × 0.645). Peripheral resistance vessels must therefore have dilated in response to the alarm stimulus.

d. Darcy's law tells us that flow = pressure gradient/resistance **(Figure 1.5)**. Since the 1.29-fold rise in blood pressure is too small to cause a 6-fold rise in forearm blood flow, we can conclude that the resistance vessels in the forearm dilated, lowering local vascular resistance 4.65-fold (1.29 × 4.65 = 6). What probably caused the vasodilatation? Human muscle has no vasodilator innervation and reduced sympathetic vasoconstrictor activity cannot increase flow this much. The most likely cause is the release of adrenalin by the adrenal medulla as part of the alerting (fear–fight–flight) reaction. Adrenaline causes β_2-adrenoceptor-mediated vasodilatation in muscle **(Table 14.1)**.

e. The only possible explanation for a fall in hand blood flow despite an increase in perfusing pressure is local vasoconstriction, raising the resistance to flow in the hand. This is in keeping with a rise in circulating adrenaline, since adrenaline causes α-adrenoceptor mediated vasoconstriction in cutaneous resistance vessels **(Table 14.1)**.

CHAPTER 15

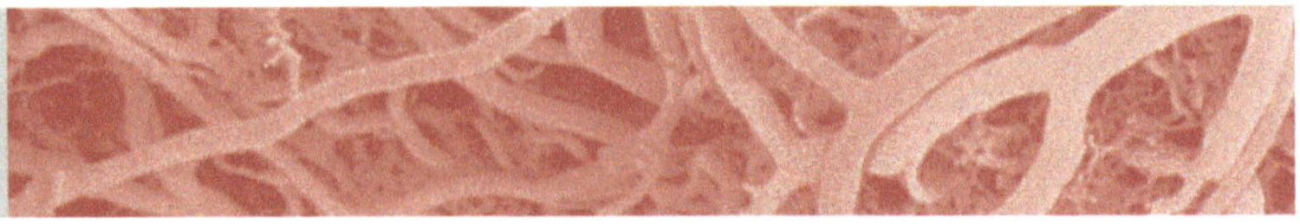

Specialization in individual circulations

T F

15.1 In a healthy woman the local oxygen demand sometimes exceeds delivery by the bloodstream to

a. skeletal muscles during exercise.
b. the myocardium during exercise.
c. the skin during hot weather.
d. the uterus during labour.
e. the cerebral cortex during exercise.

15.2 The vascular resistance of

a. ventricular myocardium increases as cardiac output increases.
b. skeletal muscle falls during dynamic exercise.
c. the cutaneous circulation is raised in cold weather.
d. the motor cortex increases during voluntary movement.
e. the cerebral circulation is lower than that of the pulmonary circulation.

The coronary circulation

15.3 In the coronary circulation of a healthy ventricle,

a. the myocardial capillary density is several times greater than in skeletal muscle.
b. the coronary venous O_2 concentration is about the same as in the right ventricle.
c. the blood flow is almost directly proportional to the cardiac output.
d. the blood flow is higher during ventricular ejection than during diastole.
e. the blood flow can be increased by adrenaline.

15.4 In the human coronary circulation during exercise,

a. increased O_2 transfer is achieved mainly through increased O_2 extraction rather than increased blood flow.
b. blood flow is increased by sympathetic cholinergic nerves.
c. increased cardiac sympathetic fibre activity raises coronary perfusion.
d. autoregulation is suppressed.
e. a rise in interstitial adenosine may contribute to vasodilatation.

15.5 When a major human coronary vessel is obstructed by thrombosis,

a. abundant arterio-arterial anastomoses greatly limit the ischaemic area.
b. local hypoxia and acidosis cause downstream vasodilatation.
c. a sharp pain is experienced over the heart on the left side of the chest.
d. the ECG often shows ST segment elevation.
e. the plasma level of myocardial lactic dehydrogenase falls.

T F

15.6 Angina pectoris

a. is mediated by chemosensitive ventricular nociceptor fibres that travel in the cardiac sympathetic nerves.
b. is usually triggered by exercise.
c. can be triggered by mental stress.
d. can occur in a resting, non-stressed patient.
e. is associated with ST segment elevation during an exercise test.

Here is a 'choose the right word' question for a change.

15.7 The treatment of angina

Angina is caused by ______ in the coronary arteries. For many years it has been treated by sublingual ______, which dilates mainly the ______ and ______. The ______ reduces cardiac filling pressure (preload), while the ______ reduces systolic pressure (afterload). These two changes reduce ______ and thus O_2 demand. Nitrodilators may also dilate ______, enhancing blood flow to the ischaemic zone. ______, such as propranolol, are used prophylactically to reduce myocardial O_2 demand by reducing ______ and ______. Similarly, ______, such as nifedipine, reduce cardiac work and O_2 demand. A new, purely chronotropic drug, ______, slows the pacemaker and thus reduces myocardial O_2 demand. Other drugs that may be prescribed include ______ to reduce plasma ______, a major risk factor for atheroma, and ______, to reduce platelet aggregation as a prophylaxis against ______.

Choose the best answer from the table, using a word as often as required, or not at all.

thrombosis	systemic capillaries	cardiac volume	high density lipoprotein
atheroma	systemic arteries	heart rate	salt
media hypertrophy	systemic veins	contractility	statins
atropine	coronary collaterals	myocardial work	Ca^{2+} channel blockers
ivabradine	venodilatation	cholesterol	β-adrenergic blockers
ACE inhibitors	arterial relaxation	digoxin	low-dose aspirin

T F

The skeletal muscle circulation

See also questions 13.5, 13.9 and 13.10.

15.8 Blood flow through human skeletal muscle

a. can be reduced by the baroreflex.
b. increases four-fold when cardiac output increases four-fold during exercise.
c. is increased partly by parasympathetic vasodilator fibres.
d. is promoted partly by the venous muscle pump during leg exercise.
e. is reduced by sympathetic vasomotor fibres after a haemorrhage.

15.9 When a skeletal muscle is exercised,

a. the diffusion distance for O_2 is reduced by capillary recruitment.
b. the O_2 saturation of the local venous blood can fall to 20% or less.
c. anaerobic metabolism can result in lactate accumulation.
d. the muscle may swell due to increased capillary filtration.
e. intermittent claudication is a symptom of venous thrombosis.

To add variety and promote a quantitative approach, here is a simple, numerical problem.

15.10 Oxygen delivery to skeletal muscle. Human leg muscles receive a resting blood flow of 400 ml min^{-1}. Arterial blood contains 200 ml O_2 per litre and the muscle venous blood contains 150 ml O_2 per litre at rest.

a. What is the metabolic rate of the resting leg muscles, expressed as O_2 consumption? (Hint – think Fick!)

b. If cycling raises the muscle blood flow to 4 litre min^{-1}, and the venous O_2 content falls to 90 ml O_2 per litre, what is the new metabolic rate of the leg muscles? By what factor has it increased?

T F

Cutaneous circulation

15.11 The flow of blood though skin is

a. governed mainly by the contractile tone of the subpapillary venous plexus.
b. controlled in part by the hypothalamus.
c. reduced by sympathetic activity after a haemorrhage.
d. reduced during the Lewis triple response.
e. raised by disorders that raise blood viscosity.
f. increased by adrenaline.

15.12 Cutaneous perfusion

a. is increased when core temperature rises.
b. is reduced when ambient temperature falls.
c. can be increased in acral skin by contraction of arterio-venous anastomoses (AVA).
d. is increased by a fall in sympathetic activity in acral skin.
e. is increased by a fall in sympathetic cholinergic activity in non-acral skin.
f. can increase paradoxically after 5–10-min exposure to cold.

15.13 Blood flow through the skin

a. can be increased by sensory C-fibre activity.
b. is increased during the alerting (fear–flight–fight) response.
c. is reduced by sympathetic-mediated vasoconstriction during heart failure.
d. is increased in skin below heart level due to the pull of gravity.
e. increases above normal when a period of physical compression is terminated.
f. shows an exaggerated response to cooling in Raynauld's disease.

The cerebral circulation

15.14 The human cerebral circulation

a. delivers >10% of the resting cardiac output to an organ that is only ~2% of total body weight.
b. arises from anastomosing arteries surrounding the sella turcica.
c. has an unusually large fraction of its total resistance located in the large arteries.
d. branches to provide a similar capillary density to skeletal muscle.
e. has arteries that are innervated by perivascular nociceptive C fibres.

T F

15.15 In the cerebral circulation,

a. vasoconstriction can be caused by hyperventilation.
b. glucose permeates the capillary wall through the intercellular clefts.
c. general anaesthetics permeate the capillary wall through the cell membrane.
d. increased local neuronal activity raises local blood flow.
e. serotonin (5-hydroxytrytamine) can evoke arterial vasospasm.

15.16 Cerebral vascular perfusion is

a. reduced by local hypoxia.
b. reduced during postural hypotension.
c. reduced in the steady state during standing because carotid blood flow is uphill, against gravity.
d. increased when interstitial K^+ concentration is raised by neuronal activity.
e. reduced during hypotension by baroreflex activation of sympathetic vasomotor nerves.

15.17 With regard to the effect of arterial pressure on the brain,

a. cerebral perfusion is directly proportional to arterial pressure.
b. the myogenic response is poorly developed in cerebral resistance vessels.
c. severe hypertension can disrupt the blood–brain barrier.
d. severe hypertension can cause cerebral oedema.

15.18 In the brain

a. the anterior cerebral artery supplies most of the blood perfusing the motor cortex.
b. a subarachnoid haemorrhage can cause a stroke by triggering vasospasm.
c. a large cerebral tumour can raise arterial blood pressure.
d. a large cerebral tumour can raise the heart rate.
e. vasoconstriction is associated with the headache phase of a migraine.
f. substance P and calcitonin gene-related peptide contribute to pathological cerebral artery dilatation.

Pulmonary circulation

15.19 In the pulmonary circulation of a resting human,

a. the arterial blood flow over several heart beats equals the total systemic flow over the same period.
b. the vascular resistance equals the systemic peripheral resistance.
c. the pulmonary veins contain blood with an O_2 saturation of ~75%.
d. the arterial pressure averages 14–17 mmHg.
e. pulmonary hypertension leads to left ventricular hypertrophy.

15.20 Regarding blood–gas exchange in the human lungs,

a. the diffusion distance from alveolar gas to pulmonary capillary plasma is ~5 μm.
b. the capillary density per gram tissue is higher than in any other organ.
c. the alveolar gases equilibrate with the blood in <1 s at rest.
d. blood flow increases in regions of the lung with a low partial pressure of O_2.

T F

e. the ideal ventilation/perfusion ratio for alveoli in a resting human is ~0.8.
f. right ventricular output can be calculated from measurements of gas exchange and blood gas content.

15.21 Regarding the pressure–flow relation of the pulmonary circulation,
a. pulmonary artery pressure increases as flow increases during exercise.
b. pulmonary artery pressure falls at high altitudes.
c. pressure and blood flow are greater in the base of the lungs than in the apex during standing.
d. hypoxic pulmonary vasoconstriction is mediated by a rise in pulmonary vascular myocyte cytosolic Ca^{2+} concentration.
e. hypoxic pulmonary vasoconstriction tends to increase the inequalities in the ventilation/perfusion ratios of alveoli.

15.22 Regarding fluid exchange in the lungs,
a. pulmonary capillary pressure is approximately one-third of systemic capillary pressure at heart level.
b. lung lymph has a low colloid osmotic pressure.
c. lung airspaces are kept 'dry' by epithelial sodium channels (ENaC) and basolateral Na^+–K^+ pumps.
d. dyspnoea can arise from pulmonary vascular distension when left atrial pressure increases.
e. pulmonary oedema develops when left atrial pressure reaches 10 mmHg.

15.23 Cyanosis can result from
a. severe anaemia.
b. impaired O_2 uptake caused by pulmonary oedema.
c. an uneven distribution of ventilation–perfusion ratios within the lungs.
d. a patent foramen ovale.
e. carbon monoxide poisoning.

15.24 When a patient experiences a pulmonary embolism,
a. the embolus has usually arisen from an atheromatous plaque.
b. surgery of the pelvis or leg is a common predisposing event.
c. pressure falls in the pulmonary trunk.
d. left ventricular stroke volume rises.
e. central venous pressure rises.

Answers

15.1 a. **T** – During heavy exercise, especially if isometric, the muscle contractions not only raise O_2 consumption but also compress the intramuscle blood vessels, reducing perfusion. Anaerobic metabolism develops, leading to lactate accumulation, a burning pain and a large O_2 debt.

b. **F** – Coronary blood flow keeps pace with myocardial O_2 demand beautifully in healthy subjects **(Figure 6.20)**.

c. **F** – Skin has a low metabolic rate and its blood flow is well in excess of demand, especially in hot weather, when cutaneous perfusion is greatly increased.

d. **T** – The powerful uterine contractions during labour utilizes more O_2 than the compressed circulation can deliver, leading to ischaemic contraction pains.

e. **F** – Grey matter (mainly neurons) has a high metabolic rate, but a correspondingly high blood flow, which increases in proportion to O_2 demand **(Figure 15.1b)**.

15.2 a. **F** – Myocardial vascular resistance falls as cardiac output increase, raising the coronary blood flow **(Figure 6.20)**.

b. **T** – The large fall in vascular resistance, not the modest rise in blood pressure, is the main factor increasing the perfusion of active muscle.

c. **T** – Cutaneous vasoconstriction reduces cutaneous blood flow in cold weather, thereby reducing heat loss **(Figure 15.2a,c)**.

d. **F** – Local neuronal activity triggers cerebral vasodilatation, increasing local cerebral perfusion **(Figure 15.1b)**.

e. **F** – The pulmonary circulation is a low resistance circulation, as proved by the low pressure head required to drive the entire cardiac output through it **(Figures 1.6 and 6.23)**. Formally, this is proved by Darcy's law: resistance = pressure difference/flow.

15.3 a. **T** – The high myocardial capillary density increases the area for gas exchange and shortens the diffusion distances **(Figure 15.3)**.

b. **F** – Coronary sinus blood has a very low O_2 concentration, whereas mixed venous blood is still approximately three-quarters saturated in a resting human **(Figure 6.24)**.

c. **T** – Coronary flow is linked to myocardial O_2 consumption through metabolic vasodilators **(Figure 6.20)**.

d. **F** – Although coronary artery pressure is higher during systole than diastole, the intramural (inside-the-wall) blood vessels are squeezed by the contracting myocardium, so perfusion is low. Most of the coronary perfusion occurs during diastole, when the vessels are not compressed **(Figure 15.4)**. Unfortunately, diastole gets shorter as heart rate increases **(Figure 2.4)**.

e. **T** – Coronary resistance vessels strongly express β-adrenoceptors, which are G_s-coupled to the vasodilator cAMP system.

15.4 a. **F** – Coronary sinus blood has a very low O_2 concentration, even at rest; so O_2 extraction can increase only slightly during exercise **(Figure 6.24)**. Most of the increased O_2 transfer is due to increased coronary blood flow. The Fick principle tells us that O_2 uptake = blood flow × (arterio-venous O_2 difference).

b. **F** – Coronary vessels are innervated by sympathetic vasoconstrictor fibres, not cholinergic dilator fibres.

c. **T** – Cardiac sympathetic fibre activity raises the cardiac output and work, which evokes a powerful metabolic vasodilatation **(Figure 13.9)**. The metabolic vasodilators outweigh the direct vasoconstrictor action of sympathetic vasomotor fibres on coronary resistance vessels.

d. **F** – Metabolic hyperaemia and autoregulation can and do co-exist **(Figure 13.9)**.
e. **T** – Adenosine is one of the candidate metabolic vasodilators. It is formed by the degradation of released AMP by 5′-nucleotidase.

15.5 a. **F** – Human coronary arteries are 'end arteries', with few functionally useful arterio-arterial anastomoses, unlike the dog **(Figure 15.5)**. Consequently, the ischaemic area is extensive.
b. **T** – Vasodilatation around the poorly perfused edge of the infarct helps to limit its extent.
c. **F** – Cardiac pain is dull and crushing in nature, and located in a band across the whole chest, often radiating into the arms and neck. This is attributed to afferent pathway convergence in the spinal cord.
d. **T** – ST segment elevation is common in the first few hours **(Figure 5.8)**.
e. **F** – Myocardial lactic dehydrogenase is released by dying myocytes, *raising* the plasma level. Due to the expression of this enzyme, myocytes can normally burn lactate as a metabolic fuel.

15.6 a. **T** – Curiously, these afferent fibres accompany the cardiac sympathetic fibres to reach the spinal cord.
b. **T** – The stenosed artery prevents coronary blood flow from increasing sufficiently to match the increased myocardial O_2 demand during exercise.
c. **T** – Mental stress increases sympathetic drive to the heart and raises blood pressure. Both factors increase cardiac work and therefore O_2 demand, triggering angina **(Figure 15.6)**.
d. **T** – This 'variant' or Prinzmetal angina is caused, not by increased O_2 demand, but by reduced O_2 delivery at rest, resulting from an episode of coronary artery vasospasm.
e. **F** – Angina usually causes subendocardial ischaemia, which results in ST depression **(Figures 5.8a and 15.6)**.

15.7 Angina is caused by **atheroma** in the coronary arteries. For many years it has been treated by sublingual **glyceryl trinitrate**, which dilates mainly the **systemic veins** and **systemic arteries**. The **venodilatation** reduces cardiac filling pressure (preload), while **arterial relaxation** reduces systolic pressure (afterload). These two changes reduce **myocardial work** and thus O_2 demand. Nitrodilators may also dilate **coronary collaterals**, enhancing blood flow to the ischaemic zone. **Beta-adrenergic blockers**, such as propranolol, are used prophylactically to reduce myocardial O_2 demand by reducing **cardiac contractility** and **heart rate**. Similarly, **Ca^{2+} channel blockers**, such as nifedipine, reduce cardiac work and O_2 demand. A new, purely chronotropic drug, **ivabradine**, slows the pacemaker and thus reduces myocardial O_2 demand. Other drugs that may be prescribed include **statins** to reduce plasma **cholesterol**, a major risk factor for atheroma; also **low-dose aspirin** to reduce platelet aggregation as a prophylaxis against **thrombosis**.

15.8 a. **T** – Sympathetic vasoconstrictor activity to muscle resistance vessels is controlled by the baroreflex **(Figure 6.21)**. Since muscle is the largest mass of tissue in the body, its vascular resistance has a major effect on arterial blood pressure.
b. **F** – A four-fold rise in cardiac output indicates near-maximal exercise. The active muscle blood flow increases 20-fold or more, because an increasing *proportion* of the cardiac output goes to the active muscle **(Figure 13.1)**. Inactive muscle perfusion decreases, during to sympathetic vasoconstrictor activity.
c. **F** – Muscle blood vessels have a sympathetic noradrenergic vasoconstrictor innervation, but no parasympathetic innervation.

d. **T** – The calf muscle pump lowers local venous pressure, which increases the pressure difference (artery to vein) driving blood through the active leg muscles **(Figure 8.27)**.
e. **T** – Baroreflex-mediated vasoconstriction in skeletal muscle helps support the arterial blood pressure after a haemorrhage.

15.9 a. **T** – Arteriolar dilatation increases the number of well-perfused capillaries (capillary recruitment). This reduces the radius of the Krogh cylinder of muscle supplied by each capillary **(Figure 10.7)**.
b. **T** – Oxygen extraction can reach 80–90%, cf. 25% in resting muscle.
c. **T** – The lactate represents the O_2 debt.
d. **T** – Arteriolar dilatation raises capillary pressure **(Figures 8.21 and 11.7)**. This raises the capillary filtration rate (Starling's principle of fluid exchange).
e. **F** – Intermittent claudication (ischaemic limb pain after walking a short distance) is caused by stenosis of a major leg *artery*, by atheroma, often in a smoker or diabetic.

15.10 a. The Fick principle, which is simply a version of the law of conservation of mass, tells us that *O_2 consumption = blood flow × (arterial concentration − venous concentration)* **(Figure 7.3)**. At rest, therefore, $0.4\,l\,min^{-1} \times (200\,ml\,l^{-1} - 150\,ml\,l^{-1}) = 20\,ml\ O_2\,min^{-1}$.
b. During cycling, $4.0\,l\,min^{-1} \times (200\,ml\,l^{-1} - 90\,ml\,l^{-1}) = 440\,ml\ O_2\ min^{-1}$. Muscle metabolic rate has increased 22-fold.

15.11 a. **F** – As in all tissues, venous resistance is negligible compared with arteriolar resistance. It is the arterial resistance vessels that regulate flow through non-acral skin, along with arteriovenous anastomoses in acral skin **(Figure 15.7)**.
b. **T** – The temperature-regulating centre in the hypothalamus controls the sympathetic *cholinergic* vasodilator outflow to blood vessels and sweat glands in the skin of the limbs and torso **(Figure 15.8, lower panel)**.
c. **T** – During hypovolaemia the baroreflex increases sympathetic *noradrenergic* vasoconstrictor outflow to the skin arterial and venous vessels – hence the patient's pallor.
d. **F** – The Lewis triple response is a local redness at the site of trauma (vasodilatation), a wheal (inflammation oedema) and a spreading flare (vasodilatation) mediated by the nociceptive C fibre axon reflex **(Figure 14.4)**.
e. **F** – A rise in blood viscosity increases the resistance to flow (Poiseuille's law, **Figure 8.19**); compare the curves for Ringer's solution (saline, low viscosity) and blood in **Figure 8.20**. Myeloma can raise the viscosity of plasma, impairing fingertip perfusion. Polycythaemia raises the viscosity of whole blood **(Figure 8.13)**.
f. **F** – Skin vessels express mainly α-adrenoceptors, so adrenaline contracts skin vessels (cf. dilates muscle vessels). Adrenaline is often mixed with local anaesthetic for the skin; the resulting local cutaneous vasoconstriction prevents the anaesthetic from being washed away quickly.

15.12 a. **T** – Hypothalamic temperature sensors control the sympathetic cholinergic outflow to non-acral skin and the sympathetic noradrenergic fibres innervating arterio-venous anastomoses in acral skin. Cutaneous vasodilatation increases sharply as core temperature rises **(Figure 15.2b)**, causing heat loss.
b. **T** – Skin resistance vessels vasoconstrict in response to local cooling, reducing perfusion and heat loss **(Figure 15.2a,c)**.
c. **F** – Contraction of AVAs reduces skin blood flow and heat loss. Dilatation of AVAs increases the flow of hot blood through the skin, increasing heat loss **(Figure 15.7)**.

d. **T** – At room temperature the arterio-venous anastomoses are tonically constricted by the tonic sympathetic noradrenergic fibre activity. A fall in sympathetic activity therefore increases the blood flow in acral skin **(Figure 15.8, upper panel)**.

e. **F** – Sympathetic cholinergic fibres cause cutaneous vasodilatation and sweating, and thus increase heat loss. If these nerves are blocked, there is little to no heat-induced vasodilatation **(Figure 15.8, lower panel)**.

f. **T** – Episodes of paradoxical cold vasodilatation restore flow to severely vasoconstricted, cold skin for short periods **(Figure 15.2c)**.

15.13 a. **T** – Nociceptive C fibres can release the vasodilator neuropeptides, substance P and calcitonin gene-related peptide (CGRP). This mediates the spreading flare response to skin trauma **(Figure 14.4)**.

b. **F** – The alerting response increases sympathetic vasoconstrictor fibre discharge to skin – we go pale with fear.

c. **T** – Sympathetic activity is high during heart failure, reducing cutaneous perfusion.

d. **F** – Gravity has no direct effect on flow through a rigid siphon **(Figure 8.25)**. Skin blood flow actually decreases below heart level, due to a veni-arteriolar contractile response to the gravitation-induced rise in local vascular pressures **(Figure 11.6)**.

e. **T** – This response, called reactive or post-ischaemic hyperaemia, helps resupply the tissue with O_2 and nutrients, and remove accumulated metabolites **(Figure 13.12)**.

f. **T** – The mechanisms underlying the exaggerated, extreme vasoconstriction remain unclear.

15.14 a. **T** – Cerebral blood is ~13–14% of the resting cardiac output **(Figure 1.3)**. This is necessitated by the exceptionally high O_2 demands of cerebral neurons, which account for ~18% of human resting O_2 consumption.

b. **T** – The sella turcica (Turkish saddle) is the bony cavity in which the pituitary gland sits. It is surrounded by the arterial circle of Willis, from which the cerebral arteries arise **(Figure 15.9)**.

c. **T** – Cerebral arterioles are unusually short, so the large arteries account for ~40% of the vascular resistance.

d. **F** – Grey matter has ~10 times more capillaries per unit area than skeletal muscle, i.e. 3000–4000/mm^2, similar to myocardium. This improves O_2 transport to the neurons.

e. **T** – The perivascular nociceptors are thought to mediate vascular headaches and migraine.

15.15 a. **T** – Hyperventilation causes hypocapnia (low arterial CO_2). Cerebral vessels are very sensitive to CO_2, which dilates them **(Figure 13.6)**.

b. **F** – Cerebral capillaries have unusual, tightly sealed intercellular junctions, creating the blood–brain barrier. Although D-glucose crosses the wall through the intercellular clefts of most capillaries, it cannot do so in the brain. Transport is by facilitated, GLUT-1 carrier-mediated diffusion through the endothelial cells.

c. **T** – The membrane is mainly lipid, and general anaesthetics are lipid-soluble, so they diffuse for blood to neuron very quickly. There is no blood–brain barrier for lipid soluble solutes.

d. **T** – For example, movement increases blood flow in the motor cortex **(Figure15.1)**.

e. **T** – Release of the vasoconstrictor, serotonin, from platelets and perivascular nerves is thought to contribute to the vasospasm triggered by cerebral haemorrhage, leading to a haemorrhagic stroke.

15.16 a. **F** – Hypoxia causes cerebral vasodilatation, which increases flow and O_2 delivery **(Figures 13.7 and 15.10)**.

b. **T** – On standing, venous pooling in the lower body reduces stroke volume, which in turn reduces cerebral blood flow temporarily. This can cause the occasional transient dizziness that is familiar to most of us.
c. **F** – Cerebral flow is indeed reduced by 10–20% in the steady state during standing, but not for the spurious reason given; flow in a rigid siphon (artery–capillaries–vein) is not affected by orientation **(Figure 8.25)**. Flow is reduced by (1) cerebral vasoconstriction (caused by reduced CO_2 and increased sympathetic activity) and (2) gravity-related collapse of unsupported draining veins **(Figures 6.9b and 8.26)**.
d. **T** – Cerebral resistance vessels show marked metabolic vasodilatation. This is mediated in part by a rise in interstitial K^+ concentration, brought about by increased neuronal activity **(Figure 15.11)**.
e. **F** – The role of the baroreflex is to safeguard cerebral perfusion, not strangle it! Other circulations are strangled (vasoconstricted) to *preserve* cerebral and myocardial perfusion during hypotension. Cerebral vessels are little affected by sympathetic activity or circulating catecholamines, because they express relatively few α-adrenoceptors.

15.17 a. **F** – The cerebral circulation shows excellent autoregulation, i.e. near-constant flow despite changes in blood pressure over the physiological range **(Figure 13.6)**.
b. **F** – The myogenic response is very well developed in cerebral vessels **(Figure 13.2)**. It is largely responsible for the excellent cerebral autoregulation.
c. **T** – This can be seen in the retina, which develops as an extension of the brain in the embryo. Severe hypertensive retinopathy is characterized by dots and blots (microhaemorrhages) and exudates (oedema).
d. **T** – Hypertensive encephalopathy is a serious condition. In eclamptic toxaemia of pregnancy, severe hypertension can precipitate fits.

15.18 a. **F** – The primary motor and sensory cortex, located around the central sulcus, are perfused by the *middle* cerebral artery **(Figure 15.9)**. Most thrombo-embolic strokes involve the middle cerebral artery, so they cause contralateral paralysis (hemiplegia).
b. **T** – The release of serotonin, endothelin and neuropeptide Y causes arterial vasospasm, which leads to a haemorrhagic stroke (cerebral ischaemia).
c. **T** – The expanding tumour forces the brainstem against the wall of the foramen magnum. This raises the activity of presympathetic neurons in the vasomotor centres, leading to a rise in blood pressure (part of Cushing's reflex) **(Figure 8.17)**.
d. **F** – The rise in blood pressure (see question c) stimulates the baroreceptors, which causes a reflex *brady*cardia. This is called Cushing's reflex **(Figure 8.17)**.
e. **F** – The headache phase is associated with *dilatation* of the major cerebral vessels. The dilatation and local inflammation stimulate nociceptive C fibres in the arterial adventitia.
f. **T** – These vasodilator neuropeptides are released from the nociceptive C fibres around the major arteries.

15.19 a. **T** – Right ventricle output equals left ventricle output, due to the operation of Starling's law of the heart **(Figure 6.8)**. Imbalances are transient, e.g. during inspiration/expiration, standing.
b. **F** – Resistance is the pressure difference needed to drive unit flow (Darcy's law). Pressures are low in the pulmonary circulation **(Figures 1.6 and 6.23)**, so resistance must be low. Pulmonary vascular resistance is approximately one-sixth of systemic vascular resistance, because pulmonary resistance vessels are short and numerous.

c. **F** – Pulmonary veins contain blood draining from the alveoli, so the O_2 saturation is almost 100% **(Figure 1.4)**.
d. **T** – The low arterial pressure is the result of the low resistance to flow.
e. **F** – Pulmonary arterial hypertension causes *right* ventricular hypertrophy, and eventually failure.

15.20 a. **F** – This thickness would greatly impair O_2 transfer. The alveolar membrane is extremely thin – only ~0.3 μm **(Figure 15.12)**.
b. **T** – Capillary packing is extraordinarily dense in the alveoli **(Figure 15.12)**.
c. **T** – The transit time for blood in a pulmonary capillary is ~1 s in a resting human. CO_2 and O_2 equilibrate long before the end of the capillary is reached (**Figure 10.6**, curves 1–2, flow-limited exchange).
d. **F** – Hypoxia causes local pulmonary vasoconstriction (hypoxic pulmonary vasoconstriction, HPV) **(Figure 15.13)**. HPV reduces the perfusion of underventilated alveoli and thus helps to normalize the ventilation/perfusion ratios and prevent hypoxaemia.
e. **T** – In a resting 70 kg human, the alveolar ventilation is ~4 $l\,min^{-1}$ and blood flow (cardiac output) is ~5 $l\,min^{-1}$, so the ratio is 0.8.
f. **T** – This is the Fick method. Cardiac output = pulmonary blood flow = oxygen consumption per minute/arteriovenous difference in oxygen content **(Figure 7.3)**.

15.21 a. **T** – The increase in right ventricular output during exercise raises pulmonary artery pressure **(Figure 6.23)**.
b. **F** – High altitude causes hypoxia, which causes vasoconstriction in the pulmonary circulation (unlike the vasodilator response of systemic vessels). This depresses the pressure–flow curve **(Figure 15.14)** and can lead to cardiac failure.
c. **T** – Gravity raises blood pressure in the base, distending the passive pulmonary vessels. Conversely, vessels in the apex collapse during diastole **(Figure 15.15)**. This results in ventilation/perfusion inequality between base and apex during standing.
d. **T** – Hypoxia inhibits certain K^+ channels in the vascular myocyte membrane, causing depolarization and Ca^{2+} entry. Over a longer interval, hypoxia also activated vascular rho kinase, which increases vascular sensitivity to Ca^{2+}.
e. **F** – HPV is a clever way of *normalizing* the alveolar ventilation/perfusion ratios, and thus optimizing gas exchange **(Figure 15.13)**.

15.22 a. **T** – This keeps the tension low in the very thin alveolar–endothelial membrane, and slows the rate of fluid filtration into the lungs.
b. **F** – Lung lymph colloid osmotic pressure (COP) is ~70% of the plasma level. This is due to the inverse relation between capillary filtration rate and interstitial plasma protein concentration **(Figure 11.10)**. The high interstitial COP maintains capillary filtration despite pulmonary capillary pressure being lower than plasma COP **(Figure 11.11, lowest left point)**.
c. **T** – As Na^+ is absorbed from the airways through ENaC (rate-limiting step) and basolateral pump, water follows by osmosis. This is especially important in clearing fluid from the neonatal lungs at birth.
d. **T** – The rise in pulmonary venous pressure distends the lung vasculature (pulmonary congestion), making the lungs stiff and difficult to inflate.
e. **F** – Due to the safety margin against oedema **(Figure 11.17)**, left atrial pressure has to reach 20 mmHg or so before clinical pulmonary oedema appears (cough, dyspnoea, crepitations). This can happen in severe left ventricular failure and mitral stenosis.

15.23 a. **F** – Cyanosis is only detectable when there is at least 50 g/litre of deoxyhaemoglobin in the blood. This is unlikely to be the case if the patient has a very low haemoglobin concentration. Blood normally contains 150 g haemoglobin per litre.

b. **T** – Thickening of the diffusion barrier by oedema fluid slows oxygen diffusion into the pulmonary capillary blood (Fick's law of diffusion). This raises circulating deoxyhaemoglobin concentration.

c. **T** – A severe ventilation/perfusion inequality causes hypoxaemia and cyanosis **(Figure 15.13, lower middle panel)**.

d. **F** – Pressure is higher in the left than the right atrium **(Table 2.1)**, so blood leaks from left to right through a patent foramen ovale. Consequently, deoxygenation blood does not enter the systemic circulation.

e. **F** – Carbon monoxide displaces O_2 from haemoglobin, but the monoxide–haemoglobin complex is cherry red in colour. There is thus hypoxaemia without cyanosis.

15.24 a. **F** – A pulmonary embolus can only come from the venous side of the systemic circulation; it is a detached venous thrombus. Veins do not develop atheroma, which is an arterial pathology.

b. **T** – The post-surgical immobility and increase in plasma fibrinogen predispose to venous thrombosis.

c. **F** – The embolus increases vascular resistance. Since pulmonary trunk pressure = CO × pulmonary vascular resistance, the pressure upstream of the embolus rises.

d. **F** – The rise in afterload (pulmonary arterial pressure) on the right ventricle reduces its stroke volume. A fall in right ventricular stroke volume leads to a fall in left ventricular stroke volume.

e. **T** – When the output of a pump changes, the input pressure (CVP) changes in the opposite direction **(Figure 6.14)**.

CHAPTER 16

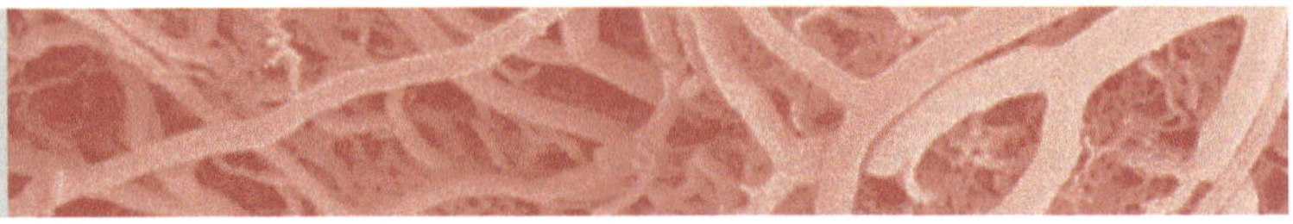

Cardiovascular receptors, reflexes and central control

T F

16.1 Arterial baroreceptors

a. respond primarily to stretch, not pressure.
b. are located chiefly in the aortic and carotid bodies.
c. can be stimulated by a rise in pulse pressure with no rise in mean pressure.
d. reflexly attenuate fluctuations in the mean arterial pressure.
e. have afferent fibres in both the trigeminal and vagus nerves.

16.2 The activity of carotid baroreceptor afferent fibres (action potentials)

a. ceases completely below blood pressures in the range 50–100 mmHg.
b. is pulsatile at normal blood pressures.
c. elicits a 'pressor' reflex.
d. causes a reflex tachycardia.
e. causes a reflex decrease in sympathetic vasoconstrictor fibre activity.
f. causes a reflex rise in cardiac contractility.

16.3 The baroreflex

a. is an example of a positive feedback control system.
b. reduces systemic arterial blood pressure.
c. causes a reflex tachycardia on moving from lying to standing.
d. is reset to a lower operating point during exercise.
e. can be stimulated by massaging the neck just below the angle of the jaw.

16.4 Baroreceptor unloading during hypovolaemia reflexly

a. helps to maintain the cardiac output.
b. increases the total peripheral resistance.
c. minimizes the fall in central venous pressure via sympathetic-mediated venoconstriction.
d. promotes capillary absorption of interstitial fluid.
e. promotes renal fluid retention by inhibiting the renin–angiotensin system.
f. promotes renal fluid retention by stimulating vasopressin secretion.

16.5 Cardiac afferents

a. that are mechanosensitive and are located in ventricular myocardium mediate the pain of a heart attack.
b. in the venoatrial region elicit a reflex tachycardia and diuresis when cardiac filling pressure is elevated.
c. that are chemosensitive and are located in ventricular myocardium mediate the pain of angina pectoris.
d. unlike baroreceptor afferents, do not relay in the nucleus ambiguus solitarius of the medulla oblongata.

T F

16.6 An acute increase in extracellular fluid volume in a human

a. can stimulate both arterial baroreceptors and venoatrial stretch receptors. ☐ ☐
b. elicits a reflex vasoconstriction in the skin, muscle and renal circulations. ☐ ☐
c. elicits a reflex fall in circulating vasopressin. ☐ ☐
d. elicits a rise in circulating atrial natriuretic peptide. ☐ ☐
e. elicits a reflex activation of the renin–angiotensin system. ☐ ☐

16.7 In the long-term control of arterial blood pressure,

a. the cardiopulmonary stretch receptors help normalize arterial blood pressure. ☐ ☐
b. blood pressure is influenced by extracellular fluid volume. ☐ ☐
c. the renal regulation of body salt mass is pivotal. ☐ ☐
d. body water mass is coupled to body salt mass via vasopressin. ☐ ☐
e. the kidneys regulate extracellular fluid volume, but not red cell mass. ☐ ☐

16.8 Regarding the reflex regulation of the cardiovascular system,

a. carotid chemoreceptors cause reflex peripheral vasodilatation during asphyxiation. ☐ ☐
b. lung stretch receptors excited by inflation cause a reflex tachycardia. ☐ ☐
c. skeletal muscle mechanoreceptors (group III afferents) reflexly inhibit cardiovagal tone. ☐ ☐
d. skeletal muscle metaboreceptors (group IV afferents) reflexly raise blood pressure during isometric exercise. ☐ ☐
e. facial cold receptors cause a reflex tachycardia. ☐ ☐

16.9 In the central control of the cardiovascular system,

a. sensory integration begins in the nucleus tractus solitarius of the medulla. ☐ ☐
b. a projection from medullary expiratory neurons to the nucleus ambiguus (cardiac vagal motorneurons) contributes to sinus arrhythmia. ☐ ☐
c. a projection from the nucleus tractus solitarius to the hypothalamus reflexly influences sympathetic vasoconstrictor outflow. ☐ ☐
d. the cerebral cortex can raise cardiac output during exercise by 'central command'. ☐ ☐
e. presympathetic neurons in the rostroventrolateral medulla are organized topographically. ☐ ☐
f. spinal transection raises blood pressure, by interrupting the net inhibition of spinal preganglionic sympathetic neurons by descending bulbospinal fibres. ☐ ☐

16.10 The alerting response to sudden stress (fear–flight–fight response)

a. involves the dilatation of resistance vessels in skeletal muscle. ☐ ☐
b. includes cutaneous venodilatation. ☐ ☐
c. causes a fall in blood pressure. ☐ ☐
d. involves a rise in heart rate. ☐ ☐
e. is organized by the limbic system and periaqueductal grey matter. ☐ ☐
f. is impaired in many patients with hypertension. ☐ ☐

Finally, here is a data interpretation problem.

16.11 The regulation of heart rate and blood pressure at the onset of static exercise.

In a study of the human response to exercise, a subject was asked to squeeze an object in the hand with maximum voluntary force for 4 s. Within two heartbeats of starting the exercise, heart rate had increased from 68 min^{-1} to 80 min^{-1}. Mean arterial pressure increased from 98 to 110 mmHg by the end of the 4 s. Afferent input from the muscles of the arm was then blocked by injections of local anaesthetic into the axillary and radial nerves, and the study repeated. The heart rate increased less, from 68 to 72 min^{-1} by the second beat; blood pressure increased from 96 to 102 mmHg by the end of the 4 s effort.

a. How could the heart rate be monitored so accurately that it was possibly to detect an increase within two beats of starting the exercise?
b. Which branch of the autonomic nervous system is more likely to account for a change in heart rate in under 2 s?
c. What can be inferred from the reduced cardiac response to static exercise after muscle afferent block by local anaesthetic?
d. What types of muscle receptor might mediate the exercise pressor response?
e. Did afferent blockade completely block the tachycardia at the onset of exercise? How might the result be interpreted?

Answers

16.1 a. **T** – Baroreceptors are spray endings that sense distension of the vessel wall **(Figure 16.1**, inset). If distension is prevented by a plaster cast, a rise in pressure does not stimulate the baroreceptors. Normally, a rise in pressure distends the wall and increases firing frequency **(Figure 16.2a)**.

b. **F** – Peripheral *chemo*receptors are located in the carotid and aortic bodies. Arterial baroreceptors are located mainly in the walls of the carotid sinus and aortic arch **(Figure 16.1)**.

c. **T** – Arterial baroreceptors respond to pulse amplitude as well as mean pressure **(Figure 16.3b,c)**.

d. **T** – Baroreceptors trigger a negative feedback loop **(Figure 16.4)**. The net effect of the loop is to reduce the fluctuation in arterial pressure **(Figure 16.5a upper trace)**.

e. **F** – Afferent fibres from carotid sinus baroreceptors travel in the glossopharyngeal (ninth cranial) nerve. Aortic baroreceptor fibres travel in the vagus (tenth cranial nerve) **(Figure 16.1)**.

16.2 a. **T** – Baroreceptors have a threshold below which they are silent. The threshold is typically ~60 mmHg for A fibres and ~100 mmHg for C fibres **(Figure 16.3a)**.

b. **T** – Baroreceptors are dynamically sensitive, and are temporarily silenced as blood pressure falls **(Figure 16.2, fibre 2)**. Consequently, their firing pattern in response to the normal, pulsatile arterial pressure is itself pulsatile **(Figure 16.2, fibre 3)**.

c. **F** – 'Pressor' means 'causes a rise in pressure'. The baroreflex is 'depressor', i.e. baroreceptor activation causes a reflex depression of arterial blood pressure **(Figure 8.16)**, via the pathways in **Figures 16.4**.

d. **F** – Baroreceptor stimulation causes a reflex bradycardia **(Figure 8.16 and 6.21)**.

e. **T** – There is reflex fall in sympathetic vasomotor activity **(Figure 6.21)**. This reduces total peripheral resistance, which helps bring a raised blood pressure back down to normal.

f. **F** – The baroreflex *reduces* cardiac sympathetic nerve activity **(Figure 6.21)**. This lowers cardiac contractility and heart rate.

16.3 a. **F** – The baroreflex is an example of *negative* feedback, i.e. a rise in the sensed variable (blood pressure) causes changes in motor fibre output that lower the sensed variable **(Figure 16.4)**.

b. **T** – There is a reflex fall in sympathetic activity and rise in cardiac vagal inhibition **(Figure 6.21)**. This lowers the blood pressure **(Figures 8.16 and 16.3c)**.

c. **T** – Blood pressure in the carotid sinus falls on standing, because the sinus is above heart level (effect of gravity, **Figure 8.3**). Also arterial pulse pressure falls on standing, due to venous 'pooling' in the lower limbs, reducing cardiac filling pressure and hence stroke volume. The resulting unloading of baroreceptors, especially in the carotid sinus, triggers the reflex tachycardia.

d. **F** – The baroreflex is reset to operate at a moderately *higher* pressures during exercise **(Figure 16.6)**. This helps stabilize the raised blood pressure during exercise.

e. **T** – Massaging the carotid sinus, which is located just under the angle of the jaw, stimulates the sinus baroreceptors. The resulting reflex can sometimes arrest a supraventricular tachycardia.

16.4 a. **T** – Cardiac sympathetic activity is reflexly increased, and cardiac parasympathetic activity is reduced. This boosts heart rate and contractility. So haemorrhage evokes a tachycardia **(Figure 8.11)**.

b. **T** – A reflex rise in sympathetic vasomotor activity promotes contraction of peripheral resistance vessels, raising peripheral resistance. This helps preserve the mean arterial pressure **(Figure 8.11)**.

c. **T** – There is a reflex increase in sympathetic venomotor activity **(Figure 8.11)**. The central venous pressure (CVP) is an important determinant of stroke volume (Starling's law of the heart).

d. **T** – The sympathetic-mediated constriction of precapillary resistance vessels, along with the fall in venous pressure, reduces capillary pressure **(Figure 11.7)**. This allows plasma colloid osmotic pressure to predominate for a while **(Figure 11.4b)**, causing the absorption of interstitial fluid **(Figure 8.11)**.

e. **F** – Baroreceptor unloading *activates* renin secretion **(Figure 14.7)**. This leads to higher circulating levels of the vasoconstrictor peptide angiotensin II and the salt-retaining steroid aldosterone.

f. **T** – Reflex vasopressin secretion causes renal anti-diuresis, and also helps raises peripheral resistance via its vasoconstrictor action **(Figure 14.6)**.

16.5 a. **F** – These unmyelinated afferents travel in the vagus **(Figure 16.7)** and cause a depressor reflex, similar to the baroreflex. Being mechanoreceptors, they do not sense ischaemia.

b. **T** – Myelinated atrial afferents signal atrial distension and contraction **(Figure 16.7)**. The evoked reflex (tachycardia, diuresis) helps prevent over-distension. These receptors may also contribute to reflex peripheral vasodilatation when human CVP is raised.

c. **T** – These unmyelinated afferents travel with the cardiac sympathetic nerves to the spinal cord, then up the spinothalamic tract **(Figure 16.7)**. They are stimulated by many substances released by ischaemic myocardium (bradykinin, K^+, acid, prostaglandins, 20-HETE) and thus mediate the pain of both angina and heart attack.

d. **F** – *All* cardiovascular afferents relay in the nucleus tractus solitarius of the brainstem **(Figure 16.8)**.

16.6 a. **T** – An increase in extracellular fluid volume raises plasma volume and therefore cardiac filling pressure, which stimulates venoatrial receptors. A large increase in filling pressure tends to raise the stroke volume (Starling's law) and pulse pressure, thus stimulating arterial baroreceptors too.

b. **F** – An increase in plasma volume elicits a reflex *vasodilatation*, which helps lower the vascular pressures.

c. **T** – An inhibitory synapse in the central relay pathway (nucleus tractus solitarius via the caudal ventrolateral medulla to the magnocellular neurons) reduces vasopressin secretion when extracellular fluid (ECF) volume increases **(Figure 14.6)**.

d. **T** – Atrial natriuretic peptide (ANP)-secreting atrial myocytes respond directly to stretch.

e. **F** – The renin-secreting juxtaglomerular cells of the renal afferent arteriole are *inhibited* by a rise in arterial pressure and tubular NaCl load, and by reduced sympathetic activity **(Figure 14.7)**. The resulting fall in circulating aldosterone concentration promotes natriuresis and diuresis.

16.7 a. **T** – Denervation of the arterial baroreceptors alone raises blood pressure a little; but denervation of the baroreceptors *and* cardiopulmonary receptors raises blood pressure markedly **(Figure 16.5b)**.

b. **T** – Plasma is part of the extracellular fluid compartment. A rise in plasma volume raises the cardiac filling pressure, which raises stroke volume through the Frank–Starling mechanism. This raises arterial blood pressure.

c. **T** – In the long term the mean blood pressure is proportional to body water mass, which is directly proportional to body salt mass **(Figure 16.9)**. Renal salt handling is crucial, therefore, to the long-term regulation of blood pressure.

d. **T** – The salt-to-water ratio determines extracellular fluid osmolarity, which is sensed by central osmoreceptors that regulate vasopressin (ADH) secretion **(Figure 14.6)**. If body salt mass rises, the temporary increase in osmolarity cause ADH secretion and hence renal water retention, until water mass increases sufficiently to restore normal osmolarity.

e. **F** – The kidneys secrete the hormone erythropoietin, which stimulates red cell production and release by the bone marrow.

16.8 a. **F** – Carotid body and aortic body chemoreceptors are excited by hypoxia and hypercapnia (asphyxia), but they cause a reflex peripheral *vasoconstriction*. This 'pressor' reflex helps maintain the arterial blood pressure perfusing the brain during asphyxia.

b. **T** – The lung inflation reflex contributes to sinus arrhythmia and the tachycardia of asphyxia.

c. **T** – Group III muscle mechanoreceptors contribute to the very rapid increase in heart rate at the onset of exercise.

d. **T** – Group IV muscle metaboreceptors are stimulated by K^+ ions, lactic acid and other agents in under-perfused muscle. Their afferent input reflexly raises sympathetic vasomotor and cardiac activity, contributing to the exercise pressor response **(Figure 16.10)**. This reflex is especially strong in isometrically contracting muscle.

e. **F** – Facial cold receptors reflexly increase cardiac vagal activity, causing a marked *bradycardia*. This is part of the diving reflex; facial submersion in cold water greatly slows the human heart, and that of diving mammals even more so.

16.9 a. **T** – When the inputs from several sources converge on one neuron (e.g. a baroreceptor input and a venoatrial receptor input), the output of the neuron depends on the combined input. This is called sensory integration.

b. **F** – Sinus arrhythmia is a regular tachycardia associated with *inspiration* **(Figure 4.3a)**. This is largely due to an inhibitory projection from the *inspiratory* neurons to the vagal motorneurons **(Figure 16.11)**. The tachycardia helps compensate for the fall in left ventricle stroke volume during inspiration, caused by reduced venous return into the left heart as the pulmonary circulation expands.

c. **T** – The parvocellular neurons of the hypothalamic paraventricular nucleus and depressor area receive a projection from the nucleus tractus solitarius, and send projections to the medullary presympathetic vasomotor neurons **(Figure 16.12)**.

d. **T** – Central command, along with the muscle mechanoreceptor reflex, accounts for the very rapid increase in heart rate on starting exercise **(Figure 16.12)**.

e. **T** – The most rostral part of the ventral vasopressor area controls renal sympathetic outflow; other zones control limb sympathetic outflow. This enables discrete control of sympathetic outflow – outflow can increase to one tissue and at the same time decrease to another tissue, e.g. during the alerting response.

f. **F** – There are both inhibitory and excitatory descending fibres, but the net bulbospinal drive is excitatory **(Figure 16.8)**. Spinal transection thus *reduces* peripheral sympathetic vasomotor activity and causes hypotension.

16.10 a. **T** – The increase in muscle blood flow anticipates fight or flight.
b. **F** – The alerting response evokes cutaneous veno*constriction* ('startle' response, **Figure 6.15**). We grow pale with fear.
c. **F** – Blood pressure rises. This is important for doctors to recognize; a tense patient will have a raised blood pressure – 'white coat hypertension'.
d. **T** – The alerting tachycardia is evident in question 14.12, which describes a human study.
e. **T** – The central long axis (amygdala of limbic system, perifornical hypothalamus and the periaqueductal grey matter) generate this co-ordinated, stereotyped alerting responses **(Figure 16.12)**. The output of the central long axis modulates the nucleus tractus solitarius, cardiac vagal motor neurons **(Figure 16.11)** and rostral vasopressor neurons to produce the characteristic cardiac and vasomotor changes.
f. **F** – Hypertensive subjects often show an exaggerated *rise* in blood pressure in response to stress, as do their offspring. This may contribute to the establishment of chronic hypertension.

16.11 a. Beat-by-beat heart rate can be obtained from a continuous ECG recording, by measuring each R–R interval. Alternatively, a continuous recording of the pulse, based on an ear oximeter or finger/wrist monitor, could be used to measure the beat-to-beat interval.
b. The extreme rapidity of the change in heart rate is typical of a disinhibition of the pacemaker by reduced vagal activity. The effect of the vagal parasympathetic fibres on heart is very quick **(Figure 4.2)**, whereas the effect of increased sympathetic drive is of slower onset **(Figure 4.6)**.
c. The results indicate that afferent information from the contracting muscles contributes to a reflex that raises heart rate and blood pressure during static exercise. In other words, there are work receptors in skeletal muscle that help drive appropriate cardiac changes during exercise **(Figure 16.4)**.
d. Muscle work receptors (ergoreceptors) are of two kinds – mechanosensitive group III afferents and chemosensitive group IV afferents. Muscle mechanoreceptors reflexly inhibit vagal tone, so they probably account for the almost immediate change in heart rate. Muscle chemosensitive afferents (metaboreceptors) are important contributors to the developing pressor response **(Figure 16.10)**.
e. No. The most likely factor driving the persistent albeit lesser tachycardia is 'central command', i.e. a signal from the motor areas of the brain to the cardiovascular autonomic centres in the lower brain **(Figure 16.12)**.

CHAPTER 17

Co-ordinated cardiovascular responses

T F

17.1 When a healthy subject moves from a supine to a standing position,

a. gravity causes a backflow of venous blood into the legs, leading to venous pooling.
b. the jugular veins in the neck collapse.
c. the central venous pressure (CVP) increases.
d. there is a sustained fall in arterial pulse pressure.
e. the circulating blood volume decreases slowly.

17.2 On standing up,

a. carotid sinus baroreceptor activity declines.
b. peripheral resistance falls.
c. the heart rate falls.
d. mean arterial pressure dips (transient hypotension).
e. mean arterial pressure in the steady state is higher than the supine value.
f. postural dizziness can be treated with the α-blocker phentolamine.

17.3 Forced expiration against a closed glottis, e.g. during childbirth, elicits

a. an instantaneous rise in arterial blood pressure on starting the manoeuvre.
b. a sustained increase in right ventricle stroke volume.
c. an increase in aortic pulse pressure.
d. a transient increase in venous return on ceasing the manoeuvre.
e. a temporary slowing of the heart on ceasing the manoeuvre.

17.4 During upright, dynamic exercise, such as running or cycling,

a. O_2 uptake from the alveolar gas increases as pulmonary blood flow increases.
b. cardiac output is increased mainly through a rise in stroke volume.
c. cardiac β_1-adrenoceptors are stimulated.
d. the end-diastolic volume of the ventricles is increased.
e. the end-systolic volume of the ventricles is increased.
f. heart rate is raised quickly at the onset of exercise via reduced vagal activity.

17.5 The cardiovascular changes during exercise include

a. a fall in gastrointestinal blood flow.
b. a rise in renal blood flow.
c. a rise in active muscle blood flow caused chiefly by the rise in blood pressure.
d. a greater rise in systolic blood pressure than diastolic pressure.
e. a rise in total peripheral resistance.
f. a greater increase in stroke volume during supine than upright exercise.
g. a greater increase in blood pressure during static than dynamic exercise.

	T	F

17.6 In the microcirculation of exercising skeletal muscle,

a. O_2 transfer is enhanced by capillary recruitment.
b. the average O_2 concentration in the capillary in increased, relative to rest, due to the increased blood flow.
c. CO_2 removal is enhanced by a fall in diffusion distance.
d. glucose transfer is enhanced by active transport across the endothelium.
e. glucose transfer is enhanced by a fall in interstitial glucose concentration.
f. increased capillary fluid filtration can reduce the circulating plasma volume.

17.7 The cardiovascular adjustments during exercise can be initiated partly by

a. central command by the cerebral cortex.
b. central resetting of the baroreflex to a lower operating point.
c. feedforward from muscle metaboreceptors.
d. feedforward by the alerting response.
e. a rise in circulating catecholamines in cardiac transplant patients.

For additional questions on exercise, see questions 13.5, 13.9, 13.10 and 15.9.

17.8 Dynamic, endurance training leads to

a. a rise in resting stroke volume.
b. a rise in resting heart rate.
c. a rise in maximum heart rate.
d. a rise in maximal O_2 transport capacity, $\dot{V}_{O_{2max}}$.
e. a fall in blood volume.
f. angiogenesis in the trained muscle groups.

17.9 The cardiovascular changes after a substantial meal include:

a. an increase in gastrointestinal mucosal blood flow.
b. an increase in cardiac output by ~20%.
c. a fall in blood flow to the limbs.
d. a fall in vagal parasympathetic drive to pancreatic blood vessels.
e. postprandial hypertension in patients with autonomic dysfunction.

17.10 Breath-hold immersion of the face in cold water evokes

a. a rise in heart rate.
b. a fall in limb blood flow due to peripheral vasoconstriction.
c. a fall in arterial chemoreceptor activity.
d. a reflex mediated by trigeminal nerve receptors.

17.11 The cardiovascular changes associated with normal ageing include

a. arteriosclerosis, which is primarily an intimal accumulation of cholesterol.
b. increased stiffness of the elastic arteries.
c. a greater rise in diastolic blood pressure than systolic pressure.
d. a rise in mean blood pressure due to an increase in total peripheral resistance.
e. a fall in the maximum heart rate during exercise.
f. increased responsiveness of the myocardium to β-adrenoceptor stimulation.

Data interpretation problems involving integrated cardiovascular responses: Alerting response, question 14.12; Exercise (CVS changes at onset), question 16.10. Endurance-trained athletes (improved CVS performance), question 17.12, below.

17.12 The enhanced cardiovascular performance of endurance-trained athletes.

Cardiovascular and pulmonary function were measured during maximal exercise in untrained university students and Olympic athletes. Maximal oxygen uptake $\dot{V}_{O_{2max}}$ increased from $3.3\,l\,min^{-1}$ in untrained students to $5.0\,l\,min^{-1}$ in the athletes and maximum cardiac output from 20 to $30\,l\,min^{-1}$, but maximum heart rate fell from 192 to $182\,min^{-1}$.

a. Did the increase in $\dot{V}_{O_{2max}}$ require an increase in the arteriovenous difference in O_2 concentration? (Hint – consider the Fick principle.)

b. By how much did training increase the maximum stroke volume of the heart?

c. If the ejection fraction is similar for student and athlete, what might cause the increase in stroke volume?

Answers

17.1 a. **F** – Semilunar valves in peripheral veins prevent any substantial reversal of flow, as was shown by William Harvey almost 400 years ago. The venous 'pooling' is caused by the gravity-induced rise in venous pressure **(Figure 8.3)**. This distends the veins **(Figure 6.9)**; but the 'pooled' blood reaches the veins by forward flow from the capillaries, as usual.

b. **T** – Venous pressure above heart level falls, due to the effect of gravity **(Figure 8.3)**. The fall in transmural pressure causes the jugular veins to collapse **(Figures 6.9 and 8.24)**.

c. **F** – CVP falls, because the peripheral venous pooling reduces the intrathoracic blood volume **(Figure 6.9)**.

d. **T** – The fall in CVP, acting via Starling s law of the heart, reduces stroke volume by ~40% **(Figure 17.1)**. This in turn reduces the pulse pressure **(Figure 7.2)**.

e. **T** – Capillary pressure is greatly increased in the tissues below heart level **(Figure 11.6)**. This raises the capillary filtration rate, which reduces the plasma volume by ~12% over half an hour.

17.2 a. **T** – The carotid sinus is located well above heart level during orthostasis, so its transmural pressure falls **(Figure 8.3)**. Also, the pulse pressure falls on standing **(Figure 17.1)** and baroreceptors are sensitive to pulse pressure **(Figure 16.3)**.

b. **F** – Total peripheral resistance increases by 30–40% on standing **(Figure 17.1)**. The resistance increase is brought about by a baroreflex-mediated increase in sympathetic vasomotor activity to the resistance vessels of muscle, splanchnic and renal circulations **(Figure 17.2)**. This helps to maintain arterial blood pressure: *BP* = *total peripheral resistance* (raised) × *cardiac output* (reduced).

c. **F** – The baroreflex elicits tachycardia during orthostasis **(Figures 17.1 and 17.2)**.

d. **T** – The fall in stroke volume reduces arterial pressure transiently, before the reflex tachycardia and peripheral vasoconstriction have had time to kick in. This sometimes causes transient dizziness on standing (postural hypotension), even in healthy people.

e. **T** – There is a sustained fall in carotid sinus and venoatrial receptors inputs **(Figure 17.2)**. This evokes a sustained reflex elevation of mean arterial pressure during standing **(Figure 17.1)**.

f. **F** – Postural hypotension is in fact a major side-effect of α-blockers; they prevent the compensatory rise in peripheral resistance, by blocking the effect of increased sympathetic vasomotor activity.

17.3 a. **T** – Forced expiration against a closed glottis is the Valsalva manoeuvre. In phase 1, the immediate rise in intrathoracic pressure squeezes the aorta, raising arterial pressure **(Figure 17.3a)**.

b. **F** – The rise in intrathoracic pressure squeezes the thoracic veins too, which impedes venous return; so right and left ventricular stroke volumes fall.

c. **F** – The fall in stroke volume (see above) reduces the pulse pressure **(Figure 17.3a)**.

d. **T** – The pent up peripheral venous blood surges into the right ventricle as soon as intrathoracic pressure is reduced.

e. **T** – The increase in stroke volume resulting from the sudden increase in cardiac filling (Starling's law) raises the pulse pressure, which evokes a baroreflex bradycardia **(phase 4, Figure 17.3a)**. This response is used to test autonomic function.

17.4 a. **T** – The relation between O_2 uptake and pulmonary blood flow is shown in **Figure 17.4**. The Fick principle tells us that *O_2 uptake = blood flow × arteriovenous difference in O_2 concentration*. Pulmonary O_2 uptake is an example of flow-limited exchange **(Figure 10.6, points 1, 2)**.

b. **F** – The tachycardia make a greater contribution than the increase in stroke volume **(Table 17.1)**.

c. **T** – Increased cardiac sympathetic activity stimulates β_1-adrenoceptors on the pacemaker, AV node and myocardium **(Figure 4.1)**. The activated β_1-adrenoceptors raise intracellular cAMP, leading to increases in heart rate and contractility **(Figure 3.14**, upper panel).

d. **T** – During upright exercise the venous muscle pump, along with sympathetic-mediated venoconstriction in the splanchnic and other circulations, raise central venous pressure moderately, distending the ventricle in diastole **(Figure 6.10 and Table 17.1)**. This increases stroke volume through the Frank–Starling mechanism.

e. **F** – A rise in ventricular contractility increases the ejection fraction and thus *reduces* the end-systolic volume. The heart becomes bigger at the end of diastole and smaller at the end of systole **(Figure 6.10 and Table 17.1)**.

f. **T** – Parasympathetic fibres alter the heart rate more rapidly than sympathetic fibres (compare **Figures 4.2 and 4.6,)**. This is because the acetylcholine–hyperpolarization pathway is very direct **(Figure 3.14, lower panel)**. Central command and muscle mechanoreceptors trigger the sudden reduction of vagal cardiac motorneuron activity.

17.5 a. **T** – There is sympathetic-mediated vasoconstriction of inactive circulations **(Figure 13.10)**. This helps stabilize arterial blood pressure in the face of the huge fall in vascular resistance in the exercising muscles.

b. **F** – There is sympathetic-mediated renal vasoconstriction **(Figurer 13.10)**. As with gastrointestinal vasoconstriction, this helps stabilize arterial blood pressure by partially offsetting the massive fall in resistance in the exercising muscle.

c. **F** – Most of the increase in muscle blood flow during dynamic exercise is caused by the reduced resistance to flow through the dilated arterioles of the active muscle (metabolic vasodilatation). In **Figure 13.10**, muscle blood flow increases approximately eight-fold, yet blood pressure increases only ~1.2-fold **(Figure 6.22)**. Since *flow = pressure difference/resistance*, most of the increase in flow is clearly due to a fall in muscle vascular resistance.

d. **T** – Systolic pressure increases more than diastolic **(Figure 6.22)**. This is because stroke volume and ejection velocity increase, raising the pulse pressure.

e. **F** – Total peripheral resistance (TPR) falls **(Figure 6.22)**. This is because muscle vasodilatation outweighs the vasoconstriction in other tissues. Blood pressure does not fall, despite the fall in TPR, because cardiac output rises: *BP = cardiac output × TPR*.

f. **F** – Central venous pressure and therefore stroke volume are already high at rest in the supine position. There is more scope to raise the stroke volume when starting from the relatively low stroke volume of the upright position **(Table 17.2)**.

g. **T** – Static, isometric exercise causes big increases in blood pressure **(Figure 8.15)**, so is inadvisable for patients with ischaemic heart disease. The rise in pressure is due partly to the exercise pressor reflex from muscle metaboreceptors **(Figure 16.10)**, and partly to central command.

17.6 a. **T** – Metabolic vasodilatation of the arterioles improves the uniformity of capillary perfusion (capillary recruitment, **Figure 10.7**). This boosts two factors affecting diffusion – surface area (number of capillaries perfused) and diffusion distance (Fick's law of diffusion, **Figure 10.4**).

b. **F** – Mean capillary O_2 concentration actually falls during exercise, despite the increased delivery (flow), because O_2 extraction increases relatively more than the blood flow. However, without the rise in blood flow, the O_2 level would fall catastrophically.

c. **T** – Capillary recruitment boosts CO_2 uptake by the same mechanisms as boost O_2 transfer **(Figure 10.7)**.

d. **F** – Glucose diffuses passively out of the capillaries of skeletal muscle via the intercellular clefts **(Figure 9.6)**.

e. **T** – Increased muscle consumption of glucose lowers its interstitial concentration, which increases the concentration gradients for diffusion. A fall in local venous glucose during exercise reflects the fall in interstitial glucose **(Figure 10.8)**.

f. **T** – Arteriolar vasodilatation raises capillary pressure **(Figure 11.7)**; also, interstitial osmolarity increases. These forces raise the capillary filtration rate. Plasma volume can fall by over 0.5 litre during heavy, prolonged exercise, reducing the cardiac filling pressure.

17.7 a. **T** – Attempts to exercise muscles paralysed by curare lead to tachycardia, a rise in blood pressure and baroreflex resetting **(Figure 16.6)**.

b. **F** – The baroreflex is reset to operate at a *higher* pressure during exercise **(Figure 16.6)**.

c. **F** – Muscle metaboreceptors are activated by the metabolic changes within the exercising muscle, which take a little time to develop; so metaboreceptors provide feed*back* on muscle metabolic status, not feedforward control (changes in anticipation of an event) **(Figure 16.4)**.

d. **T** – If exercise has an emotional component (e.g. start of a race), the alerting response increases heart rate and muscle perfusion in anticipation of action. The alerting response is mediated by the central long axis (amygdala, hypothalamus, periaqueductal grey) **(Figure 16.12)**.

e. **T** – Circulating adrenaline and noradrenaline increase ~10-fold during exercise, stimulating cardiac β-adrenoceptors on the transplanted, denervated heart. Greyhounds with denervated hearts can still increase their heart rates to >250 min^{-1} on the racetrack, but not when the effect of adrenaline is blocked by β-blockers.

17.8 a. **T** – The cardiac myocytes are lengthened by the addition of sarcomeres in series. This enlarges the ventricular cavity (eccentric hypertrophy) and increases the resting stroke volume by up to 50%.

b. **F** – Increased vagal tone causes a resting bradycardia. This offsets the effect of the increased resting stroke volume, so that the cardiac output remains normal at rest.

c. **F** – Maximum heart rate is not increased by training.

d. **T** – $\dot{V}_{O_{2max}}$ is increased by an increase in maximal cardiac output, which results from the bigger stroke volume.

e. **F** – There is a small *increase* in blood volume, to match the increased resting ventricle size.

f. **T** – Without the formation of additional capillaries, the hypertrophy of the skeletal muscle fibres would increase the diffusion distance from capillary to muscle, making transport by diffusion less efficient. Also, arteriolar angiogenesis increases the muscle's maximal perfusion capacity.

17.9 a. **T** – Mucosal hyperaemia is evoked by local gastrointestinal hormones (gastrin, cholecystokinin), digestion products (glucose and fatty acids) and vagal cholinergic parasympathetic fibres.

b. **T** – Postprandial tachycardia raises the cardiac output, to supply the hyperaemic mucosa and pancreas.

c. **T** – Reflex sympathetic vasoconstriction of limb resistance vessels helps to maintain total peripheral resistance, and hence blood pressure, despite the fall in splanchnic vascular resistance.

d. **F** – The firing of parasympathetic fibres in the vagus *increases*, to induce pancreatic vasodilatation. This is necessary to supply the large volume of liquid secreted by the pancreas. The pancreatic parasympathetic vasodilator transmitter is mainly VIP (vasoactive intestinal polypeptide).

e. **F** – Some elderly subjects and diabetics with poor autonomic function develop postprandial *hypotension*, due to a failure of the autonomic-mediated tachycardia and peripheral vasoconstriction that normally maintain blood pressure after a meal.

17.10 a. **F** – The diving response evokes a marked vagal bradycardia **(Figures 17.5)**. This can sometimes terminate a pathological supraventricular tachycardia. The response is very pronounced in seals, whales and diving birds.

b. **T** – Muscle perfusion is reduced by sympathetic vasoconstriction **(Figure 17.5**, inset). This maintains blood pressure (hence myocardial and cerebral perfusion) despite the marked vagal bradycardia.

c. **F** – The growing arterial hypoxaemia and hypercapnia stimulate the arterial chemoreceptors in the carotid and aortic bodies. The arterial chemoreflex contributes to the sympathetic-mediated peripheral vasoconstriction.

d. **T** – Cold receptors around the eyes, nose and nasal mucosa send afferent information along the trigeminal nerve to initiate the reflex apnoea, bradycardia and peripheral vasoconstriction. These changes conserve the O_2 store for use by the brain.

17.11 a. **F** – Arteriosclerosis is indeed the primary arterial change with ageing, but it is quite different from atheroma. Atheroma (atherosclerosis) is primarily a subendothelial deposition of cholesterol. Arteriosclerosis is a stiffening of the tunica media (not intima) due to fibrosis (collagen), with loss of intact elastin and lumen dilatation (not narrowing).

b. **T** – Arteriosclerosis increases the stiffness of the major arteries (elastance, 1/compliance). This increases the pulse pressure and hence systolic pressure, just as in hypertension **(Figure 8.10)**. Faster return of the reflected pressure wave in the stiffened arteries further augments the systolic pressure **(Figure 8.12)**.

c. **F** – Systolic pressure increases much more than diastolic **(Figure 8.14)**, due to a marked increase in the pulse pressure, which results from the increased stiffness of the elastic arteries. The raised systolic pressure (afterload on the left ventricle) raises cardiac O_2 demand.

d. **T** – Mean blood pressure increases moderately **(Figure 8.14)**, due partly to an increase in sympathetic vasomotor activity with age.

e. **T** – Maximum cardiac output falls with age, due partly to a fall in the maximum attainable heart rate. As a rough rule, maximum rate $= 220\,\text{min}^{-1} -$ age in years.

f. **F** – The responsiveness of pacemaker and myocardium to β-adrenoceptor stimulation *decreases* with age, so the ability to raise the ejection fraction and heart rate declines.

17.12 a. From the Fick principle, *oxygen uptake = cardiac output × arteriovenous concentration difference*. The increase in O_2 transport, 1.5-fold, can be explained fully by the increase in maximal cardiac output, which was likewise 1.5-fold. Therefore, the data provide no evidence for changes in blood gas values between students and athletes.

b. Since *cardiac output = heart rate × stroke volume*, the maximum stroke volume was 104 ml in the students and 165 ml in the athletes – a 1.58-fold increase (61 ml).

c. If the ejection fraction has not increased, the volume of blood in the ventricle during diastole must have increased, raising the volume available for ejection. This is brought about by enlargement of the ventricular cavity as a result of training (eccentric hypertrophy).

CHAPTER 18

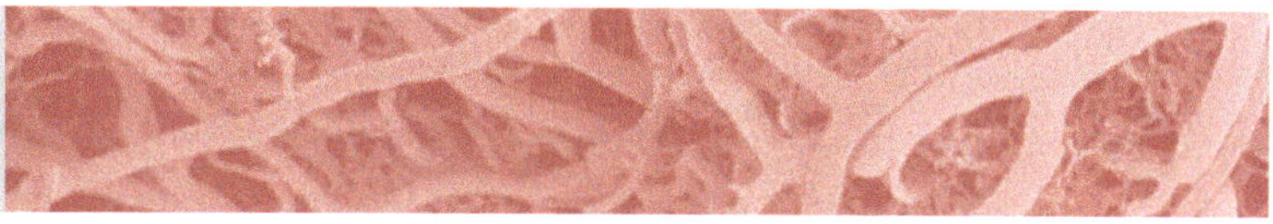

Cardiovascular responses in pathological situations

T F

18.1 At high altitudes chronic arterial hypoxaemia causes

a. stimulation of arterial chemoreceptors.
b. an increase in the arteriovenous O_2 difference.
c. depression of the cardiac output.
d. peripheral vasodilatation.
e. a fall in systemic arterial blood pressure.
f. a fall in pulmonary arterial blood pressure.

18.2 A patient in clinical shock (acute circulatory failure), due to a severe haemorrhage, usually exhibits

a. a reduced central venous pressure.
b. a low mean arterial pressure, but normal pulse pressure.
c. a pronounced tachycardia.
d. an increased cardiac output.
e. a rise in total peripheral resistance.

18.3 In response to a severe haemorrhage,

a. baroreceptor activity declines.
b. arterial chemoreceptor activity declines.
c. venoatrial mechanoreceptor activity declines.
d. the skin is pale, cold and venoconstricted.
e. the haematocrit remains normal.

18.4 The responses to hypovolaemia may include

a. a fall in circulating noradrenaline and adrenaline concentration.
b. a glucose-mediated rise in interstitial fluid osmolarity.
c. a fall in circulating vasopressin level.
d. a fall in urine production.
e. thirst mediated by a rise in circulating natriuretic peptide.

18.5 When a person faints (syncope),

a. the heart rate abruptly increases.
b. the peripheral resistance increases sharply.
c. the mean arterial pressure falls below 70 mmHg.
d. cerebral blood flow is markedly reduced.
e. the patient should not be kept upright.

T F

18.6 Clinical hypertension

a. is a chronic rise in systemic arterial blood pressure sufficient to increase morbidity and mortality.
b. increases the incidence of heart attacks, but not strokes.
c. is usually diagnosed when diastolic pressure consistently exceeds 90–95 mmHg or systolic pressure exceeds 140–160 mmHg.
d. can be caused by renal artery dilatation.
e. can be caused by adrenal cortex failure (Addison's disease).
f. is usually symptomless and without readily identifiable organic cause.

18.7 Arterial hypertension in humans

a. is often associated with a high dietary salt intake.
b. is very rare during pregnancy.
c. is characterized by a reduction in the bore of proximal resistance arteries.
d. is characterized by dilated, stiffened elastic arteries.
e. is always associated with an increase in circulating angiotensin II.

18.8 In a patient with established essential hypertension,

a. the total peripheral resistance is raised, but the cardiac output is normal.
b. systolic pressure and diastolic pressures increase by about the same amount.
c. increased wave reflection contributes to the systolic hypertension.
d. an increase in cardiac work causes left ventricular dilatation.
e. the baroreflex remains functional around a higher set point.

18.9 In the treatment of essential hypertension,

a. a reduction in dietary salt intake is not yet of proven efficacy.
b. thiazide diuretics are a common initial treatment.
c. Beta-adrenoceptor blockers reduce the sympathetic activation of renin secretion.
d. angiotensin converting enzyme (ACE) inhibitors aggravate left ventricular hypertrophy.
e. nifedipine reduces total peripheral resistance.

18.10 Chronic left ventricular failure is

a. a reduced left ventricular stroke volume in a resting subject.
b. an abnormal reduction in ventricular myocyte contractility.
c. a steeper relation between stroke work and end-diastolic pressure.
d. associated with a cardiothoracic ratio of less than 0.5.

18.11 In left ventricular failure,

a. pulmonary venous pressure decreases.
b. the compliance of the lungs is increased.
c. dyspnoea is often relieved by lying down.
d. pulmonary capillary pressure is reduced.
e. crackles (crepitations) are audible during basal lung auscultation.

T F

18.12 Failure of the right ventricle can lead to
a. visible distension of the jugular veins during orthostasis. ☐ ☐
b. facial oedema. ☐ ☐
c. pitting oedema of the lower leg. ☐ ☐
d. a right ventricular ejection fraction of ~66%. ☐ ☐
e. hepatomegaly. ☐ ☐

18.13 In a chronically failing ventricle the cardiac myocyte exhibits
a. an increased systolic Ca^{2+} transient. ☐ ☐
b. increased expression of the Na^{+}–Ca^{2+} exchanger. ☐ ☐
c. increased expression of K^{+} channels. ☐ ☐
d. increased proneness to delayed after-depolarization (DAD). ☐ ☐
e. prolonged action potentials. ☐ ☐

18.14 In patients with biventricular chronic cardiac failure,
a. the incidence of cardiac arrhythmia is markedly raised. ☐ ☐
b. there is rapid skeletal muscle fatigue during moderate physical exercise. ☐ ☐
c. ventricular dilatation increases the mechanical efficiency of contraction. ☐ ☐
d. the afterload may depress stroke volume more than in a normal heart. ☐ ☐

18.15 In the systemic circulation of patients in heart failure,
a. there is marked vasodilatation of peripheral resistance vessels. ☐ ☐
b. arterial blood pressure is often in the normal range. ☐ ☐
c. the pulse rate increases normally during exercise. ☐ ☐
d. there is marked peripheral venoconstriction. ☐ ☐

18.16 The following are raised in a patient in chronic cardiac failure:
a. peripheral and cardiac sympathetic nerve activity. ☐ ☐
b. circulating catecholamines. ☐ ☐
c. circulating angiotensin II. ☐ ☐
d. circulating endothelin. ☐ ☐
e. circulating brain natriuretic peptide (BNP). ☐ ☐

18.17 The renal response to chronic cardiac failure includes
a. reduced salt and water retention. ☐ ☐
b. reduced activation of the renin–angiotensin–aldosterone system. ☐ ☐
c. pronounced renal vasoconstriction. ☐ ☐
d. expansion of the extracellular fluid volume. ☐ ☐

18.18 Some of the physiological objectives, when treating chronic heart failure, are to
a. reduce myocardial O_2 demand. ☐ ☐
b. raise arterial blood pressure. ☐ ☐
c. reduce the radius of curvature of the ventricle. ☐ ☐
d. boost the plasma volume. ☐ ☐
e. reduce the inotropic state of the heart. ☐ ☐

T F

18.19 The pharmacological treatment of heart failure often involves

a. angiotensin converting enzyme (ACE) inhibitors. ☐ ☐
b. potassium-losing diuretics. ☐ ☐
c. inhibition of renin production by spironolactone. ☐ ☐
d. peripheral vasodilators. ☐ ☐
e. Beta-adrenoceptor blockers. ☐ ☐

18.20 Digoxin

a. inhibits the cardiac myocyte Ca^{2+} pump. ☐ ☐
b. increases the size of the myocyte systolic Ca^{2+} transient. ☐ ☐
c. causes a tachycardia. ☐ ☐
d. increases the risk of ventricular arrhythmia. ☐ ☐
e. toxicity is enhanced by hyperkalaemia. ☐ ☐

Answers

18.1 a. **T** – Hypoxaemia is detected by carotid and aortic body chemoreceptors **(Figure 16.1)**. They drive a reflex increase in breathing.

b. **F** – Arterial P_{O2} falls, so there is a smaller diffusion gradient from blood to tissue. Consequently, the amount of O_2 diffusing out of each unit volume of blood is *reduced*.

c. **F** – Heart rate and cardiac output increase **(Figure 18.1)**. This helps to maintain a normal O_2 delivery to the tissues despite the fall in arterial O_2 content (Fick's principle).

d. **T** – Hypoxia causes vasodilatation of systemic resistance vessels **(Figure 13.7)**. This reduces peripheral resistance and facilitates the increases in local blood flow and O_2 delivery **(Figure 18.1)**.

e. **T** – Peripheral vasodilatation outweighs the effect of the raised cardiac output, so systemic arterial pressure falls **(Figure 18.1)**: mean systemic arterial pressure = cardiac output × total peripheral resistance.

f. **F** – Hypoxia causes pulmonary arterial *hypertension*, due to hypoxic pulmonary vasoconstriction **(Figure 15.13)** – the opposite of hypoxic systemic vasodilatation. This is reflected in the high pulmonary perfusion pressure for a given cardiac output at high altitude **(Figure 15.14)**. Eventually, right ventricular failure can develop.

18.2 a. **T** – Hypovolaemia (low blood volume) lowers CVP, because most of the circulating blood is in the venous system.

b. **F** – The fall in cardiac filling pressure *reduces* stroke volume, and therefore pulse pressure **(Figure 8.11)**. The mean pressure may be *normal*, due to compensatory reflexes.

c. **T** – Reduced arterial baroreceptor and venoatrial stretch receptor traffic elicits a reflex tachycardia **(Figure 8.11)**. This partially compensates for the fall in stroke volume.

d. **F** – Cardiac output *falls*, because the fall in stroke volume outweighs the increase in heart rate – as during orthostasis, where there is a loss of central blood into the legs **(Figure 17.1)**.

e. **T** – A reflex increase in sympathetic vasoconstrictor activity raises systemic resistance, except in the heart and brain **(Figure 8.11)**. This helps maintain mean arterial blood pressure.

18.3 a. **T** – The fall in pulse pressure reduces baroreceptor traffic, even if mean arterial pressure does not fall (compensated haemorrhage).

b. **F** – Poor peripheral perfusion causes lactic acidosis. The fall in blood pH *stimulates* arterial chemoreceptors – hence the rapid breathing associated with clinical shock.

c. **T** – Atrial blood volume falls as cardiac filling pressure falls. Venoatrial receptors are normally stimulated by atrial distension **(Figure 16.7)**.

d. **T** – A reflex increases in sympathetic vasomotor activity and in circulating vasoconstrictor hormones (noradrenaline, adrenaline, angiotensin II, vasopressin) constricts the skin veins (causing pallor) and resistance vessels (reducing perfusion, hence the cold skin).

e. **F** – The haematocrit falls within 15–30 min, because the fall in capillary pressure allows the osmotic absorption of interstitial fluid into the circulation – the 'internal transfusion' **(Figure 8.11)**.

18.4 a. **F** – Plasma catecholamine concentration increases. This contributes to the cutaneous pallor, generalized venoconstriction and hepatic glycogenolysis.

b. **T** – Extracellular fluid osmolarity can rise by 20 mOs, following the addition of glucose by hepatic glycogenolysis, which is driven by adrenaline. The rise in extracellular osmolarity draws water from the intracellular compartment to 'top-up' the extracellular compartment and depleted plasma volume.

c. **F** – The fall in baroreceptor and venoatrial receptor traffic disinhibits the vasopressin-secreting, hypothalamic magnocellular neurons **(Figure 14.6)**. Vasopressin secretion causes an anti-diuresis and peripheral vasoconstriction.
d. **T** – Fluid excretion is reduced, due to sympathetic-mediated renal vasoconstriction (reducing glomerular filtration rate), activation of the renin–angiotensin–aldosterone system (boosting distal tubular salt reabsorption), and vasopressin (anti-diuretic hormone, boosting water reabsorption by the collecting ducts).
e. **F** – There is indeed intense thirst, but the thirst is stimulated by angiotensin II, acting on the subfornicular organ of the hypothalamus **(Figure 14.7)**.

18.5 a. **F** – There is profound bradycardia **(Figure 4.7)**. This is due to the stimulation of pacemaker muscarinic receptors by acetylcholine released from vagal parasympathetic terminals **(Figures 4.2)**.
b. **F** – There is a sharp *fall* in peripheral resistance, caused by a peripheral vasodilatation.
c. **T** – The peripheral vasodilatation and bradycardia sharply reduce the arterial blood pressure.
d. **T** – The fall in arterial blood pressure reduces cerebral perfusion and O_2 supply, causing a rapid loss of consciousness.
e. **T** – The collapsed, supine position raises central venous pressure, which boosts stroke volume during the period of bradycardia. To raise the patient would exacerbate the already low blood pressure.

18.6 a. **T** – Since the distribution of blood pressure in the population is unimodal, the morbidity/mortality criterion helps define what is 'normal' versus 'raised' and requiring treatment.
b. **F** – Hypertension increases the incidence of strokes, retinal disease, renal failure, heart attacks and cardiac failure.
c. **T** – These are the levels above which morbidity and mortality increase substantially. The lower values apply to someone under 50, the higher values to older patients.
d. **F** – A small proportion of cases are caused by renal artery *stenosis*. The low pressure beyond the stenosis activates the renin–angiotensin–aldosterone system **(Figure 14.7)**. This causes salt and water retention, resulting in hypertension **(Figure 16.9)**.
e. **F** – Adrenal cortical failure in Addison's disease causes a lack of aldosterone, which causes *hypo*tension. Excessive secretion of aldosterone by an adrenal cortex tumour (Conn's syndrome) is a rare cause of hypertension.
f. **T** – Most cases are detected through routine health checks, and show no obvious organic cause (e.g. renal artery stenosis, Conn's syndrome, phaeochromocytoma).

18.7 a. **T** – Both epidemiological and interventional studies show that a high salt intake can lead to hypertension. Blood pressure is related to body water content, which is related to body Na^+ content **(Figure 16.9)**.
b. **F** – Pre-eclamptic toxaemia (hypertension in late pregnancy) affects ~1 in 20 pregnancies.
c. **T** – The internal diameter is reduced by eutrophic inward remodelling, which increases total peripheral resistance **(Figure 18.2)**. Rarefaction (loss of vessels) also contributes to the increased resistance.
d. **T** – Elastic arteries show elastin fragmentation, dilatation and increased wall stiffness, similar to the changes of ageing. The fall in compliance raises the pulse pressure **(Figure 8.10)** and the systolic augmentation by wave reflection **(Figures 18.3 and 8.12)**.
e. **F** – Although some hypertensives show increased renin–angiotensin levels, others do not.

18.8 a. **T** – Total peripheral resistance (TPR) is raised, primarily by the narrowing of proximal resistance vessels **(Figure 18.2)**. Cardiac output is normal in established hypertension, despite the increased cardiac work.

b. **T** – The pulse pressure is greatly increased by the increased stiffness of the dilated, elastic arteries **(Figure 8.10)**. Consequently, systolic pressure increases considerably more than diastolic **(Figure 18.3)**. This increases cardiac work (area inside the ventricular pressure–volume loop).

c. **T** – The stiffer elastic artery wall conducts the pressure wave faster. Consequently, the reflected pressure wave returns earlier, during systole rather than diastole **(Figure 8.12)**. This is called systolic augmentation **(Figure 18.3)**.

d. **F** – The increase in cardiac work caused by the increased afterload (systolic hypertension) evokes concentric hypertrophy of the ventricle, with no increase in chamber diameter. Cardiac dilatation only occurs if cardiac failure develops.

e. **T** – Arterial pressure fluctuations are still buffered by the baroreflex, albeit at a higher mean pressure.

18.9 a. **F** – Reducing dietary intake to 5 g/day has been shown to lower arterial pressure by ~4 mmHg.

b. **T** – Thiazide diuretics reduce extracellular salt and water mass. A fall in salt and water lowers blood pressure **(Figure 16.9)**. Thiazide diuretics also have a mild vasodilator action.

c. **T** – Beta-blockers act on β-adrenoceptors on the renal juxtaglomerular apparatus, thus inhibiting sympathetic-driven renin secretion **(Figure 14.7)**. Beta-blockers also reduce heart rate and contractility to lower pressure; *mean arterial pressure* = *cardiac output* × *total peripheral resistance*.

d. **F** – ACE inhibitors, such as captopril, reverse the left ventricular hypertrophy evoked by hypertension. Angiotensin II is thought to be one of the growth factors driving ventricular hypertrophy.

e. **T** – Inhibitors of peripheral L-type Ca^{2+} channels lower the vascular myocyte intracellular Ca^{2+} concentration **(Figure 12.4, upper panel)**. This reduces vascular tone and lowers total peripheral resistance.

18.10 a. **F** – Stroke volume at rest is often within the normal range in mild, compensated failure **(Table 17.1 and Figure 18.5)**. This is due to the compensatory increase in contractile force evoked by ventricular distension (Frank–Starling mechanism, **Figure 18.4**).

b. **T** – Contractility is force of contraction at a given degree of distension. Reduced contractility is the primary feature of heart failure. **(Figure 18.4)**.

c. **F** – The slope of this plot (the ventricular function curve, or Starling curve) represents the contractility of the ventricle **(Figure 6.11)**. The slope is reduced in heart failure **(Figure 18.4)**.

d. **F** – A rise in filling pressure dilates the ventricles, raising the cardiothoracic ratio to >0.5 **(Figure 6.16)**.

18.11 a. **F** – Pulmonary venous pressure, the filling pressure for the left side of the heart, is *raised* **(Figure 18.4)**. The rise is caused by sump pump failure **(Figure 6.14)**, plasma volume expansion through reduced renal excretion, and peripheral venoconstriction.

b. **F** – The compliance (distensibility) of the lungs is *reduced*, due to the congestion of the pulmonary veins and pulmonary oedema (caused by increased pulmonary venous pressure). Since the stiff lungs require more effort to inflate, the patient complains of dyspnoea (difficulty in breathing).

c. **F** – Cardiac dyspnoea gets *worse* on lying down (orthopnoea). Lying down increases the pulmonary venous pressure, which aggravates the pulmonary congestion and oedema. Paroxysmal nocturnal dyspnoea wakes the supine patient during the night.
d. **F** – The rise in pulmonary venous pressure raises pulmonary capillary pressure, which of course exceeds venous pressure. Increased capillary pressure causes pulmonary oedema.
e. **T** – Air passing over the oedema fluid in the airways causes a crackly, bubbling noise.

18.12 a. **T** – In a standing, healthy human, gravity reduces jugular venous pressure to subatmospheric values in the neck **(Figure 8.3)**, so the veins are normally collapsed **(Figure 8.24)**. The rise in central venous pressure in right heart failure raises the jugular venous pressure to positive values, even when standing.
b. **F** – The oedema develops in *dependent* tissues, i.e. those below heart level, where gravity exacerbates the rise in venous pressures. Facial oedema is characteristic of the nephrotic syndrome.
c. **T** – Capillary filtration pressure is raised by the combination of increased central venous pressure and gravity. This causes pitting oedema of the feet, ankles and lower leg **(Figure 11.14)**.
d. **F** – The *normal* resting ejection fraction is 66%. Due to the reduced contractility of heart failure, the ejection fraction falls **(Figure 18.5)**.
e. **T** – The increase in systemic venous pressure distends the liver, which can become tender and palpable on examination.

18.13 a. **F** – The immediate cause of the reduced contractility of heart failure is a *decreased, sluggish* systolic Ca^{2+} transient **(Figure 18.6)**.
b. **T** – Increased expression of the Na^{+}–Ca^{2+} exchanger contributes to the fall in Ca^{2+} store size, and hence contractility **(Figure 18.6)**. The exchanger also increases the size of any afterdepolarization **(Figure 3.16)**, so it is pro-arrhythmogenic.
c. **F** – K^{+} channel expression is *reduced* **(Figure 18.6)**. This is a pro-arrhythmogenic change, because the reduced outward K^{+} current allows larger DADs, and also lengthens the action potentials in some myocytes.
d. **T** – After-depolarization is triggered by Ca^{2+} store discharge during diastole **(Figure 3.16)**. This is promoted by the high level of sympathetic activity in heart failure, and by leaky Ca^{2+} release channels (ryanodine receptors). The DAD is pro-arrhythmogenic.
e. **T** – The reduction in repolarizing outward K^{+} current, due to reduced K^{+} channel expression, prolongs the plateau. Variation in action potential duration between myocytes is pro-arrhythmogenic, because it establishes the right conditions for re-entry circuits to develop **(Figure 5.7)**.

18.14 a. **T** – The DADs and heterogeneous prolongation of the refractory period (question 18.13) can cause arrhythmia. This is a major cause of mortality in moderate heart failure.
b. **T** – Exercise intolerance is a major symptom of heart failure. It is due not only to the limited cardiac output and dyspnoea during exercise, but also abnormal Ca^{2+} handling in the skeletal muscles.
c. **F** – The increase in chamber radius *reduces* the ability of the ventricle wall to convert contractile tension into a rise in ventricular blood pressure. This is Laplace's law: *pressure generated* = 2 × *tension/radius* **(Figure 6.7)**. Excessive dilatation can also cause tricuspid/mitral valve incompetence. A goal of treatment is, therefore, to reduce cardiac dilatation.
d. **T** – The fall in contractility depresses the pump function curve (relation between stroke volume and arterial pressure or afterload **(Figure 6.3)**.

18.15 a. **F** – The cutaneous, renal and splanchnic circulations show pronounced, sympathetic-mediated vaso*constriction* **(Figure 18.7)**.
b. **T** – Blood pressure is in the normal range, except during terminal pump failure.
c. **F** – The ability to raise the heart rate during exercise is much reduced **(Figure 18.5)**. This is due to a downregulation of pacemaker β_1-adrenoceptors.
d. **T** – The increased sympathetic activity causes peripheral venoconstriction. This contributes to the rise in cardiac filling pressure, which helps maintain the resting stroke volume in compensated failure.

18.16 a. **T** – Increased sympathetic activity causes peripheral vasoconstriction (supporting blood pressure) and venoconstriction (raising filling pressure). It also increases the risk of arrhythmia.
b. **T** – Increased plasma noradrenaline and adrenaline help maintain the stroke volume in compensated failure.
c. **T** – Increased plasma angiotensin II contributes to the peripheral vasoconstriction and, via aldosterone, fluid retention **(Figure 14.7)**.
d. **T** – Increased plasma endothelin contributes to the peripheral vasoconstriction of heart failure.
e. **T** – The secretion of BNP by ventricular cells raises the circulating concentration up to 200-fold. This probably helps to limit the degree of salt and water retention in heart failure, and may be a useful biochemical marker of disease severity.

18.17 a. **F** – Salt and water retention are increased; excretion is reduced. The resulting rise in extracellular fluid volume contributes to the oedema and rise in cardiac filling pressures.
b. **F** – RAA activation is *increased* in heart failure, due to the raised renal sympathetic nerve activity.
c. **T** – Increased renal sympathetic activity causes severe renal vasoconstriction **(Figure 18.7)**. This lowers the glomerular filtration rate and contributes to fluid retention.
d. **T** – Renal retention of salt and water expands the extracellular fluid compartment.

18.18 a. **T** – Myocardial work, and therefore O_2 demand, depends on the arterial blood pressure (afterload) and stroke volume **(Figure 6.12, top)**. Therefore, reducing arterial blood pressure reduces myocardial O_2 demand and improves stroke volume.
b. **F** – The aim is to *lower* blood pressure, so that more of the contractile energy can be used in ejection, thus raising the stroke volume (see the shift from loop 3 to loop 2 in **Figure 6.12)**. Reducing blood pressure shifts the ventricle up the pump function curve **(Figure 6.3)**.
c. **T** – Reducing the ventricle radius (increasing curvature) allows wall tension to be converted into ventricular blood pressure more effectively (Laplace's law: *pressure generated* = 2 × *tension/radius*) **(Figure 6.7)**. Also, distension-induced tricuspid/mitral regurgitation benefits from reduced dilatation. In a failing heart, the gain in mechanical efficiency by reducing cardiac dilatation outweighs any negative impact of the leftward movement along the (flattened) Starling curve.
d. **F** – The plasma and extracellular fluid compartments are already over-expanded, due to the renal retention of salt and water, causing oedema and cardiac dilatation. The aim is to reverse the extracellular fluid expansion.
e. **F** – The inotropic state (contractility) needs to be *increased*, if severely depressed.

18.19 a. **T** – ACE inhibitors are usually the first-line drug for treating chronic heart failure. They reduce peripheral resistance, cardiac work and renal fluid retention, and significantly increase life expectancy.

b. **T** – Loop diuretics, such as furosemide (frusemide), are often combined with ACE inhibitors to reduce extracellular fluid volume, cardiac distension and oedema. Loop diuretics inhibit the Na^+–K^+–chloride reabsorption in the ascending loop of Henle, so they increase K^+ loss, as well as Na^+ loss. They also have some venodilator action.

c. **F** – Spironolactone is indeed used, but it is an antagonist of intracellular aldosterone receptors in the distal renal tubule; it does not affect renin production.

d. **T** – Alpha-blockers, such as phentolamine and phenoxybenzamine, combat the effect of increased sympathetic vasomotor activity. They lower total peripheral resistance and blood pressure. The fall in afterload reduces cardiac work and raises stroke volume **(Figure 6.3, point 3 to point 4)**.

e. **T** – Beta-blockers slow the heart, reduce cardiac work and reduce the incidence of arrhythmia. They increase life expectancy. But they can only be used in mild failure, because they reduce contractility.

18.20 a. **F** – Digoxin inhibits the surface membrane Na^+–K^+ pump, by ~25% **(Figure 3.6)**. The resulting rise in intracellular Na^+ reduces the inward Na^+ gradient. The reduced Na^+ gradient slows the expulsion of Ca^{2+} by the Na^+–Ca^{2+} exchanger.

b. **T** – Reduced Ca^{2+} expulsion raises the SR Ca^{2+} store. The cytosolic Ca^{2+} transient in systole is therefore increased, raising ventricular contractility **(Figure 3.15)**. This relieves symptoms, but digoxin does not increase life expectancy.

c. **F** – Digoxin causes *brady*cardia, due to a central action that increases vagal parasympathetic activity to the SA and AV nodes. For the latter reason, it tends to be used when there is concomitant heart failure and atrial fibrillation.

d. **T** – The increase in SR Ca^{2+} store increases the risk of store discharge in diastole, causing an after-depolarization – the trigger for arrhythmia.

e. **F** – Digoxin toxicity is enhanced by *hypo*kalaemia (low plasma K^+), because K^+ normally competes with digoxin to bind to the Na–K pump. Hypokalaemia may occur in cardiac failure patients taking loop diuretics, which increase K^+ loss.

Figures and Tables

CHAPTER 1

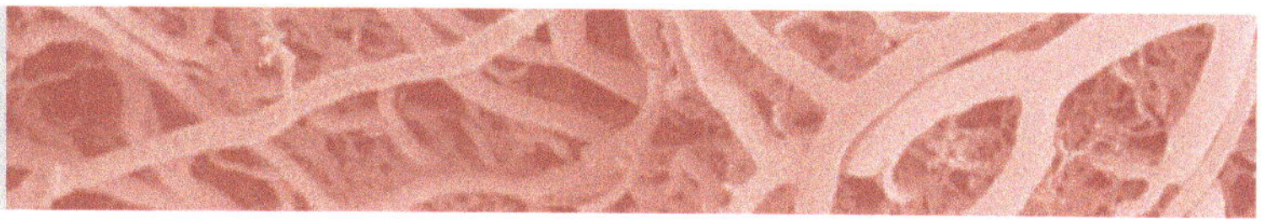

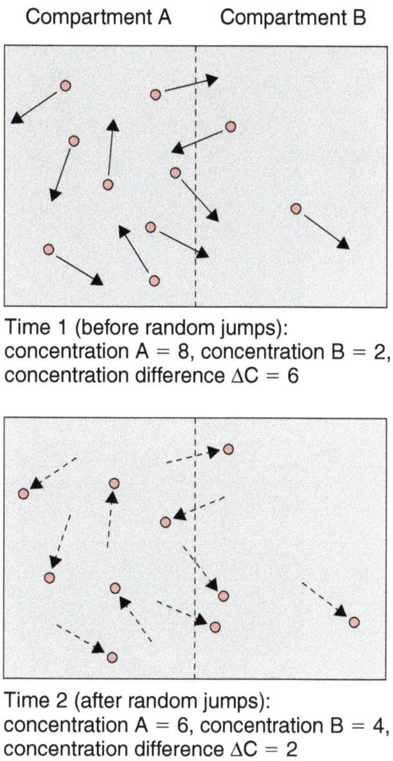

Figure 1.1 Spontaneous molecular steps in a random direction lead to a net movement of solute molecules (dots) down a concentration gradient. The probability of a randomly directed step from compartment A to B is greater than from B to A, because there are more solute molecules in A than B.

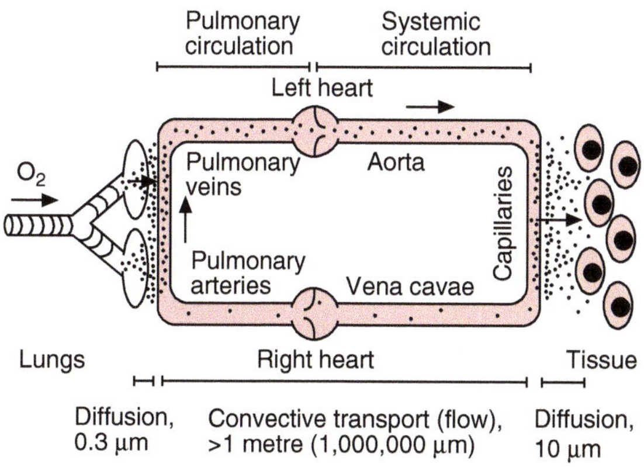

Figure 1.2 Overview of the human circulation, highlighting the relative roles of diffusion and convection in O_2 transport.

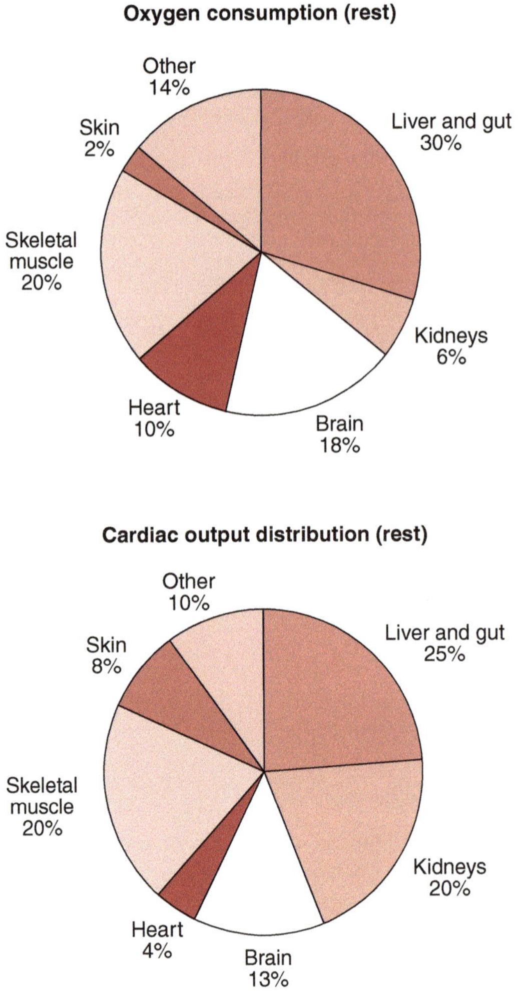

Figure 1.3 Comparison of oxygen usage and cardiac output distribution in humans at rest. (Data from Wade OL and Bishop JM. *Cardiac Output and Regional Flow*. Oxford: Blackwell, 1962.)

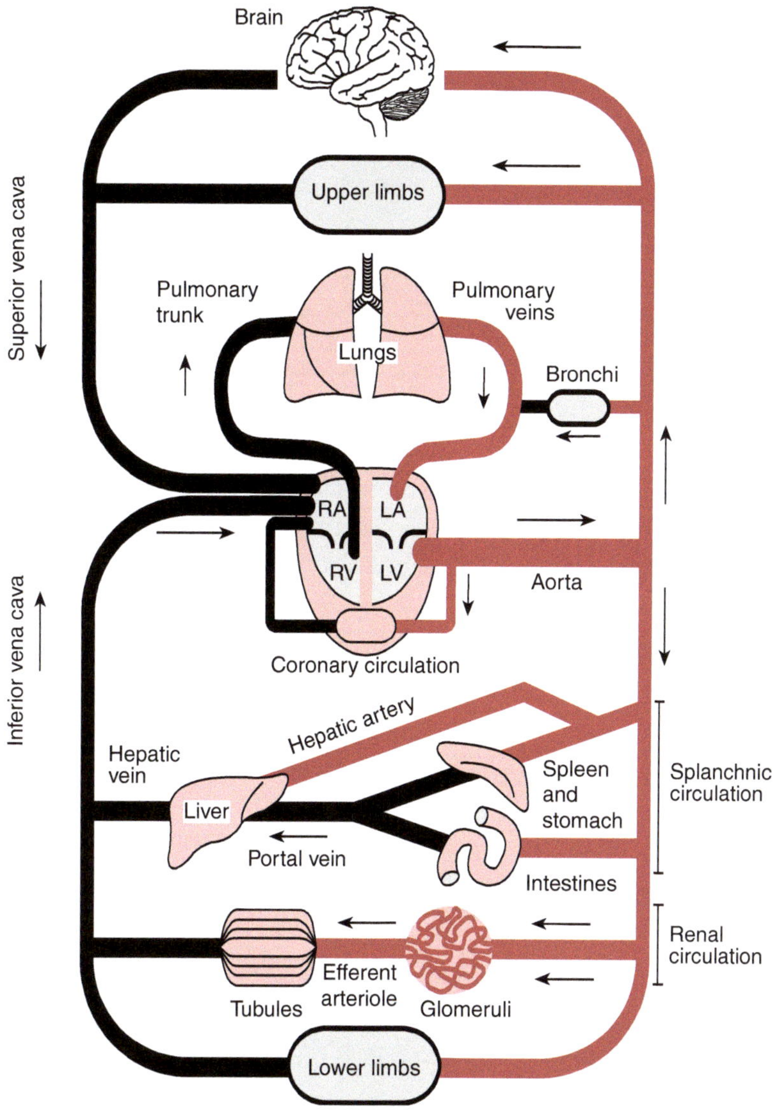

Figure 1.4 'Plumbing' of the human circulation. The systemic and pulmonary circulations are in series. The circulation to most systemic organs is in parallel (brain, myocardium, limbs, etc.), but the liver and renal tubules have an 'in series' or portal blood supply. Bronchial venous blood drains anomalously into the left atrium, slightly desaturating it. Red, oxygenated blood; black, deoxygenated blood. RA, LA, RV, LV, right and left atrium/ventricle, respectively.

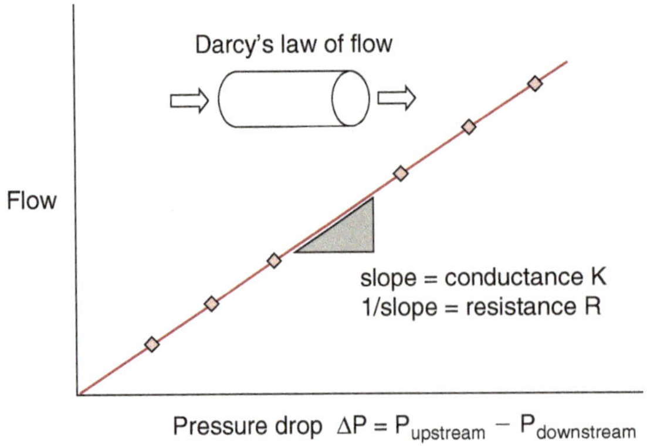

Figure 1.5 Effect of pressure difference ΔP across a tube on laminar flow. Darcy's law tells us that Flow = $\Delta P \times$ conductance K, where K is the slope. Also Flow = ΔP/resistance R, where resistance is 1/K.

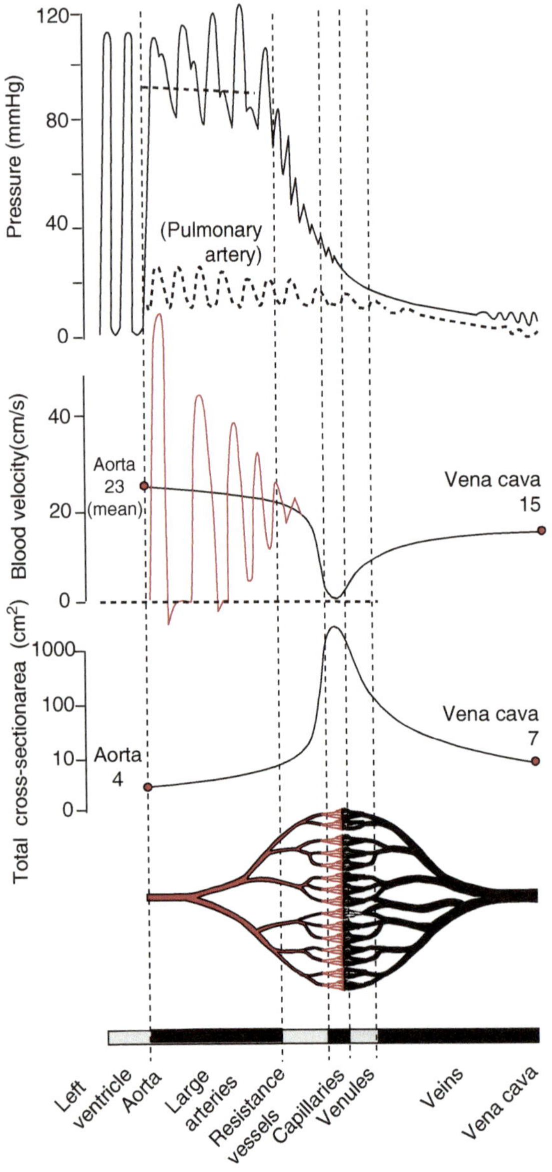

Figure 1.6 Pressure and blood velocity in systemic circulation of a resting human. *Top trace*. The drop in mean pressure across the main arteries (dashed line) is only ~2 mmHg. The large pressure drop across the terminal arteries and arterioles (diameter 30–500 μm) shows that they are the main resistance vessels. Low pulmonary pressure profile is also shown. *Middle trace*. Pulsation of blood velocity (red line) and change in mean velocity across circulation (black line). The same total blood flow passes each vertical dashed line per minute, namely the cardiac output. Mean velocity is blood flow divided by the cross-sectional area of the vascular bed. *Bottom trace*. Increase in total cross-sectional area of the circulation in microvessels.

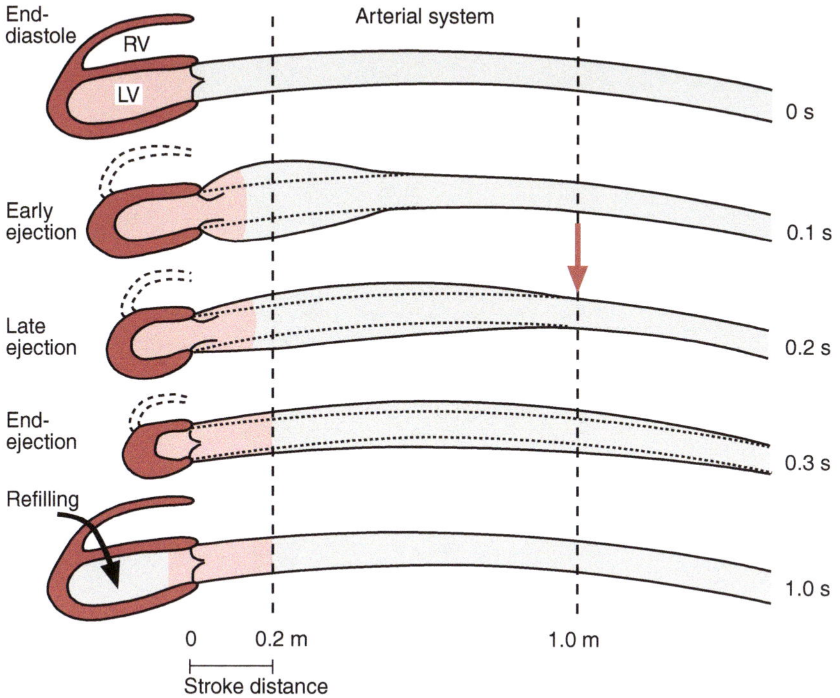

Figure 1.7 Expansion of elastic arteries to receive stroke volume, and transmission of pressure pulse along human arterial system at 5 m/s. In this example the left ventricle (LV) ejects 100 cm^3 blood into an aorta of cross-sectional area 5 cm^2. The blood advances 20 cm in one beat (*stroke distance*). The wall distension, i.e. the arterial pulse, travels much faster (1 m in 0.2 s), as marked by the red arrow.

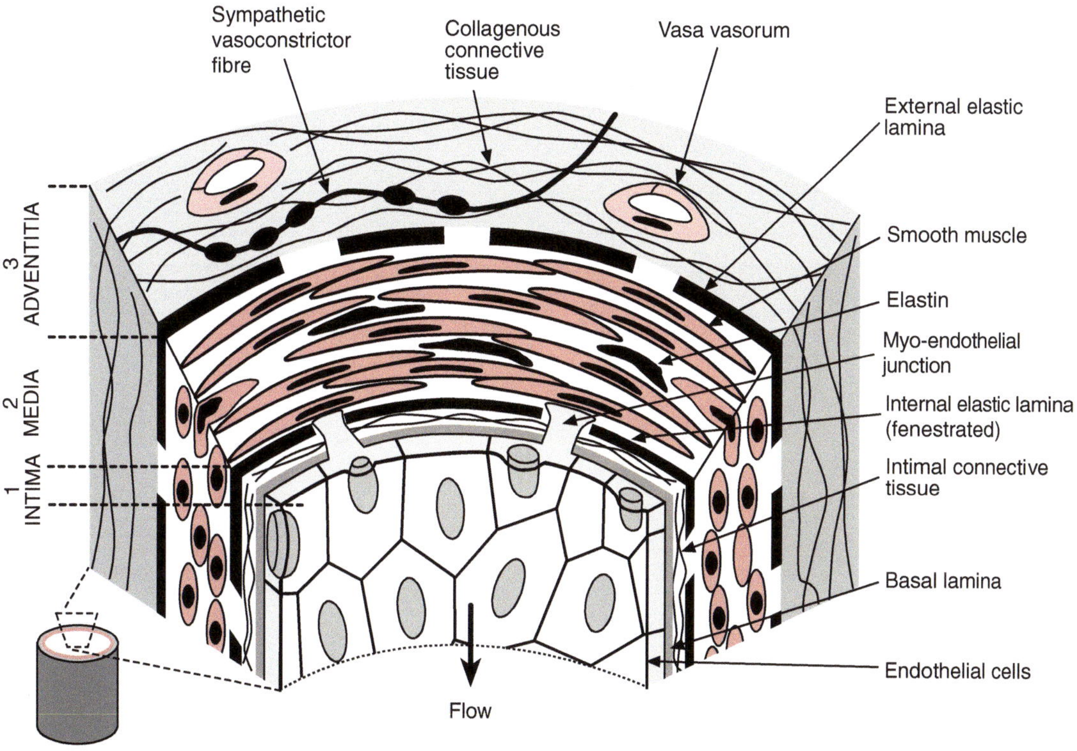

Figure 1.8 Structure of the wall of a small artery.

CHAPTER 2

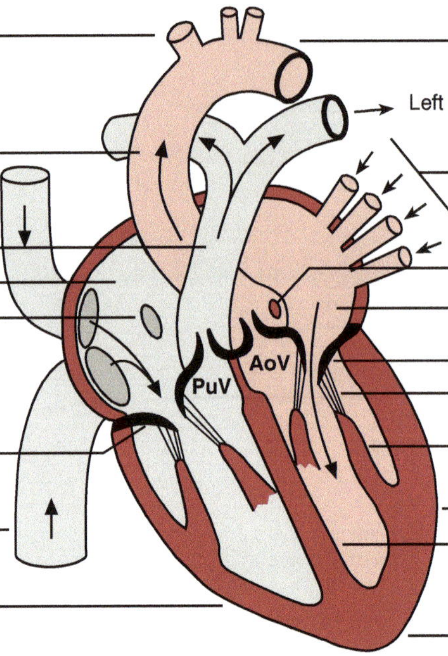

Figure 2.1 Anatomy of the human heart.

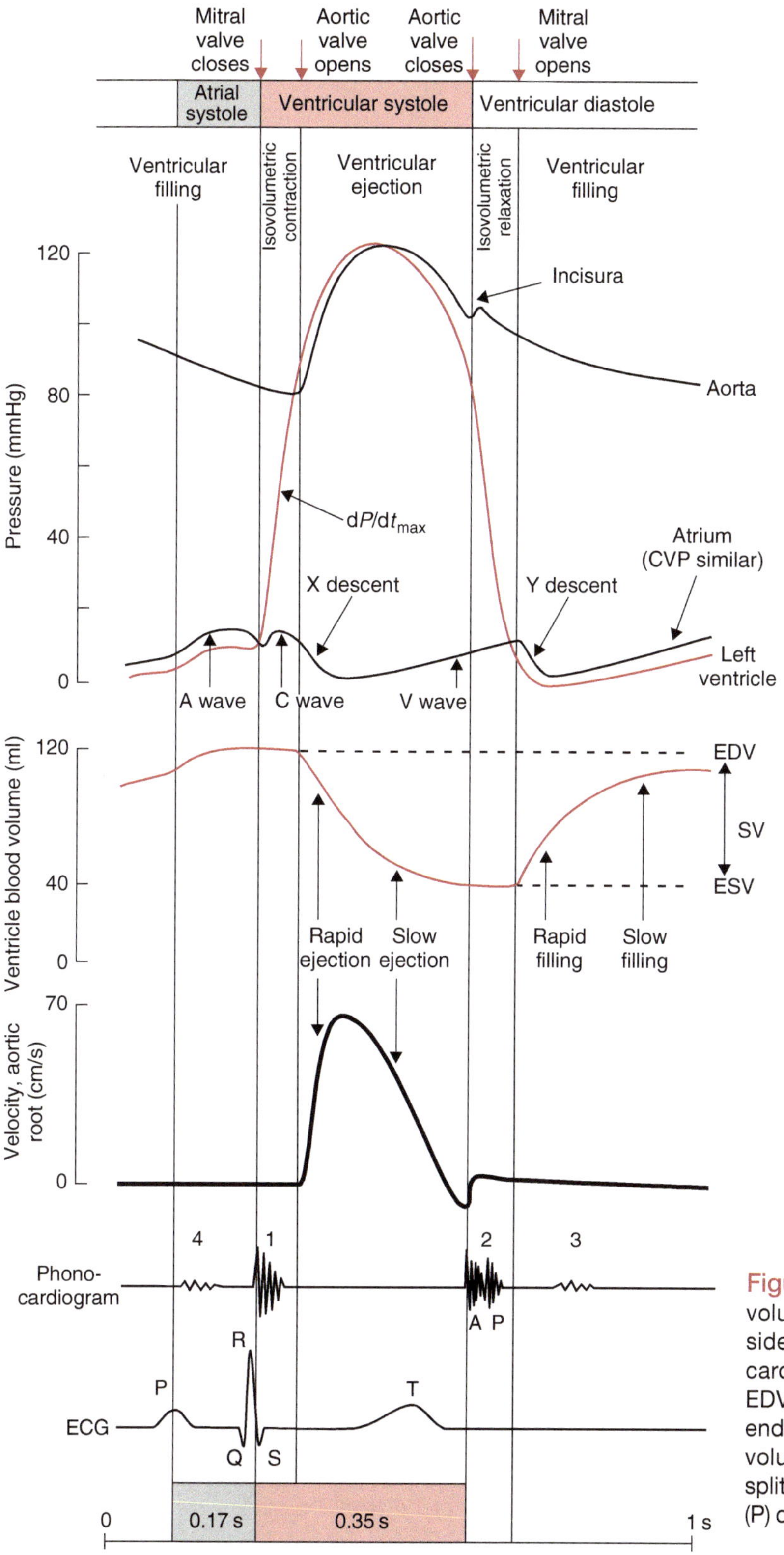

Figure 2.2 Changes in pressure, volume and flow in aorta and left side of heart during human cardiac cycle (subject upright). EDV, end-diastolic volume; ESV, end-systolic volume; SV, stroke volume. Second heart sound splits into aortic (A) and pulmonary (P) components.

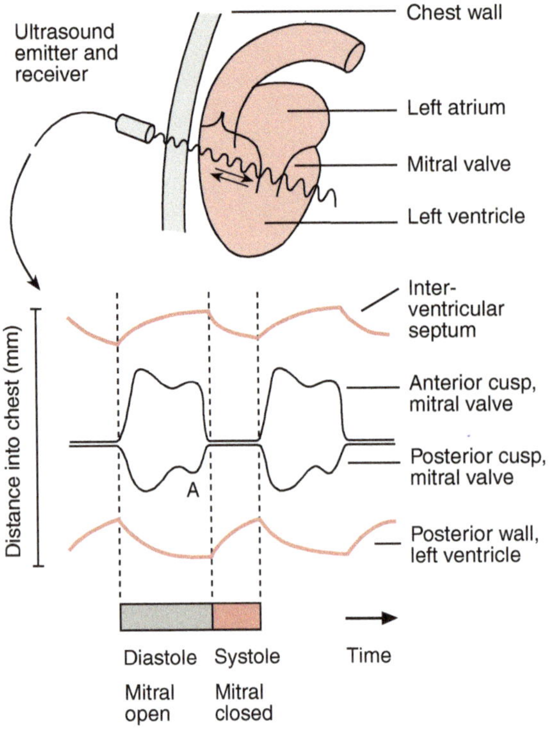

Figure 2.3 M-mode echocardiogram showing motion of mitral valve cusps and walls of the left ventricle. Note fast filling phase in early ventricular diastole, prior to atrial systole (A); also fast ejection phase in early systole.

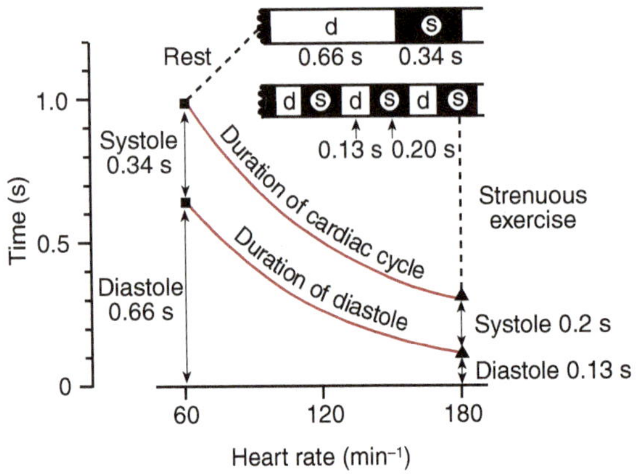

Figure 2.4 Effect of heart rate on the diastolic period available for filling. d, diastole; s, systole. Diastole is curtailed more than systole as heart rate increases.

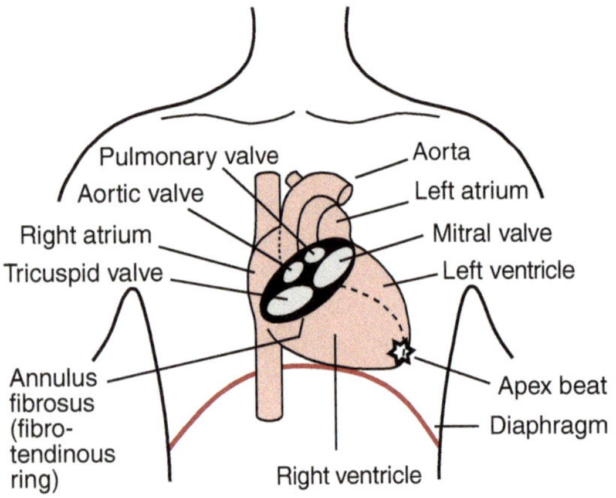

Figure 2.5 Oblique orientation of heart in human thorax. Right atrium and right ventricle form most of anterior surface. A fibrotendinous ring forms the 'base' of the heart. Tip of ventricle forms the 'apex'. Apex beat is in the fifth interspace, in line with the mid-clavicle. The four valves are grouped closely in an oblique plane behind the sternum.

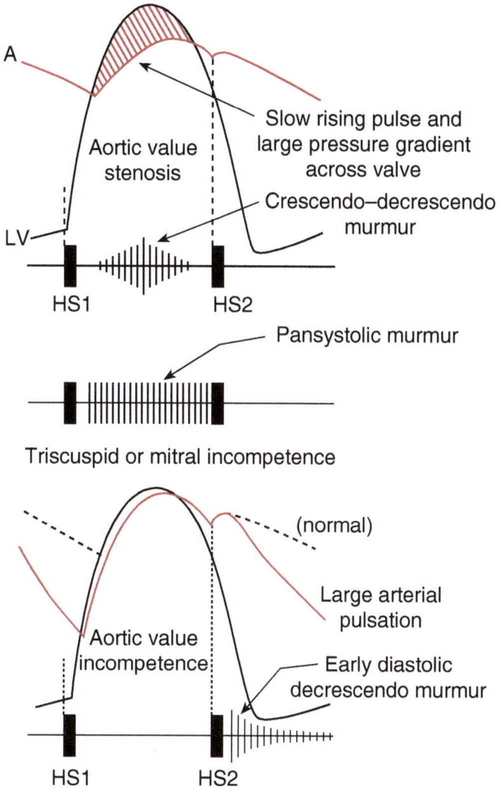

Figure 2.6 Three cardiac murmurs. (*Top*) Aortic valve stenosis creates a large pressure gradient between aorta (A) and left ventricle (LV) during ejection (hatched zone). The slow-rising arterial pulse is associated with a crescendo–decrescendo ejection murmur. (*Middle*) In tricuspid or mitral incompetence, regurgitation from ventricle to atrium during systole creates a pansystolic murmur. (*Bottom*) In aortic valve incompetence, diastolic leakage from the aorta to left ventricle causes a characteristic wide pulse pressure (systolic minus diastolic) and an early diastolic, decrescendo murmur as the pressure head decays.

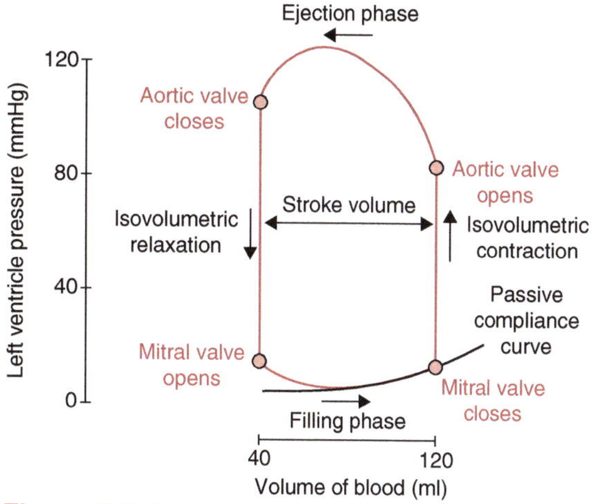

Figure 2.7 Pressure–volume loop for human left ventricle (subject resting, upright).

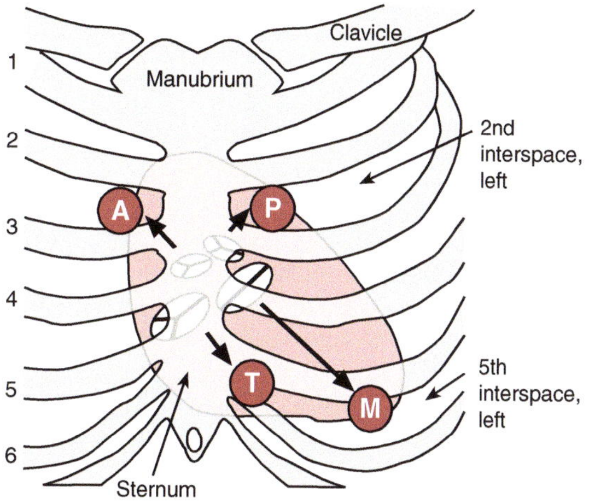

Figure 2.8 Location of cardiac valves and auscultation areas in human chest. A, aortic valve area; P, pulmonary valve area; T, tricuspid area; M, mitral area.

CHAPTER 3

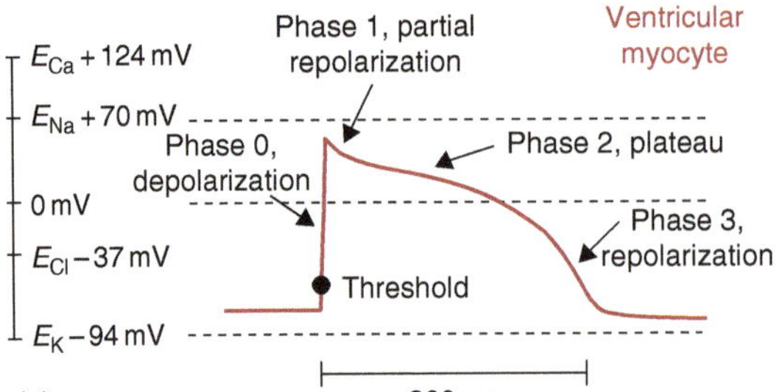

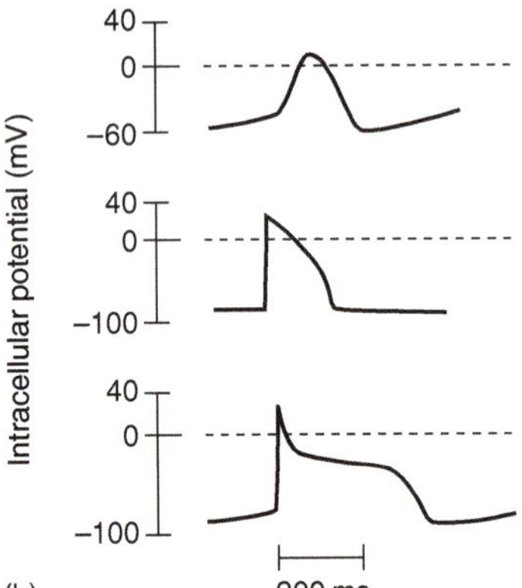

Figure 3.1 (a) Intracellular potential of a ventricle subendocardial myocyte during an action potential. Resting potential −80 mV. Ion equilibrium potentials marked for comparison. (b) Different forms of cardiac action potential. SA node and some Purkinje fibres have unstable resting potentials so they depolarise spontaneously.

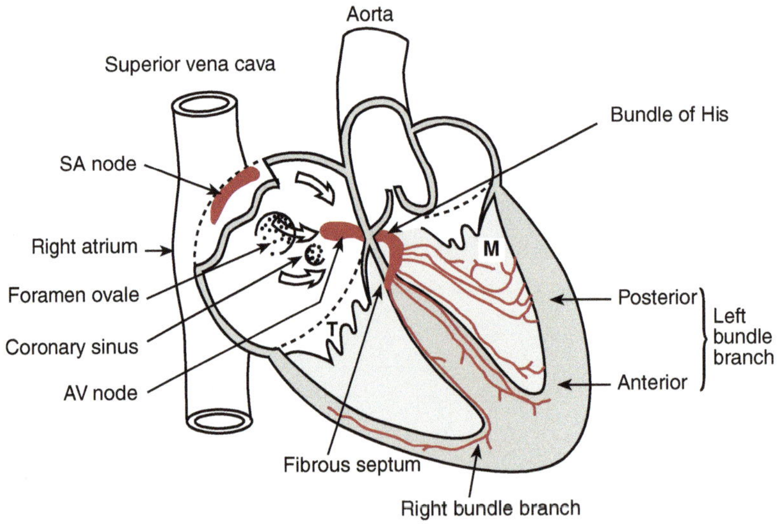

Figure 3.2 The cardiac conduction system. T, tricuspid; M, mitral.

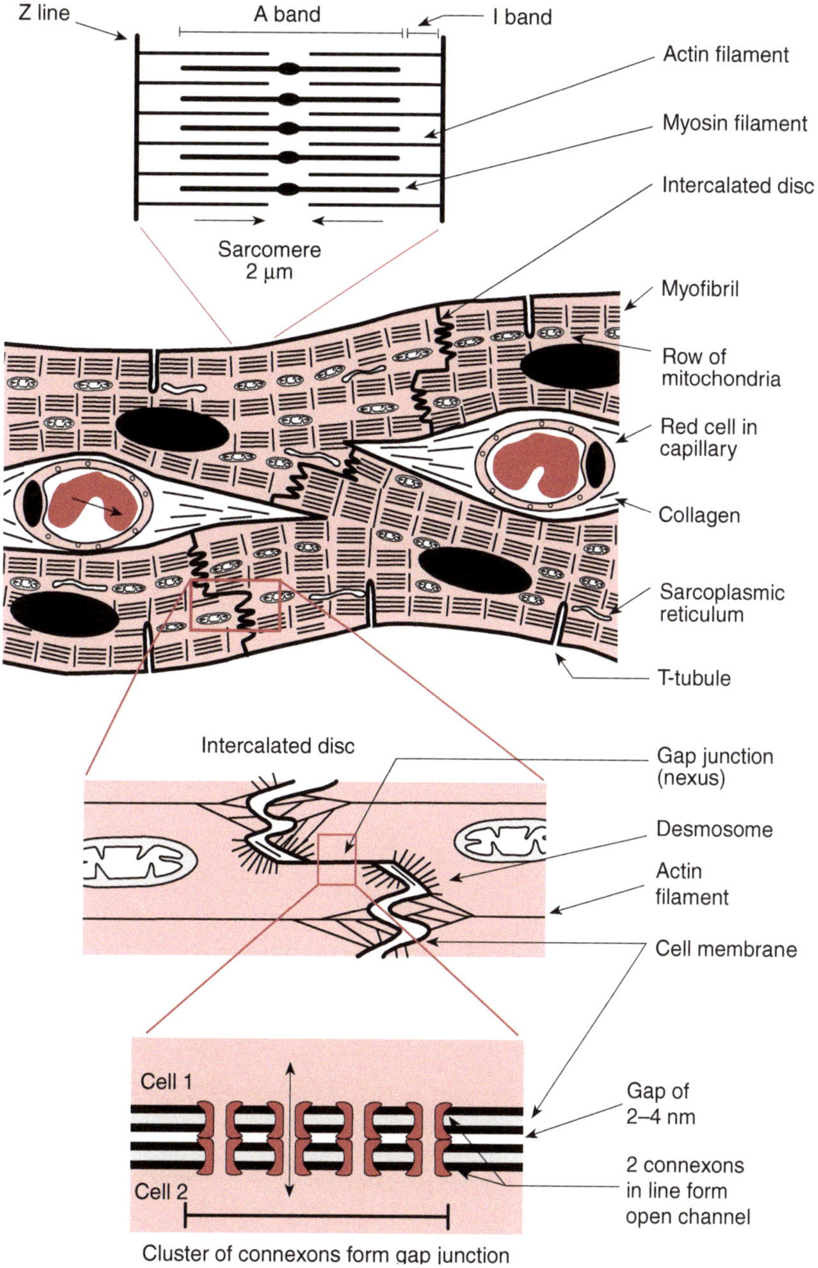

Figure 3.3 Schematic section of myocardium parallel to fibre axis.

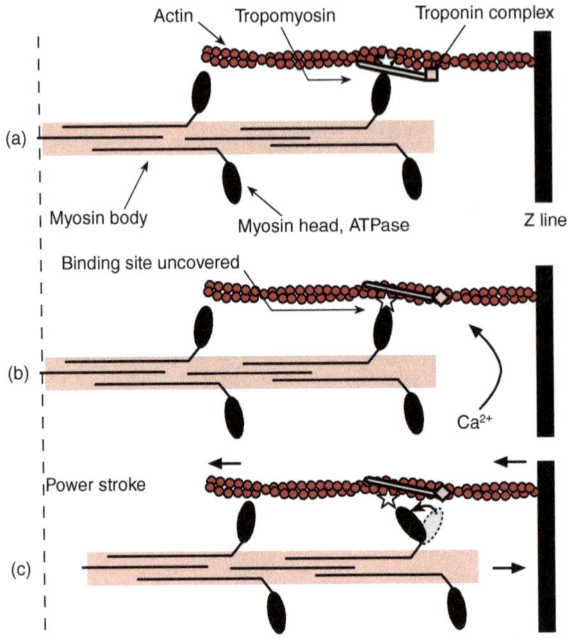

Figure 3.4 Actin–myosin contractile machinery. (a) Rest. Actin binding sites (white star) are blocked by tropomyosin. (b) Ca^{2+} displaces the troponin–tropomyosin complex, exposing actin binding sites. This allows myosin head to form a crossbridge. (c) Flexion of myosin head shifts the thin filament and Z-line towards sarcomere centre. Head then disengages and reattaches further along actin filament.

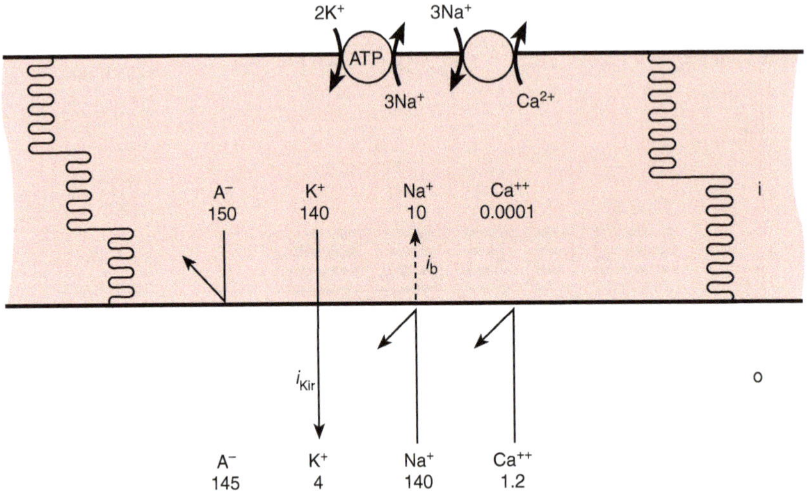

Figure 3.5 Ion gradients and currents across resting membrane (i, inside; o, outside). 'A^-' inside cell refers to impermeant intracellular anions, mainly phosphate and charged amino acids. Straight arrows show concentration gradients for ions permeating the resting sarcolemma; i_{Kir}, outward background current of K^+; i_b, inward background current (mainly Na^+). Reflected arrows indicate ions unable to penetrate the resting membrane.

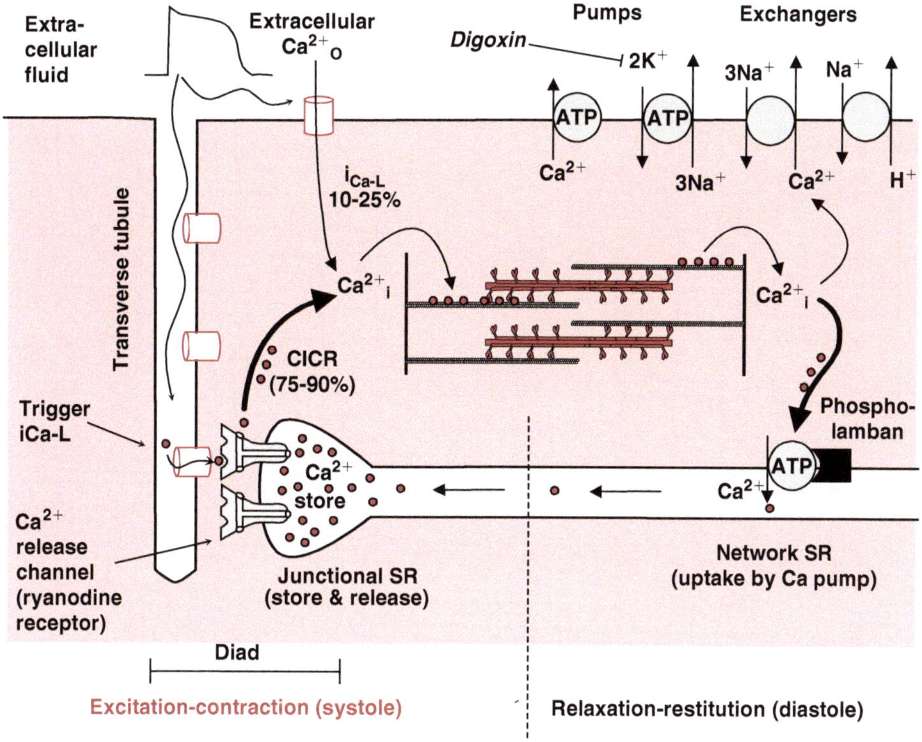

Figure 3.6 The calcium cycle during systole (left) and diastole (right). A T-tubule L-type Ca^{2+} channel and adjacent cluster of ~10 Ca^{2+}-release channels form a functional unit. SR, sarcoplasmic reticulum; CICR, calcium-induced calcium release.

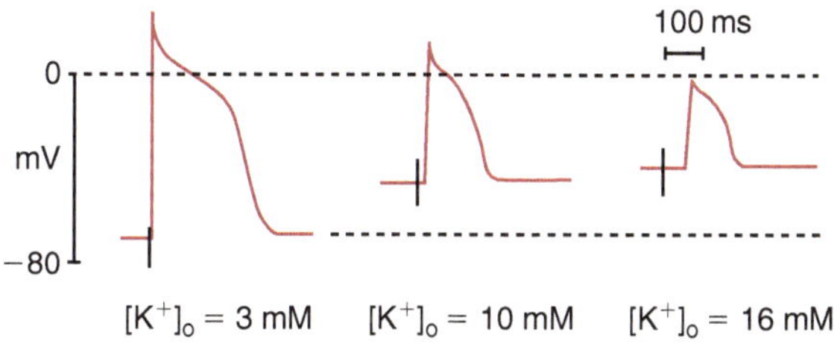

Figure 3.7 Effect of hyperkalaemia on the membrane potential of a Purkinje fibre. The spike to the left of each action potential marks stimulation by an external impulse some distance away. Note the increasing conduction time, reduced resting potential, reduced action potential size and slowed rate of rise.

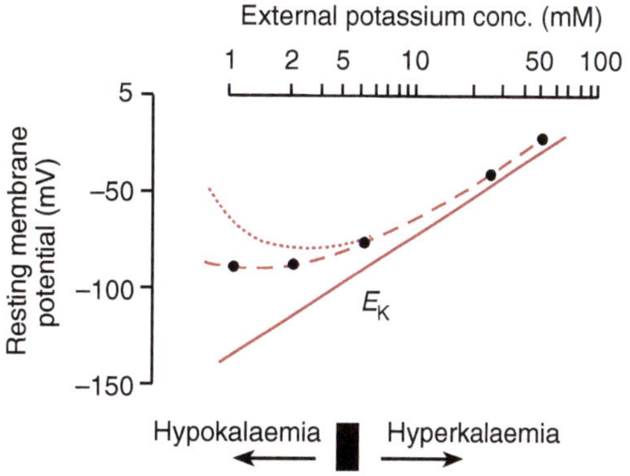

Figure 3.8 Effect of extracellular K^+ on resting membrane potential of myocyte (circles) or Purkinje fibre (dotted line). Solid line is Nernst equilibrium potential E_K. Deviation from E_K is due to inward background current i_b. Increasing deviation in hypokalaemia is due to a fall in potassium conductance g_K and reduced outward current carried by $3Na^+$–$2K^+$ pump.

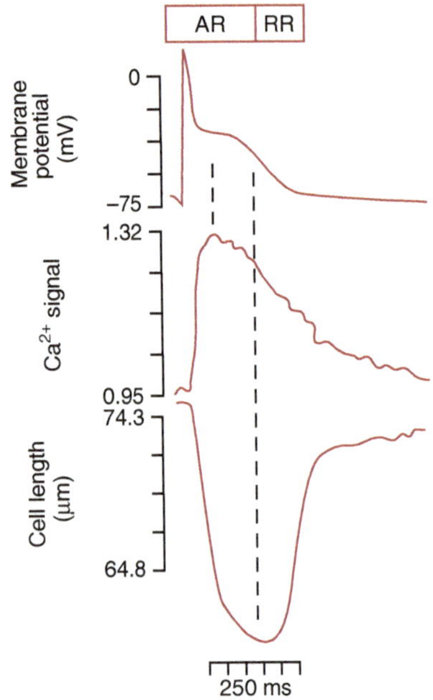

Figure 3.9 Relation between electrical, chemical and mechanical events in a single myocyte (rat). AR, RR, absolute and relative refractory periods respectively.

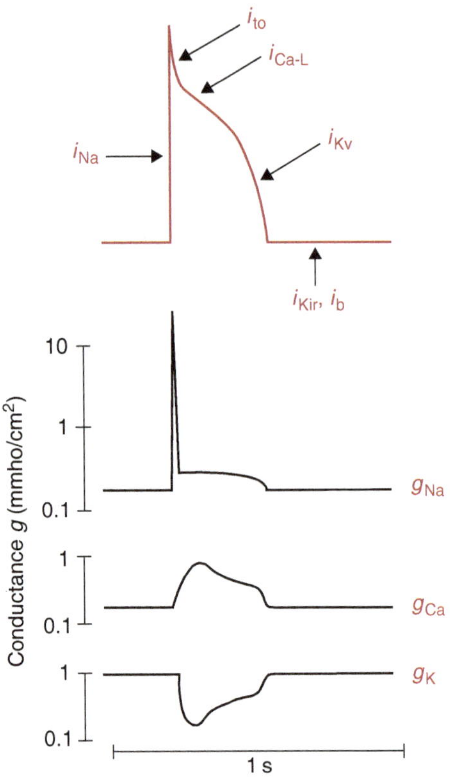

Figure 3.10 Myocyte action potential, ionic currents responsible, and changes in membrane conductances to individual ions. Note fall in K^+ conductance during action potential.

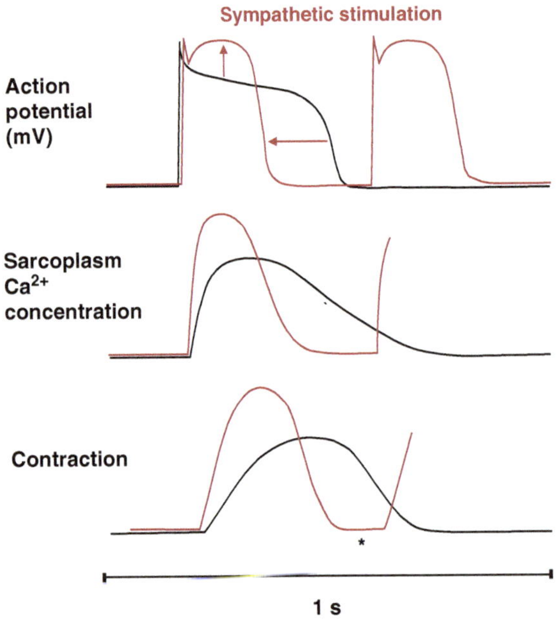

Figure 3.11 Effect of sympathetic stimulation on a ventricular myocyte. Heart rate approximately doubled in this illustration. (*Top pair of traces*) Membrane potential before (black) and after (red) sympathetic stimulation. Vertical arrow highlights increased inward Ca^{2+} current during the plateau, producing 'doming'. Horizontal arrow highlights shortening of action potential by increased outward, repolarizing K^+ current. (*Middle traces*) Increased sarcoplasmic Ca^{2+} transient and faster removal. (*Bottom traces*) The contraction is stronger, of shorter duration, and relaxation is more rapid. Despite this, the diastolic period for refilling is severely curtailed (asterisk).

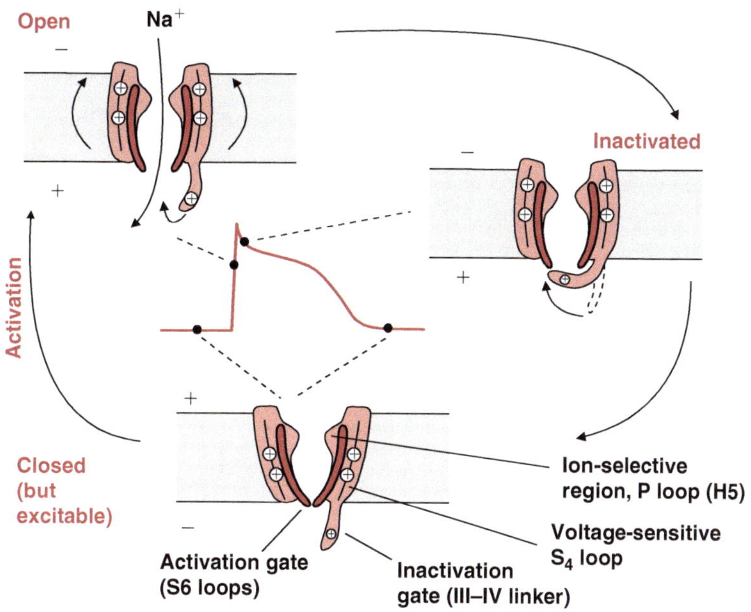

Figure 3.12 Activation–inactivation cycle of voltage-sensitive Na^+ channel. Outward displacement of the charged S4 loops by depolarization opens the activation gate (S6 loops). The slower, inactivation gate is a hinged lid. As long as the inactivation gate is closed, the myocyte is incapable of re-excitation (refractory).

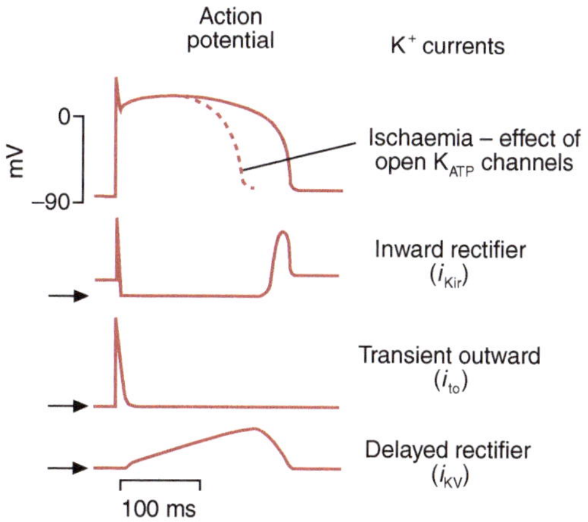

Figure 3.13 K^+ currents contributing to cardiac action potential. Arrows mark zero current. Dashed line shows effect of acute ischaemia; increased open probability of K_{ATP} channels shortens the action potential.

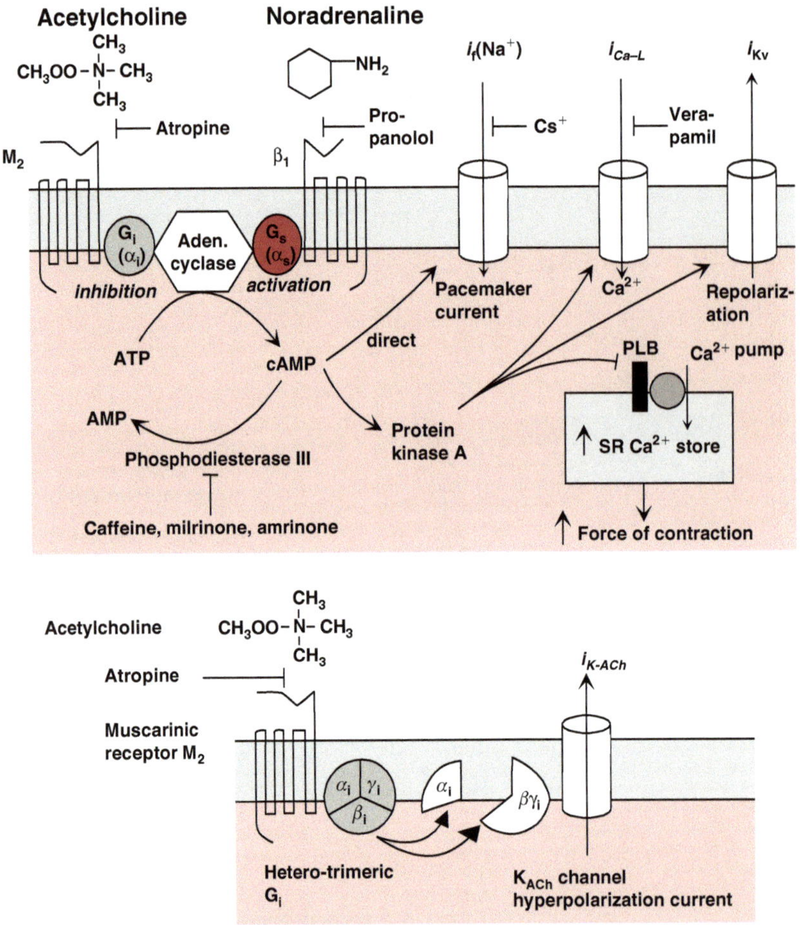

Figure 3.14 Signal transduction pathways activated by sympathetic transmitter noradrenaline and parasympathetic transmitter acetylcholine, in a myocardial or pacemaker cell. Aden. cyclase, adenylate or adenylyl cyclase; PLB, phospholamban; G_s, stimulatory guanosine triphosphate (GTP)-binding protein; G_i, inhibitory GTP-binding protein. Each G protein is a heterotrimer of α, β and γ subunits. On activation it dissociates into an α and a $\beta\gamma$ subunit (*lower panel*). The α_s subunit activates adenylate cyclase. The α_i subunit inhibits adenylate cyclase. The $\beta\gamma_i$ subunit activates K_{ACh} (K_G) channels.

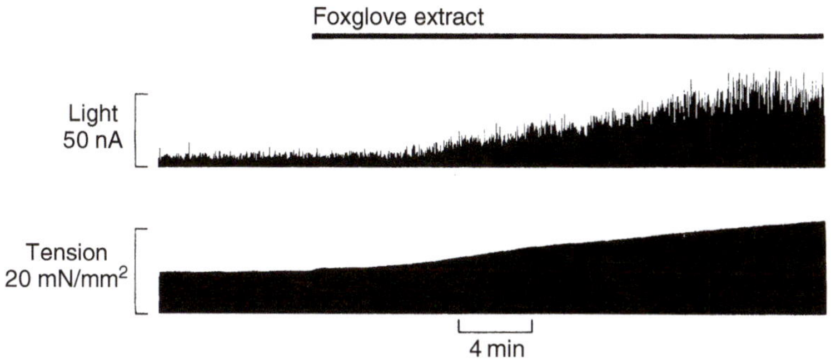

Figure 3.15 Digoxin, found in foxglove extract, increases the contractile force and intracellular Ca^{2+} concentration (light signal) in ferret papillary muscle.

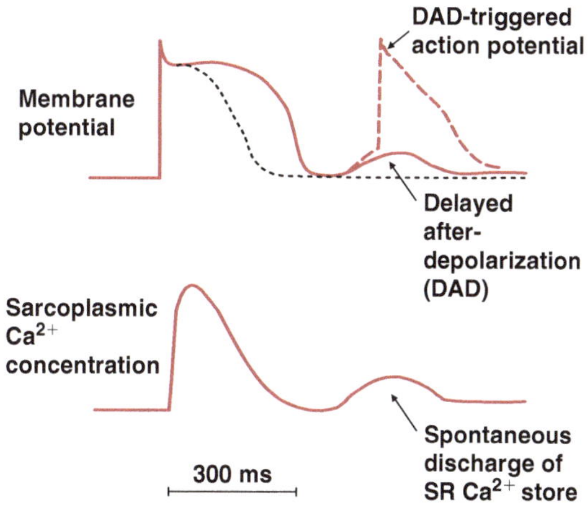

Figure 3.16 Partial discharge of overloaded internal Ca^{2+} store (*lower trace*) stimulates the electrogenic $3Na^{+}-1Ca^{2+}$ exchanger, causing a net inflow of positive charge (Na^{+}) and a delayed afterdepolarization (DAD, *upper trace*). If the DAD reaches threshold, it triggers a premature action potential (*red dashed line*). *Dotted line* shows effect of replacing external Na^{+} by Li^{+}, to inhibit the Na–Ca exchanger; the shortening of the plateau shows that exchanger current normally contributes to the late plateau; also the DAD is abolished.

CHAPTER 4

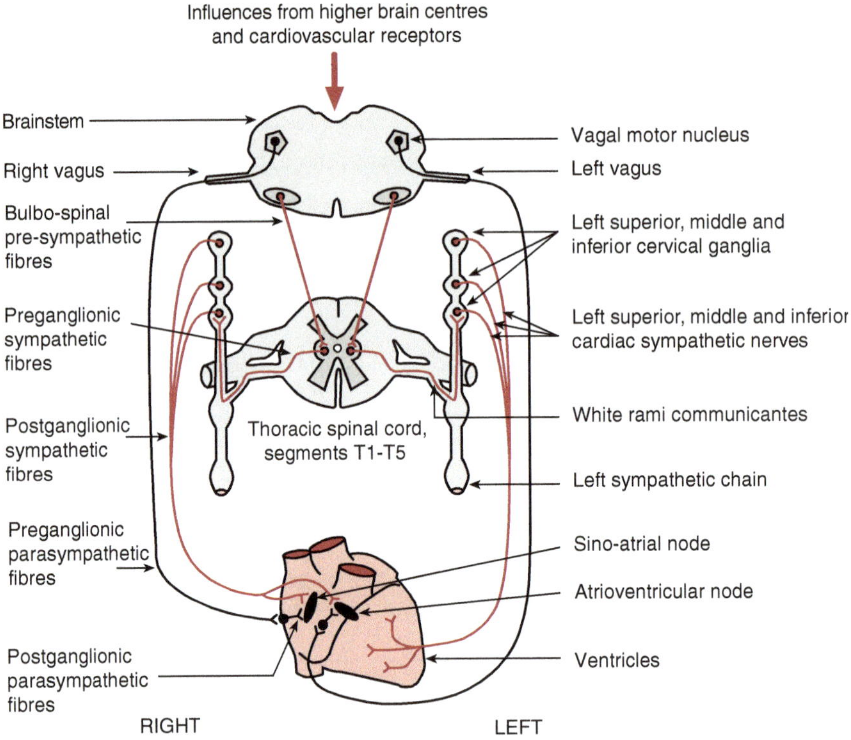

Figure 4.1 Innervation of heart by sympathetic fibres (red) and vagal parasympathetic fibres (black). The sympathetic outflow arises from the intermediolateral horns of the thoracic spinal cord segments T1–T5.

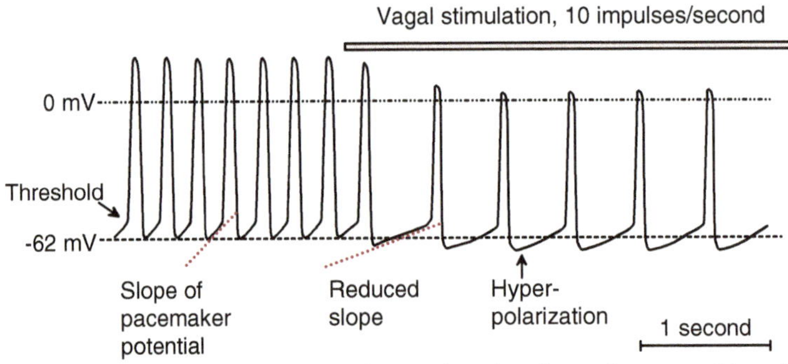

Figure 4.2 Changes in pacemaker potential and attendant bradycardia caused by stimulation of vagus. Note the brisk hyperpolarization of the resting membrane and the sustained slope reduction (dashed red line).

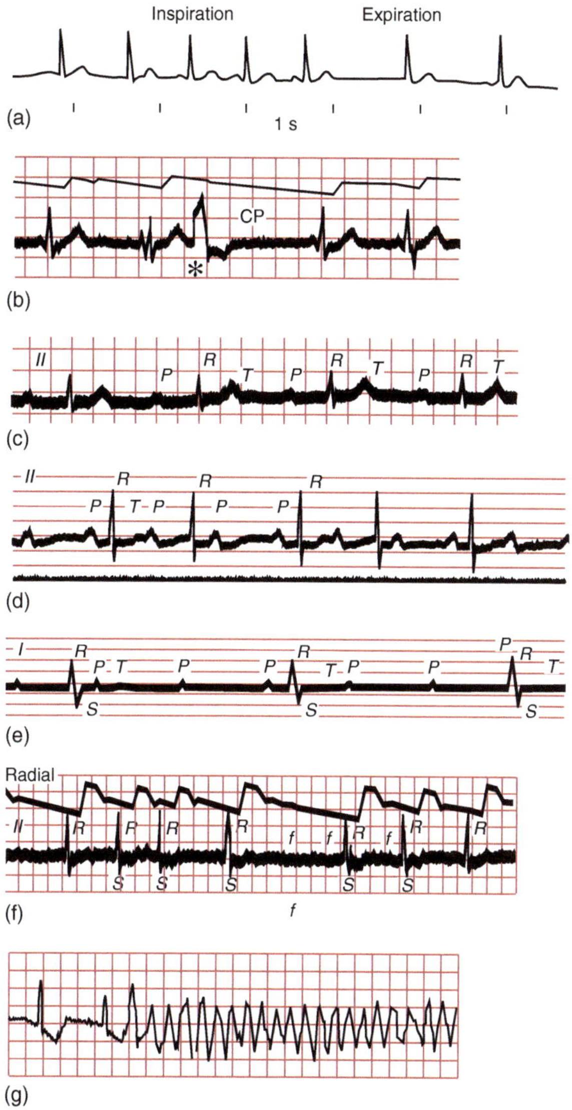

Figure 4.3 ECG recordings of arrhythmias. (a) Sinus arrhythmia in a healthy student. (b) An extrasystole (ventricular ectopic, asterisk) (CP, compensatory pause). The upper trace shows the radial pulse and missed heartbeat. (c–e) Progressive stages of heart block. (c) First-degree block, with prolonged PR interval. (d) Second-degree block; no QRS after every third P. (e) Third-degree block. QRS unrelated to P. (f) Atrial fibrillation with ‘f’ waves. (g) Ventricular fibrillation triggered during the vulnerable period (late T wave of second beat) in an ischaemic heart showing ST segment depression and T wave inversion.

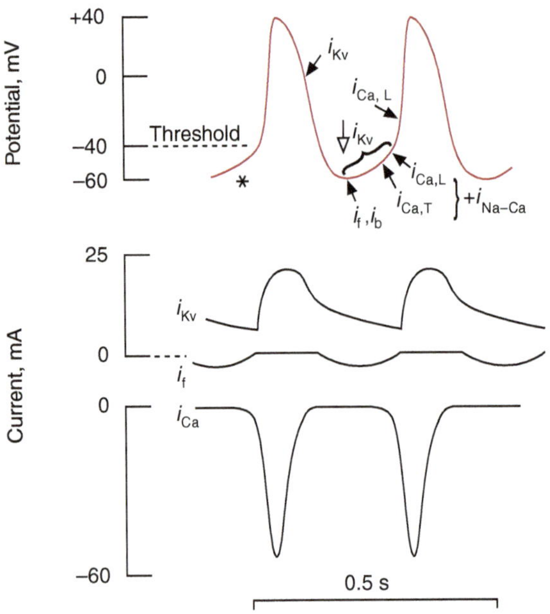

Figure 4.4 Ionic basis of pacemaker potential and action potential in sino-atrial cell. Slope of pacemaker potential (asterisk) determines time to reach threshold, and hence heart rate. Inward currents downwards, outward currents upwards. i_{Kv}, potassium current; i_f, 'funny' Na^+ current; i_b, background Na^+ current; $i_{Ca,T}$, Transient Ca^{2+} channel current; $i_{Ca,L}$, Long-lasting Ca^{2+} channel current; i_{Na-Ca}, inward current due to $3Na^+$–$1Ca^{2+}$ exchanger.

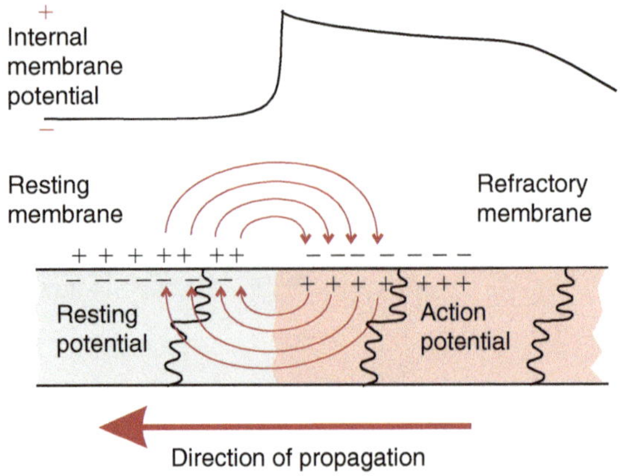

Figure 4.5 Myocardial excitation is transmitted by local currents acting ahead of the action potential. Internal current flows through the sarcoplasm and gap junctions of the intercalated disc. External current flows through the extracellular fluid. The currents discharge the membrane ahead, triggering its action potential.

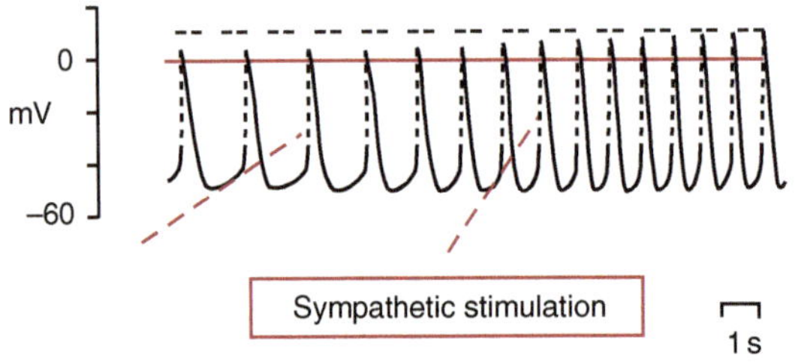

Figure 4.6 Effect of continuous sympathetic stimulation (box) on pacemaker potential. Note the relatively sluggish onset of tachycardia. The dashed, red gradients highlight the increased slope of the pacemaker potential. The upper double-dashed line draws attention to the increase in action potential size, caused by the increased inward Ca^{2+} current induced by noradrenaline-activated β-adrenoceptors.

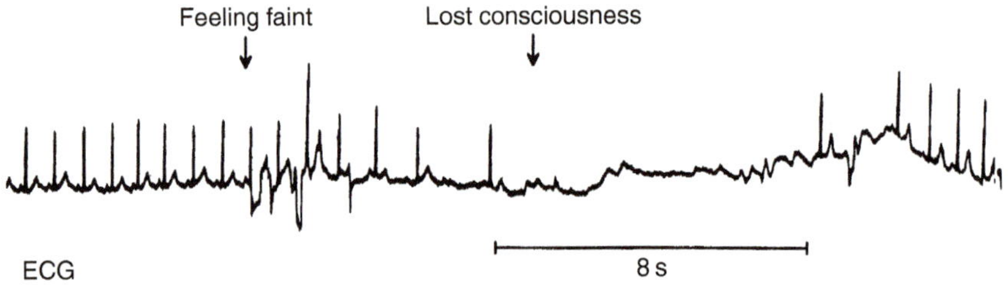

Figure 4.7 ECG recorded during a faint (vasovagal attack) in a healthy medical student. There was a period of 8 s asystole during the faint. The wobbly baseline is a movement artefact.

CHAPTER 5

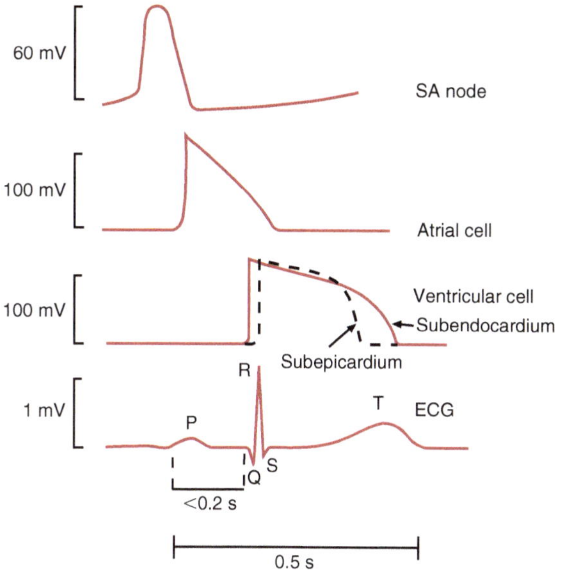

Figure 5.1 Timing of ECG waves relative to cardiac action potentials. Subepicardial myocytes (dashed trace) have ~3 times more repolarizing i_{to} K^+ channels than subendocardial myocytes, so they repolarize first. This results in an upright T wave (Figure 5.2).

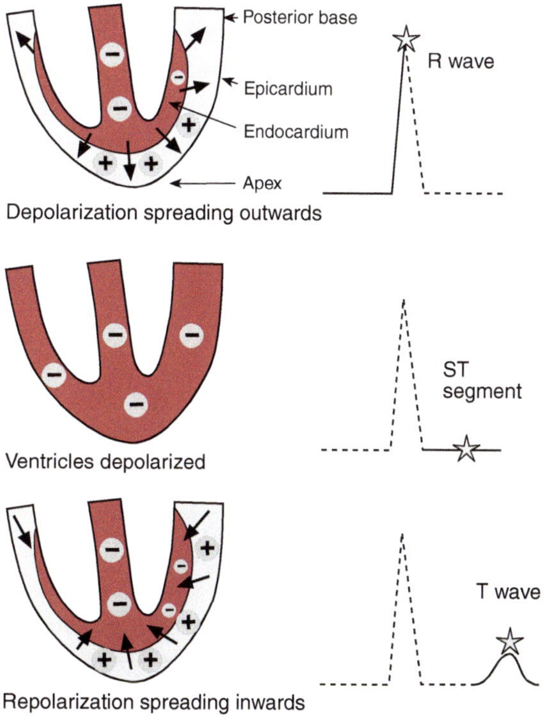

Figure 5.2 Depolarization/repolarization state of ventricles at three points in time, namely partial depolarization (red zone, R wave, *top*), full depolarization (ST segment, *middle*) and partial repolarization (grey zone, T wave, *bottom*). Signs refer to extracellular charge. Arrows show direction of advance of wave front. Since myocytes repolarize in reverse order to depolarization, the dipoles are in the same direction. Consequently, the T wave is upright.

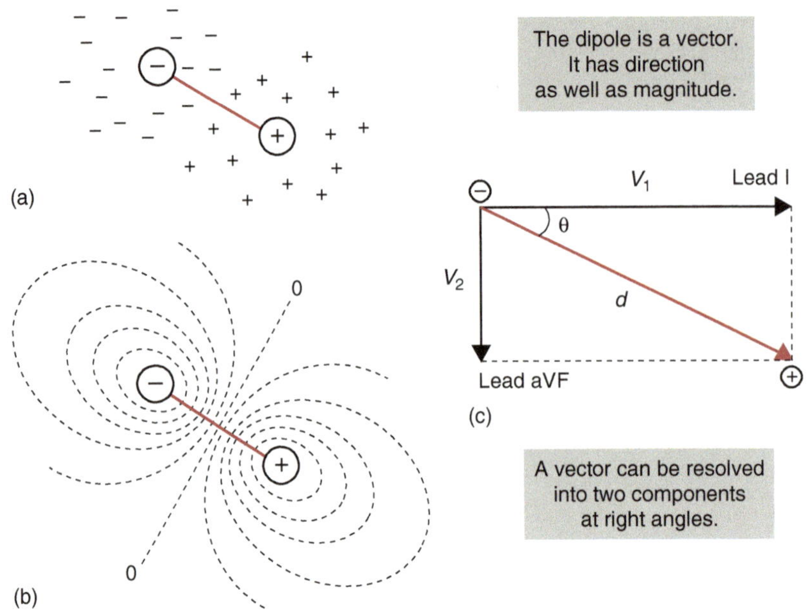

Figure 5.3 Properties of an electrical dipole. (a) Two diffuse groups of opposite charge can be represented by a dipole, i.e. two points of opposite charge, like the terminals of a battery. (b) Equipotential lines around a dipole. The zero potential runs across the middle of the dipole. (c) Resolution of dipole vector (red arrow) into two components at right angles. The length of the red arrow represents vector magnitude, d. The voltage difference V_1 detected by Lead I depends on angle θ ($V_1 = d \text{ cosine } \theta$). If V_1 and V_2 are drawn the same lengths as the R waves in Leads I and aVF, respectively, the electrical axis of the heart equals θ.

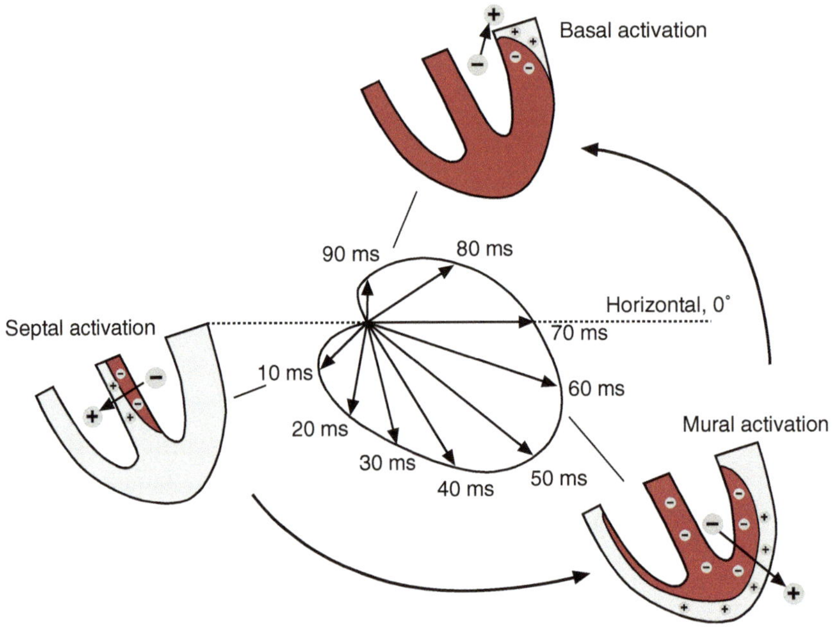

Figure 5.4 Changes in cardiac dipole (straight arrows) during ventricular excitation. Charges refer to extracellular fluid, not intracellular. Grey areas are myocytes at resting potential, so they carry a positive extracellular charge. Red areas are depolarized myocytes with negative extracellular charge. Cardiac dipole rotates anticlockwise and waxes and wanes over ~90 ms. Electrical axis here is ~40° below the horizontal.

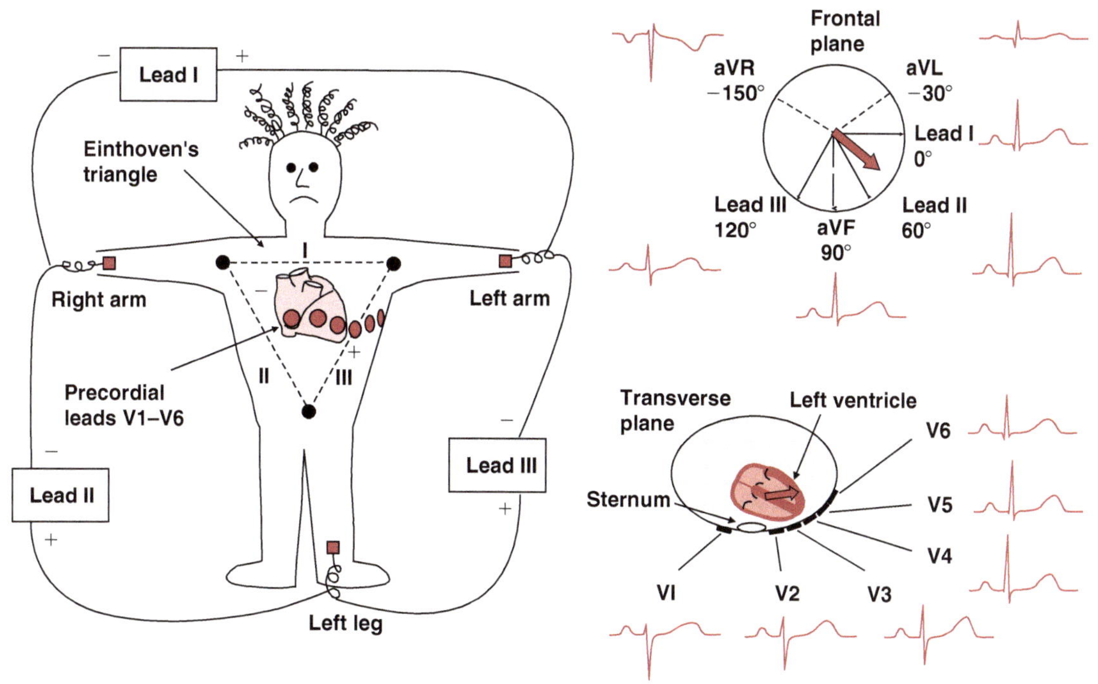

Figure 5.5 Electrode positions to record a 12-lead ECG. The bipolar limb leads (I, II and III) and unipolar limb leads (aVL, aVR and aVF) record in the frontal plane. Precordial chest leads V1–V6 record in a transverse plane. Typical records on right. Red arrows show direction of biggest potential difference during ventricular excitation (main dipole), in the frontal and transverse planes.

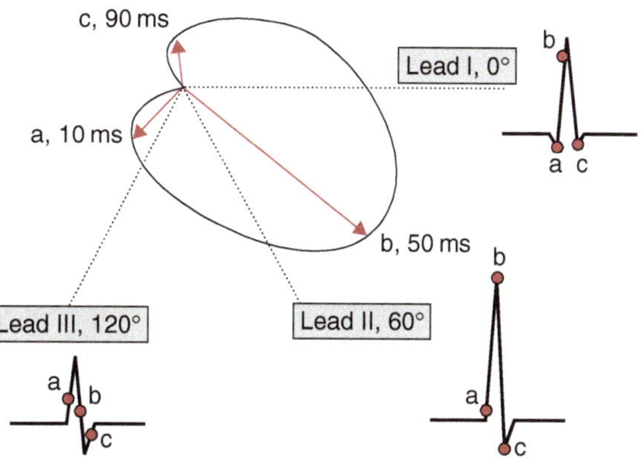

Figure 5.6 Illustration of how the changing magnitude and direction of the dipole (red arrows) create different QRS complexes in different frontal leads. The dipole is shown at three instants in time: a, b and c. The vectorial component recorded by leads I, II and III at each instant is marked by a red dot on the corresponding ECG trace.

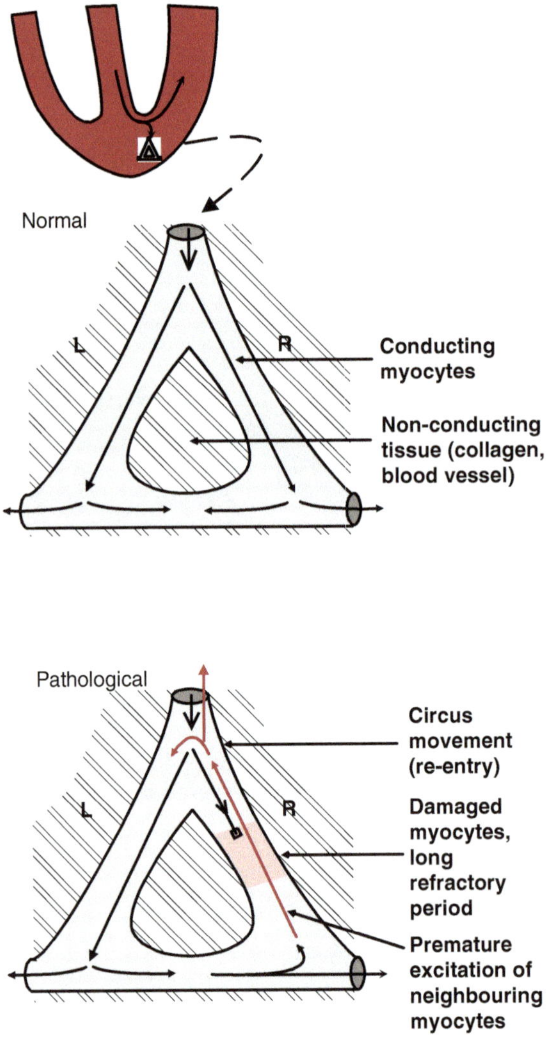

Figure 5.7 Circus (re-entry) mechanism of arrhythmogenesis. (*Top and middle*) Normal spread of excitation around non-conducting obstacles such as a blood vessel or connective tissue. (*Bottom*) Pathology, such as ischaemia or chronic heart failure, causes a long refractory period in the fibres on the right (R), and also slow conduction. As a normal excitation arrives at R, it finds the myocytes refractory from the previous impulse, so it propagates no further. By the time the slowly propagating wave has spread down L, then retrogradely up R, myocytes at R are no longer refractory. They conduct the impulse back up to the junction with L, which is re-excited (re-entry), setting up a self-perpetuating loop or 'circus'.

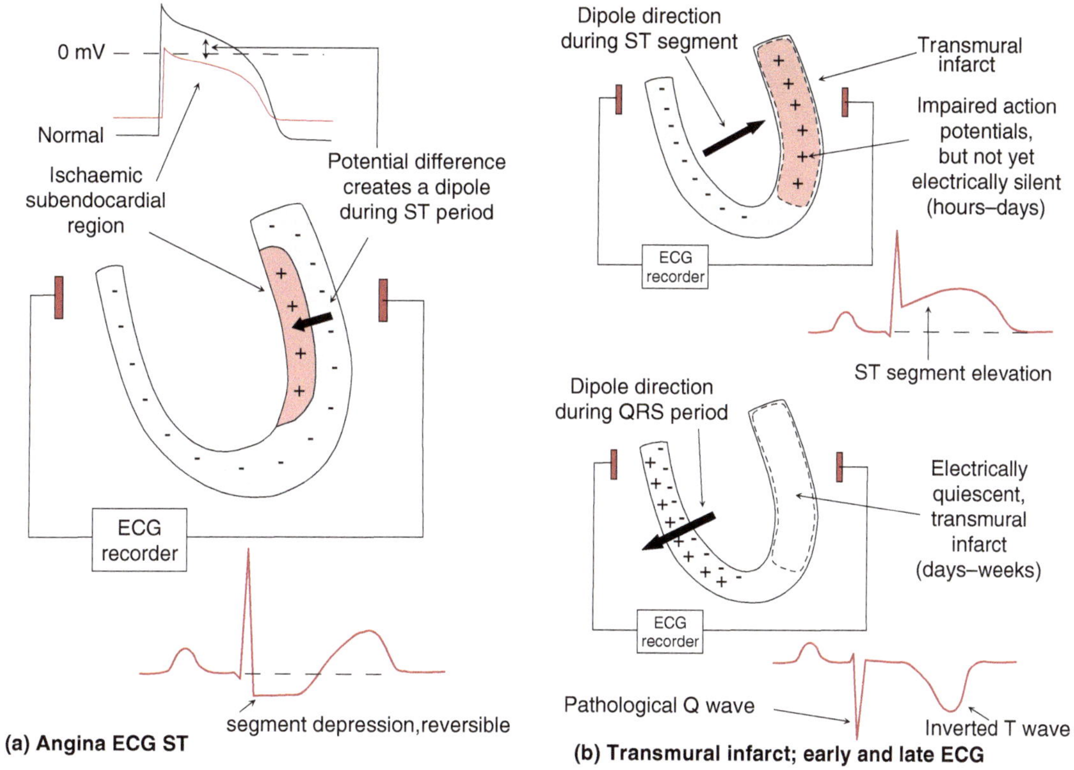

Figure 5.8 Effect of myocardial ischaemia on ventricle extracellular charge distribution and ECG. (a) ST segment depression during an angina attack. The potential difference between normal myocytes and ischaemic myocytes (usually subendocardial) creates a dipole and injury current during the ST interval (cf. normally uniform depolarization, Figure 5.8 middle) and a reversed one during the T–P interval. This depresses the ST segment relative to the baseline. The ECG reverts to normal when the angina is relieved by rest. A partial thickness, subendocardial infarct can likewise cause ST depression, but this is not relieved by rest. (b) Full thickness (transmural) infarct, caused by coronary artery thrombosis. (*Upper schematic*) Ventricle during ST interval, a few hours after infarction. The potential difference between the ischaemic and normal myocytes during ST creates a dipole and injury current, which causes ST elevation in leads facing the infarct, e.g. V1–6 for anterior infarcts, aVF and III for an inferior infarct. (*Lower schematic*) Ventricle during spread of excitation, several days later. As ischaemic cells die (necrosis), they become electrically silent, so ST elevation dwindles and is replaced by pathological Q waves and T wave inversion. Pathological Q waves are deep Q waves ($>$ 2 mm, 0.2 mV) in leads not normally showing them, persisting for years. These features are caused by the altered dipole during excitation; cf. Figure 5.7. The infarcted myocardium acts as an 'electrical window' for leads facing it.

CHAPTER 6

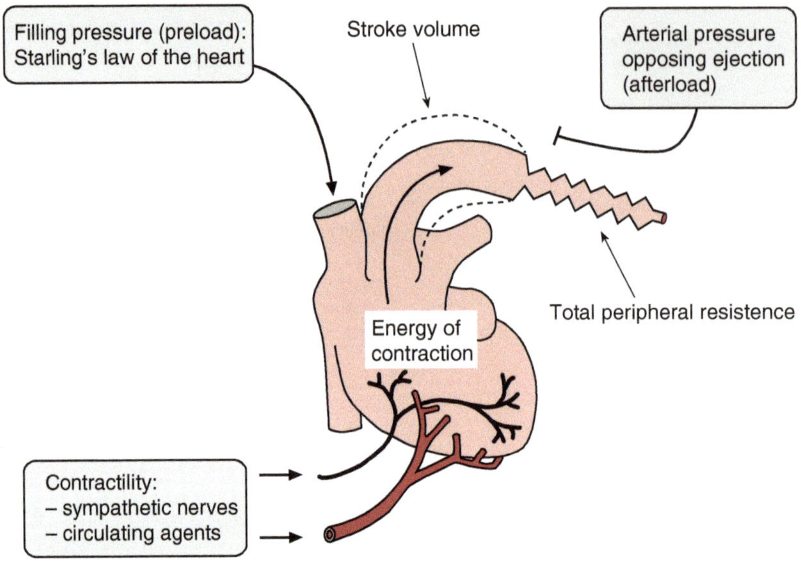

Figure 6.1 Factors affecting the stroke volume of a heart. Total peripheral resistance, which is located mainly in the arterioles and terminal arteries, is represented by the narrow tube in series with the aorta.

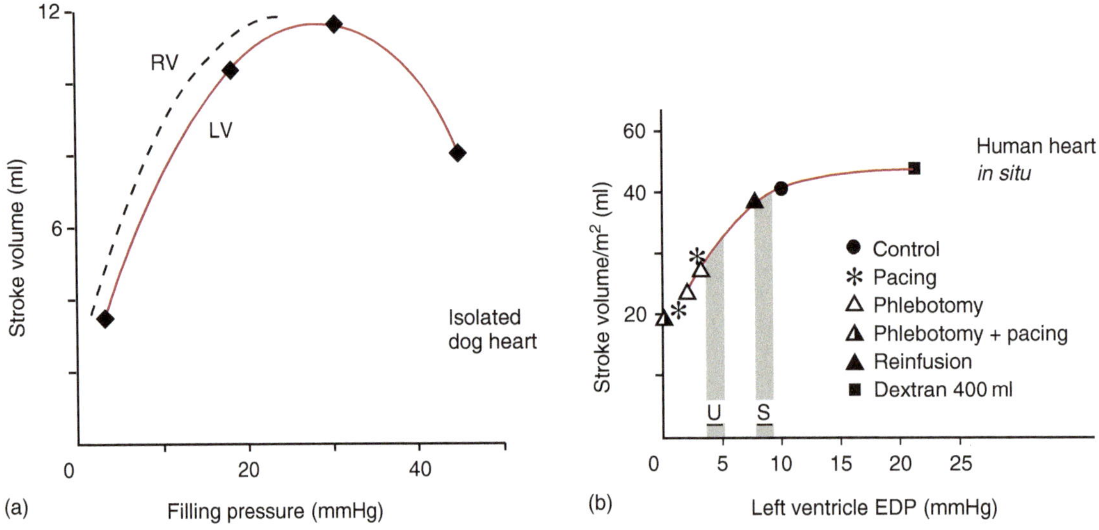

Figure 6.2 Ventricular function curves of dog (a) and human (b). (a) Effect of filling pressure (central venous pressure, dashed line; left atrial pressure, solid line) on stroke volume of isolated dog heart (Starling's data). (b) Human ventricular function curve. LV end-diastolic pressure (LVEDP) was varied *in vivo* by phlebotomy (venous bleeding) and other manoeuvres. Stroke volume is expressed per unit body surface area (stroke index). Grey bands mark normal human LVEDP when supine (S) and upright (U).

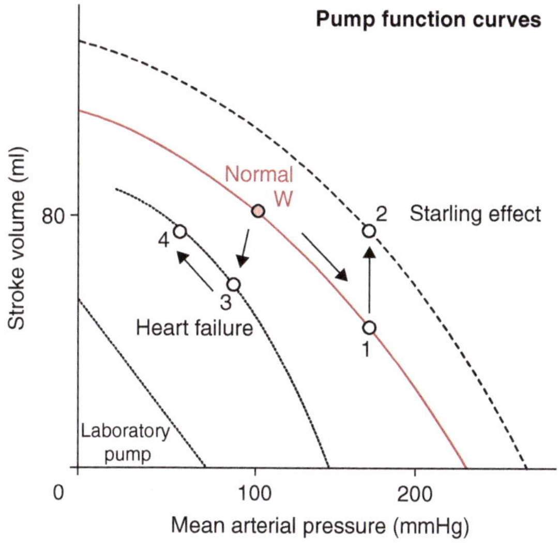

Figure 6.3 Pump function curves for normal heart, failing heart and laboratory roller pump. W, normal work point. Increasing the peripheral resistance raises pressure but depresses stroke volume (point 1). Ventricular distension can restore the stroke volume by shifting the pump function curve to a higher energy level (point 2) – the Frank–Starling mechanism. Impaired contractility (heart failure) shifts the curve to a lower energy level (point 3). The stroke volume of a failing heart can be improved by pressure-reducing drugs (point 4).

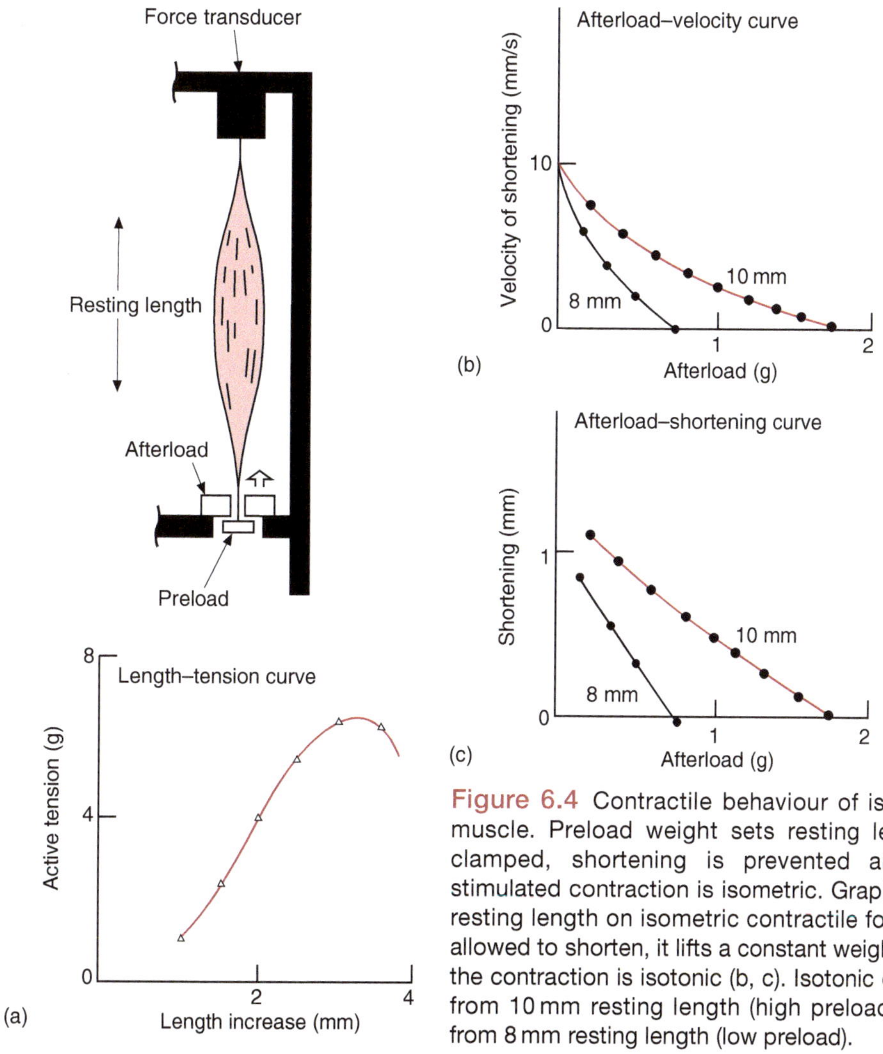

Figure 6.4 Contractile behaviour of isolated cat papillary muscle. Preload weight sets resting length. If preload is clamped, shortening is prevented and the electrically stimulated contraction is isometric. Graph (a) shows effect of resting length on isometric contractile force. If the muscle is allowed to shorten, it lifts a constant weight, the afterload, and the contraction is isotonic (b, c). Isotonic contractions starting from 10 mm resting length (high preload) are stronger than from 8 mm resting length (low preload).

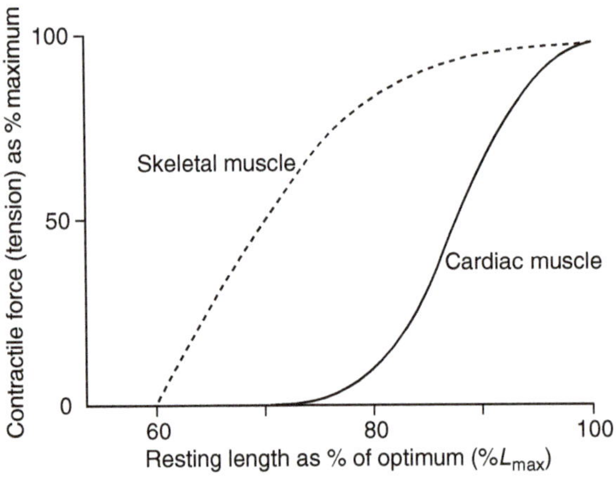

Figure 6.5 Length–tension relation of cardiac muscle compared with skeletal muscle. Cardiac muscle has a much steeper curve than skeletal muscle at physiological lengths (80–100% of L_{max}), even though the filament overlap is the same. This is because stretch increases the Ca^{2+} sensitivity of cardiac myocytes.

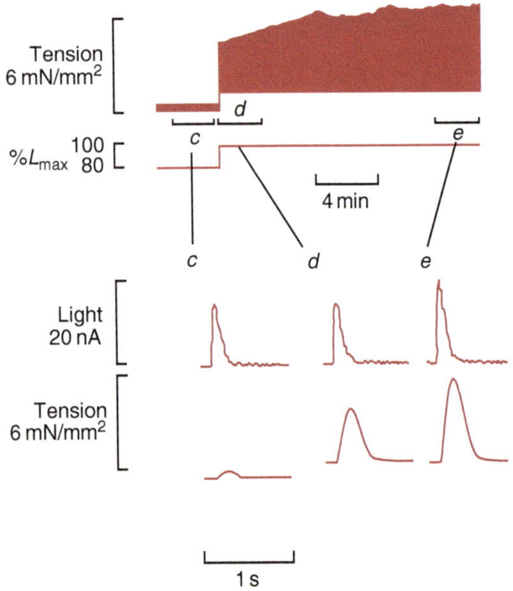

Figure 6.6 Effect of stretch ($\%L_{max}$) on isometric contractile force and Ca^{2+} transients (light signal) in isolated papillary muscle. Note immediate, large increase in force at *d* without any increase in the Ca^{2+} transient. This is followed by a smaller, slow force response and Ca^{2+} increase (the Anrep effect).

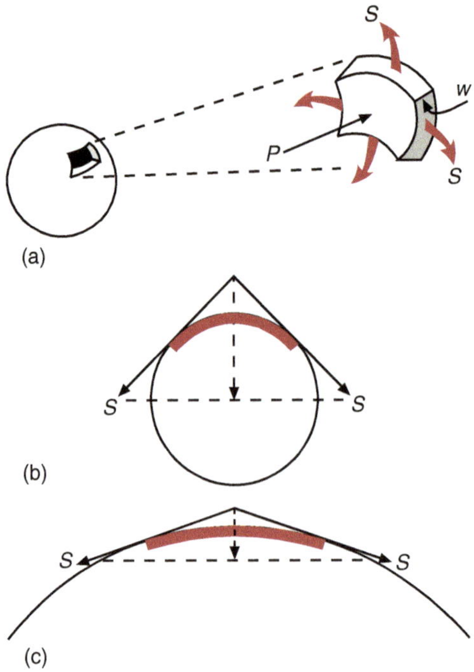

Figure 6.7 Effect of curvature of a hollow sphere on the conversion of wall stress *S* into internal pressure *P* (Laplace's law). (a) Hollow sphere with an 'exploded' segment, showing the two circumferential wall stresses. Stress is force per unit cross-sectional area, of thickness *w*. The wall stress in the ejecting heart is the afterload on the myocytes. (b) Cross section showing how the wall stresses (tangential arrows) give rise to an inwardly directed stress equal and opposite to the pressure. The thick red line represents a muscle segment exerting tension. Arrow length is proportional to stress magnitude. (c) Increasing the radius reduces the curvature, and therefore the inward component of the wall stress; so pressure falls (Laplace's law).

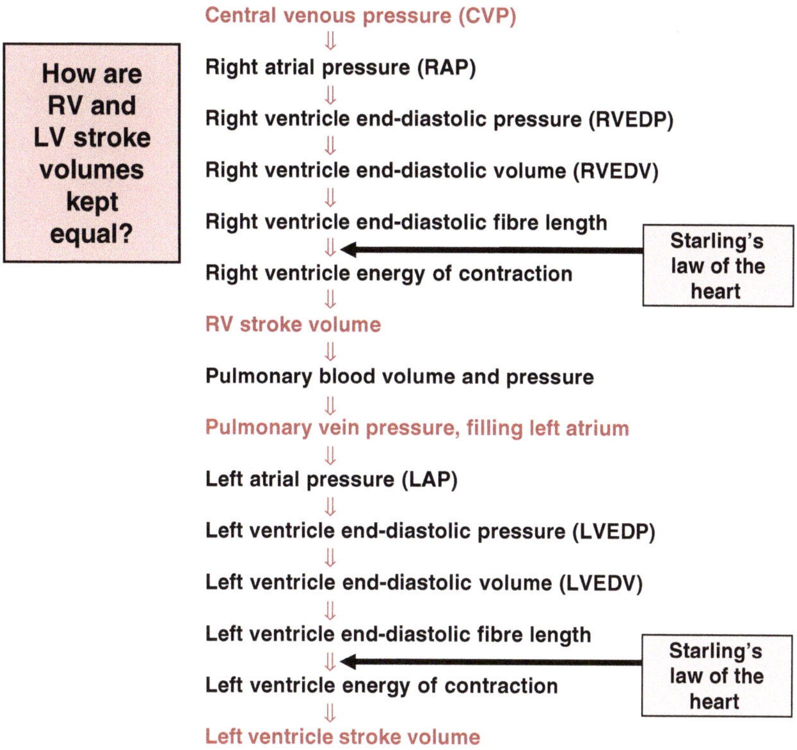

Figure 6.8 Equalization of right and left ventricular outputs by Starling's law.

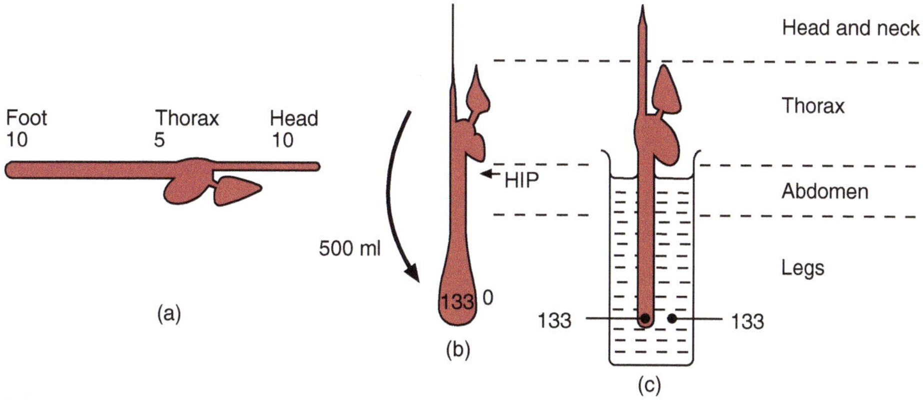

Figure 6.9 Venous blood redistribution by gravity on moving from supine (a) to standing (b). The thoracic compartment includes the central veins, heart and pulmonary blood. Numbers are cmH_2O pressure above atmospheric. HIP, hydrostatic indifferent point. (c) Immersion raises pressure around the veins, displacing the 'pooled' blood centrally and raising CVP.

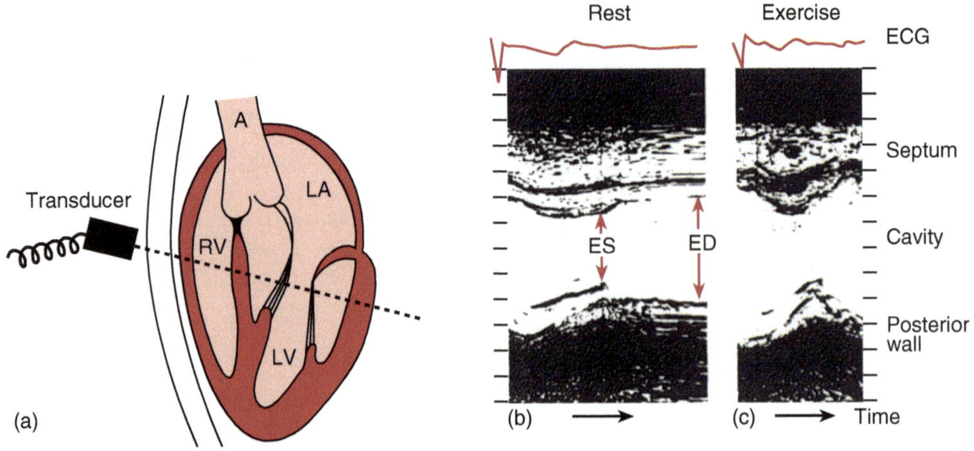

Figure 6.10 Effect of exercise on ventricular dimensions and contraction, measured by M-mode echocardiography during rest (b) and upright exercise (c). The end-diastolic dimension (ED) increased and end-systole dimension (ES) fell. The ED–ES difference, an index of stroke volume, increased by 24%.

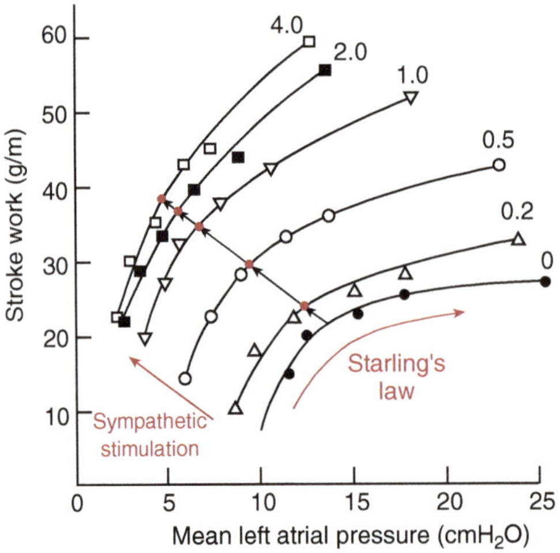

Figure 6.11 Shift in ventricular function curves (Starling curves) brought about by sympathetic stimulation (dog heart). Sympathetic activity in range 0–4 s^{-1} increased contractility. Arrows show how enhanced contractility reduces filling pressure, as well as raising stroke volume.

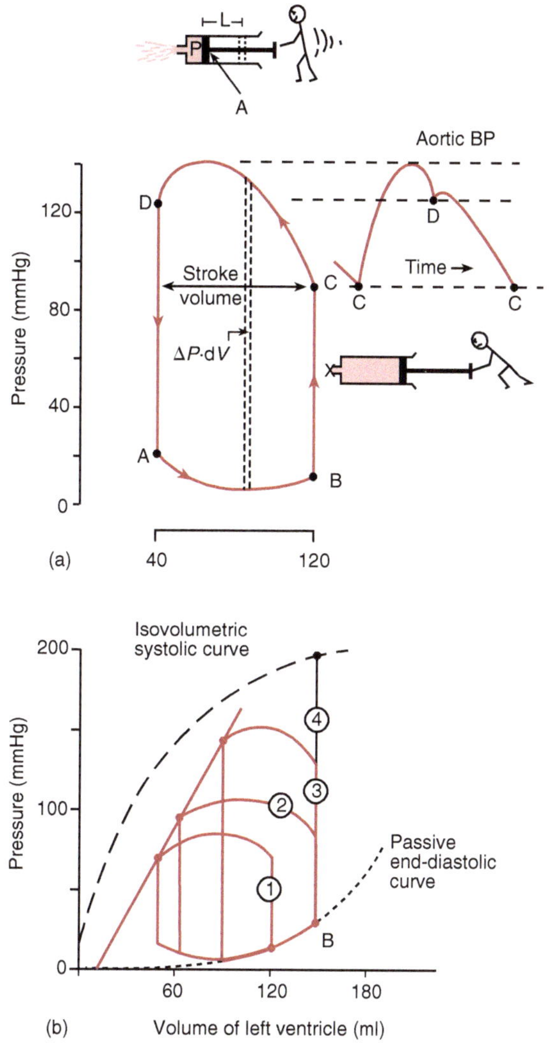

Figure 6.12 Pressure–volume loops for human left ventricle. (a) Relation to aortic pressure wave. A, mitral valve opens; AB, filling phase; B, mitral valve closes at onset of systole; BC, isovolumetric contraction; C, aortic valve opens; CD, ejection phase; D, aortic valve closes; DA, isovolumetric relaxation. Stroke work is sum of all $\Delta P \cdot dV$ strips inside the loop, i.e. total loop area. Sketches illustrate high energy expenditure and O_2 consumption by the myocardial manikin during isovolumetric contraction, achieving no external work, followed by lower energy cost of ejection. The subject is probably middle aged/elderly, since aortic pressure was 130/85 mmHg. (b) Set of pressure–volume loops for a constant contractility. Lower boundary is passive pressure–volume curve of relaxed ventricle (compliance curve). Upper boundary is systolic pressure of a purely isovolumetric contraction at increasing end-diastolic volumes (Frank–Starling mechanism). Loop 1 is basal. Raising end-diastolic volume to B increases stroke volume (loop 2), due to Starling's law. Note that end-systolic volume increases too. Raising peripheral resistance increases arterial pressure but reduces stroke volume (loop 3), due to the 'pump function' effect (Figure 6.3). A purely isovolumetric contraction (loop 4) reaches the upper boundary.

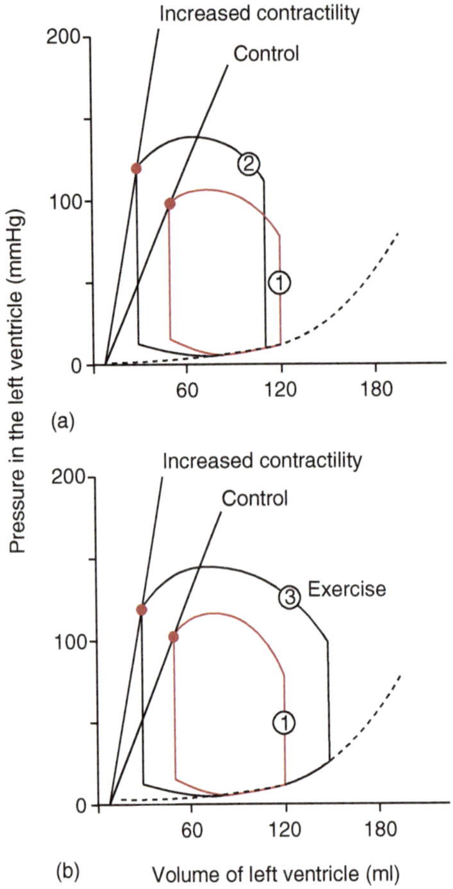

Figure 6.13 Effect of increased left ventricular contractility on human pressure–volume loop. (a) Loop 1 is basal state. Loop 2 shows effect of increased sympathetic activity. Ejection fraction is increased, so end-diastolic volume falls. Loop area (stroke work) is increased. (b) During exercise (loop 3), contractility is raised by sympathetic activity but end-diastolic volume too is raised, by peripheral venoconstriction and the skeletal muscle pump. This amplifies the increase in stroke volume.

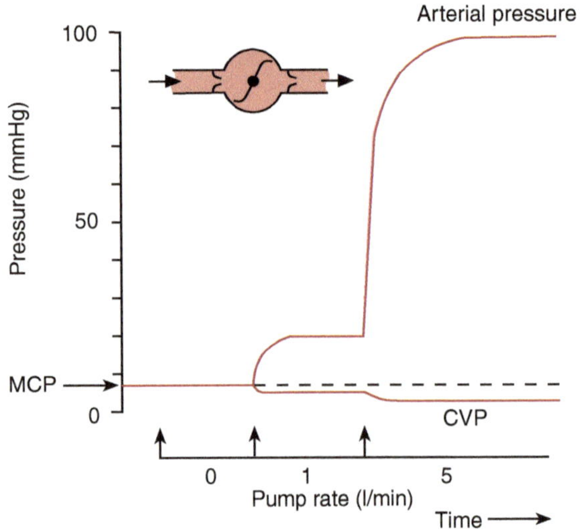

Figure 6.14 Effect of a pump on input and output pressure. At zero pumping rate, the central venous pressure (CVP) and arterial pressure equalize (mean circulatory pressure, MCP). When the pump starts, its removes fluid from the input line, so it reduces input pressure, CVP, as well as raising output pressure (arterial pressure). CVP changes less than arterial pressure, because venous compliance (volume accommodated per unit pressure change) is greater than arterial compliance.

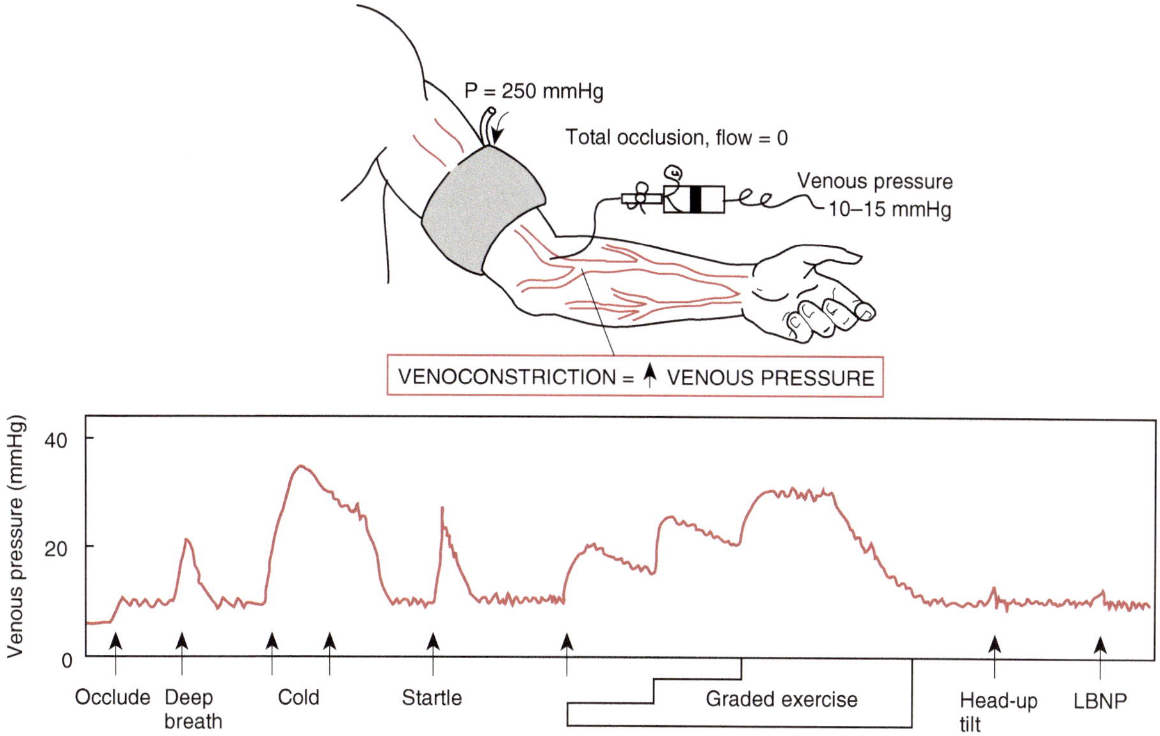

Figure 6.15 Sympathetic-mediated venoconstriction in human skin. During exercise, this helps shift blood into the thoracic veins to maintain/raise CVP

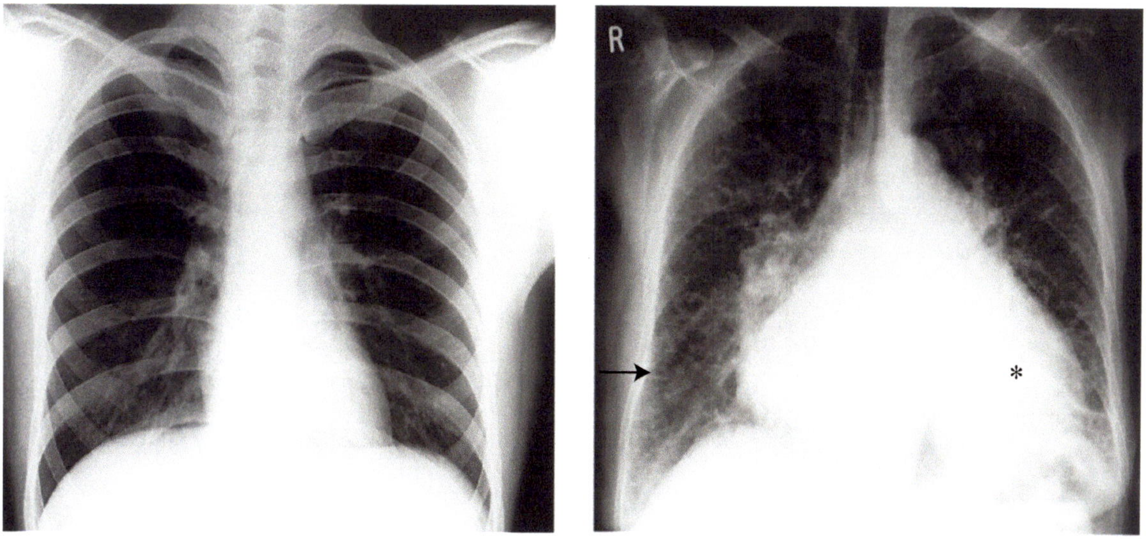

Figure 6.16 Normal chest X-ray (left) and dilated heart in patient with cardiac failure (right).

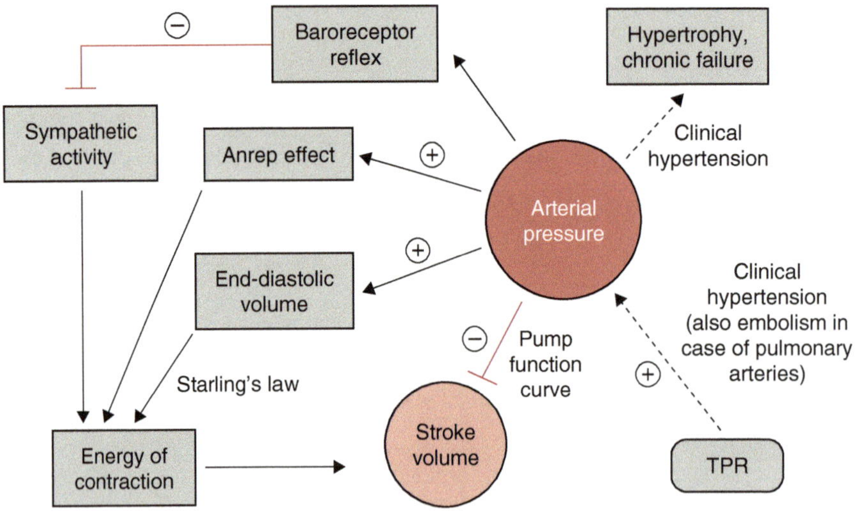

Figure 6.17 An acute rise in arterial pressure, resulting from a rise in total peripheral resistance (TPR), affects stroke volume through two negative and two positive mechanisms. TPR may be increased acutely by sympathetic vasomotor activity, or chronically by clinical hypertension.

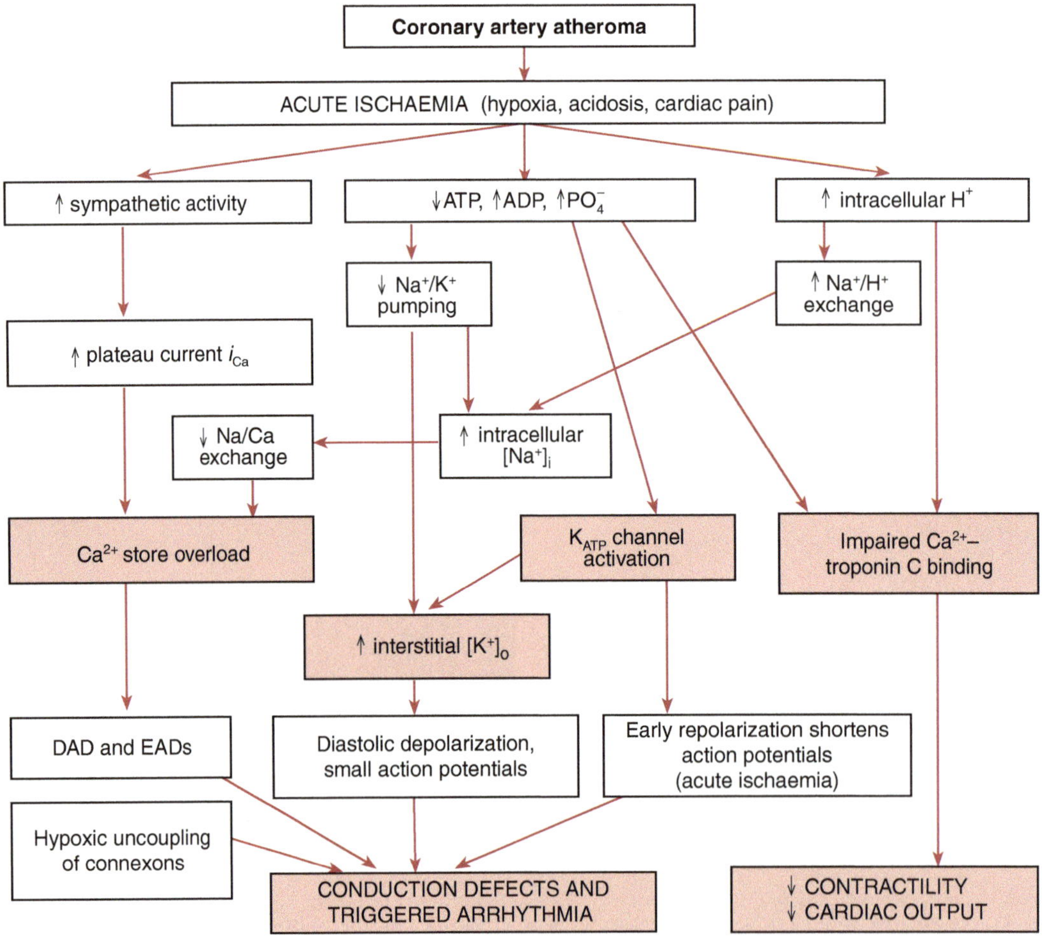

Figure 6.18 Multiple mechanisms by which acute ischaemia, due usually to coronary atheroma, impairs contractility and causes arrhythmia.

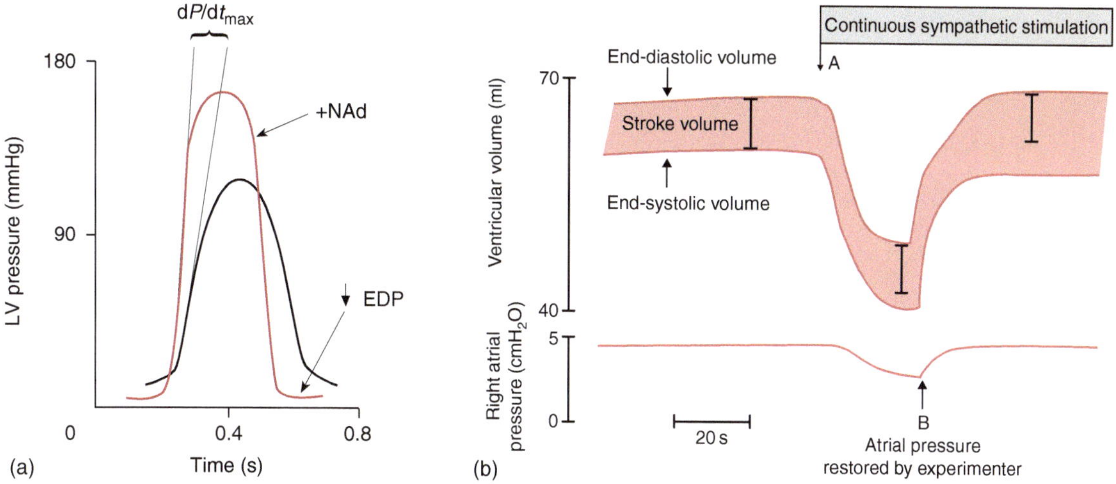

Figure 6.19 Effect of sympathetic stimulation (noradrenaline) on cardiac performance. (a) Left ventricular pressure climbs faster (dP/dt_{max}), systolic pressure increases, systole shortens, relaxation is quicker and end-diastolic pressure (EDP) falls. (b) Increased ejection fraction and stroke volume reduce filling pressure and ventricular volumes, which limits the increase in stroke volume (Starling's law). Restoring the filling pressure (B) allows the effect of contractility on stroke volume to emerge fully. Vertical bar shows size of control stroke volume.

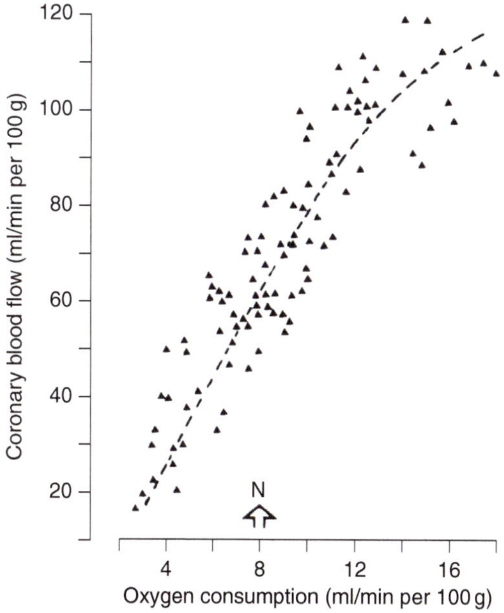

Figure 6.20 Effect of catecholamine-driven increase in cardiac output and oxygen consumption on coronary blood flow. N, normal resting value (canine).

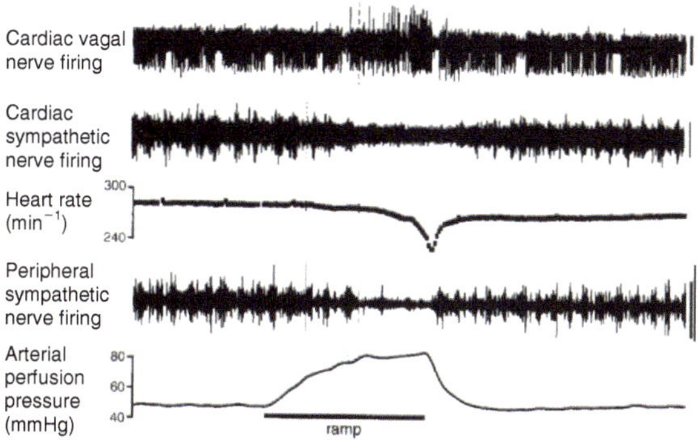

Figure 6.21 Reflex effect of an imposed rise in arterial pressure upon autonomic fibre activity and heart rate. The reflex is mediated by the arterial baroreceptors.

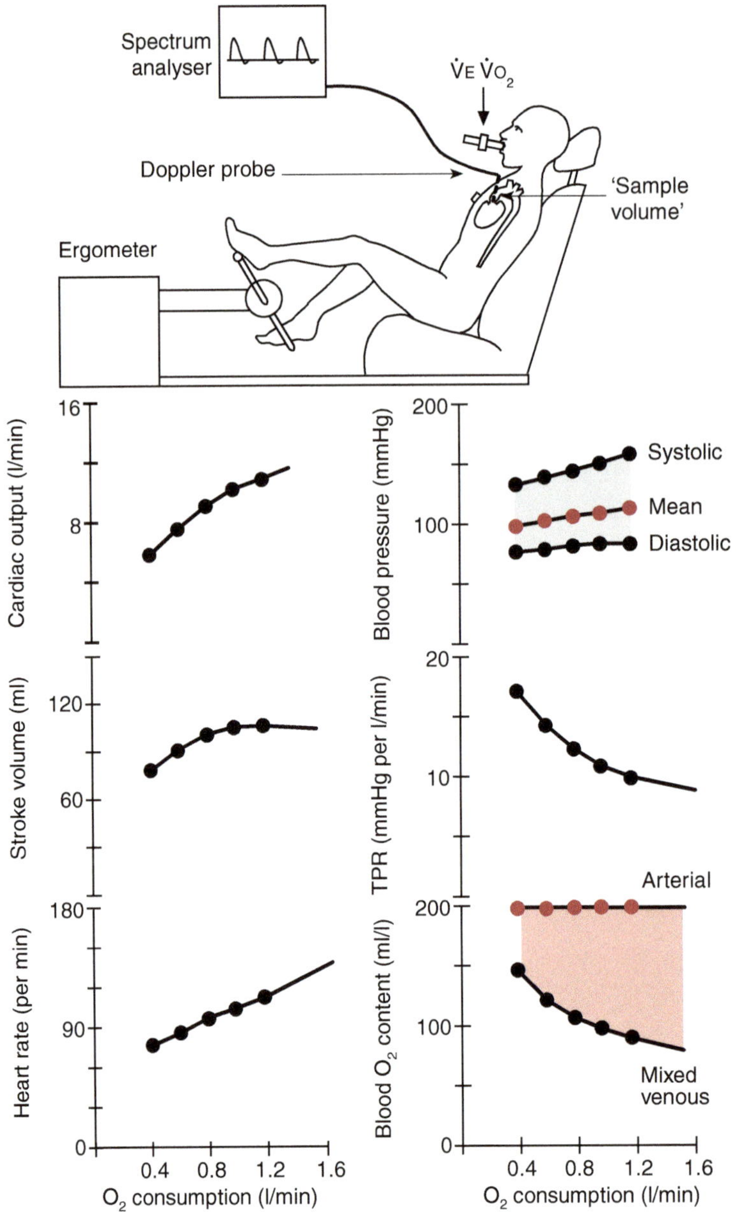

Figure 6.22 Human cardiovascular response to exercise. Stroke volume measured by pulsed Doppler method.

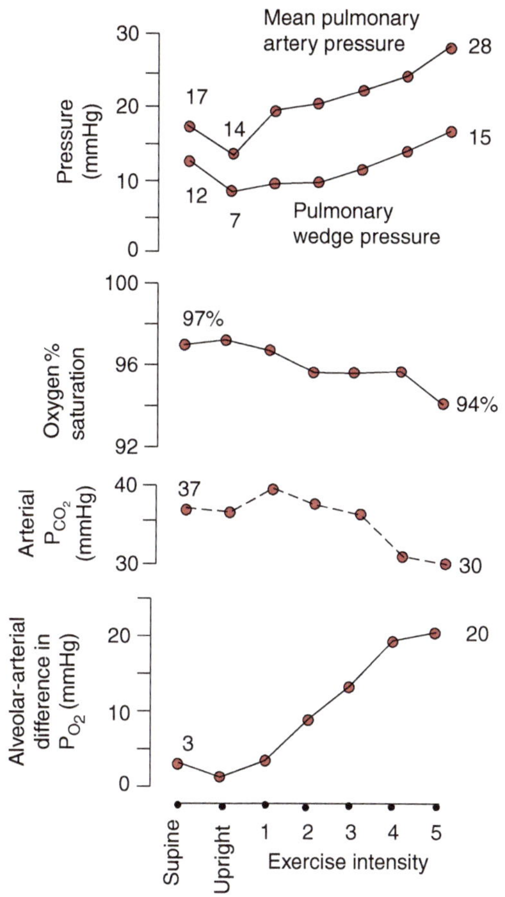

Figure 6.23 Effect of posture and exercise on pulmonary circulation.

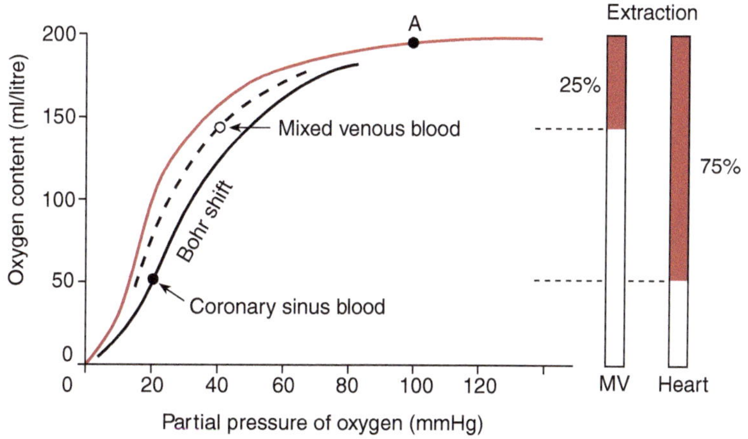

Figure 6.24 Blood oxygen transport curves, showing very high oxygen extraction by myocardium.

CHAPTER 7

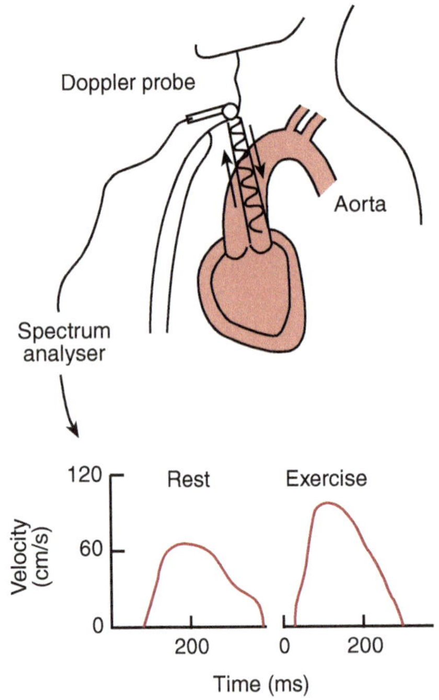

Figure 7.1 Transaortic pulsed Doppler ultrasound records aortic blood velocity at successive moments during systole. Stroke distance is area under curve.

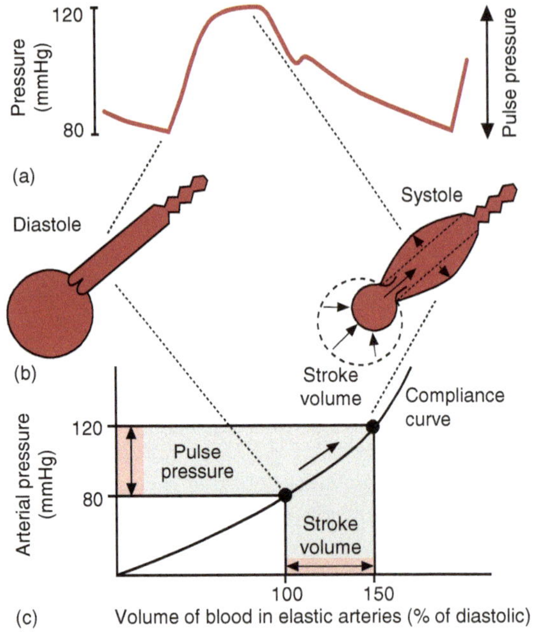

Figure 7.2 Relation between aortic pulse pressure and stroke volume.

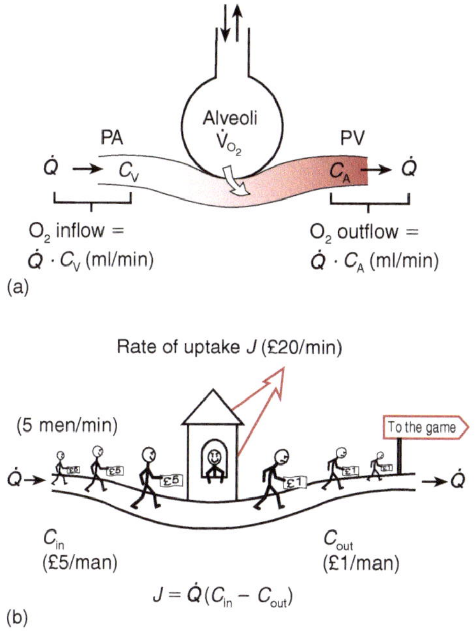

Figure 7.3 The Fick principle. (a) Applied to measure pulmonary blood flow ($\dot{Q}$). PA, pulmonary artery, blood O_2 concentration C_V. PV, pulmonary vein, oxygen C_A. Oxygen uptake rate $V_{O_2} = \dot{Q} \times (C_A - C_V)$. (b) Applied to measure flow ($\dot{Q}$) of football supporters through a gate, based on the rate of takings (J) and the 'concentration' of money in the supporters' pockets before and after the gate. In other scenarios, each individual could be a red cell giving up CO_2 to the lungs; or a volume of plasma giving up glucose to the brain; the principle has wide application.

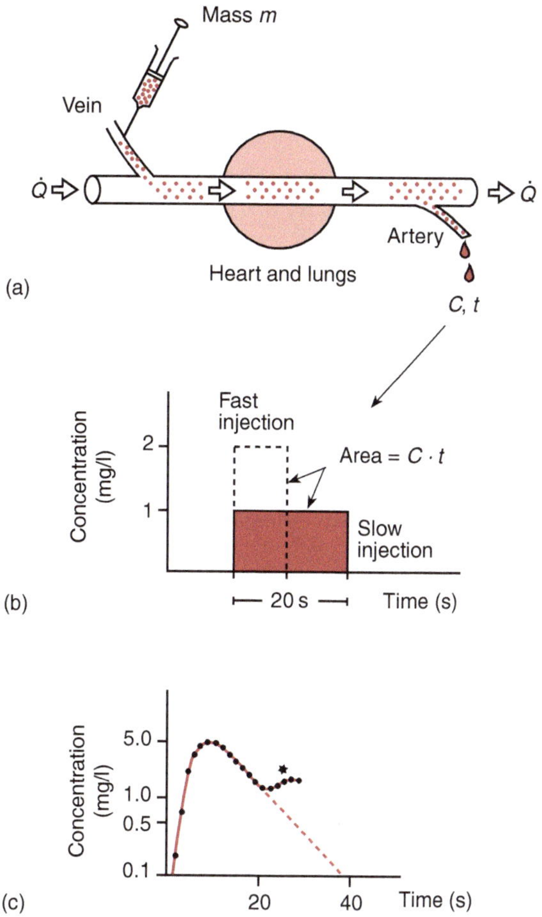

Figure 7.4 Hamilton's dye-dilution method. (a) Arterial concentration C depends on the mass of indicator injected (m) and the volume of blood in which it became diluted. (b) Idealized plot of C against time. Area $C \times t$ is 20 mg s litre^{-1} here. (The increase in concentration produced by a fast injection is offset by the shorter duration of the bolus). If m is 1 mg, the cardiac output of plasma is 1 mg/20 mg s litre^{-1} = 0.05 l/s, or 3 l/min. For a haematocrit of 0.4, the cardiac output of blood is 5 l/min. (c) In reality, the concentration peaks, decays and has a recirculation hump. Fortunately, when C is plotted on a logarithmic scale, the early decay is linear. This allows extrapolation past the recirculation hump (asterisk). Area under the extrapolated curve is used to calculate the cardiac output.

CHAPTER 8

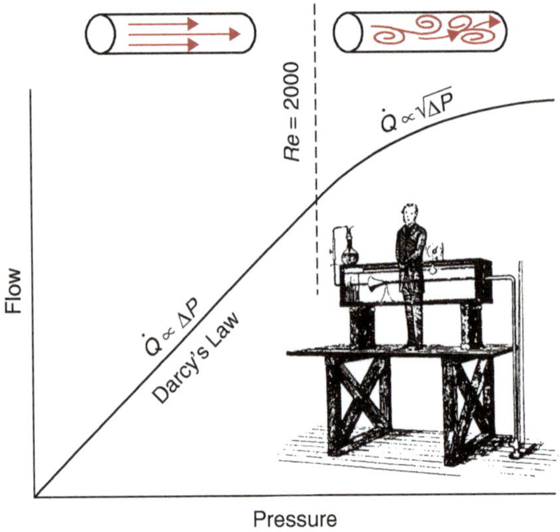

Figure 8.1 Pressure–flow relation for a Newtonian fluid in a rigid tube. Darcy's law is the straight line through the origin. This breaks down when turbulence begins. Inset shows Sir Osborne Reynolds' apparatus for studying the onset of turbulence. The flow-pattern (top) was visualized by injecting dye into the fluid.

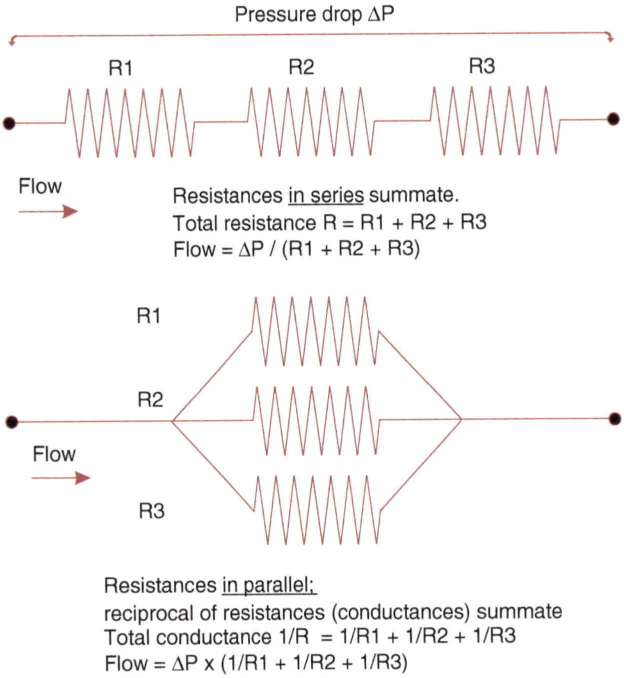

Figure 8.2 Basic rules of hydraulics. When vessels are linked in series (e.g. feed artery–terminal artery–arteriole), each adds to the resistance to the flow; net resistance is high. When vessels are linked in parallel, as in a capillary bed, their flow-transmitting capabilities (conductances) add up, so the net resistance is low.

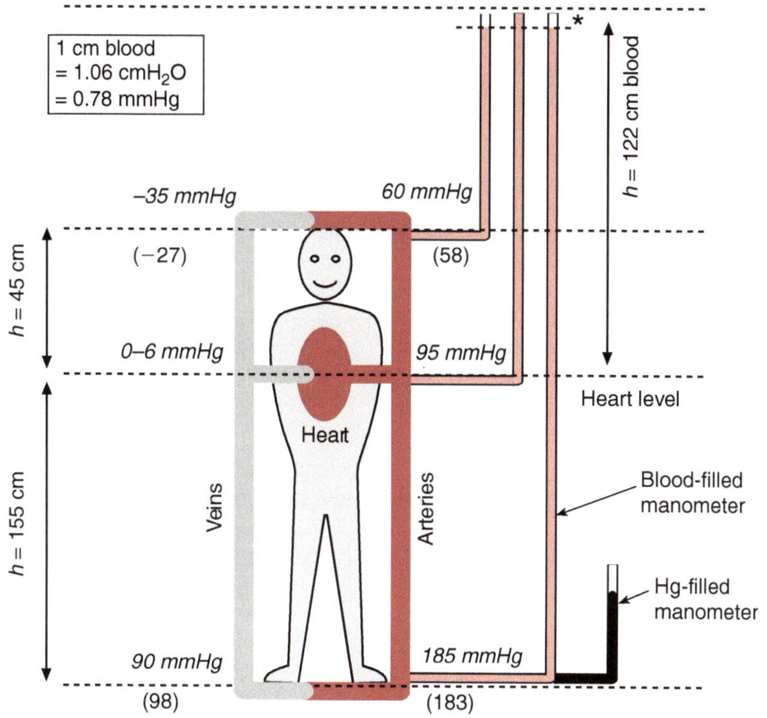

Figure 8.3 Effect of gravity on arterial and venous pressure in a standing human. Pink manometers are filled with blood, black (lower right) with mercury. Pressures in italics are central pressure plus pressure due to vertical fluid column. Pressures in brackets represents actual values for flowing blood, which are modified slightly by the arterial and venous resistances.

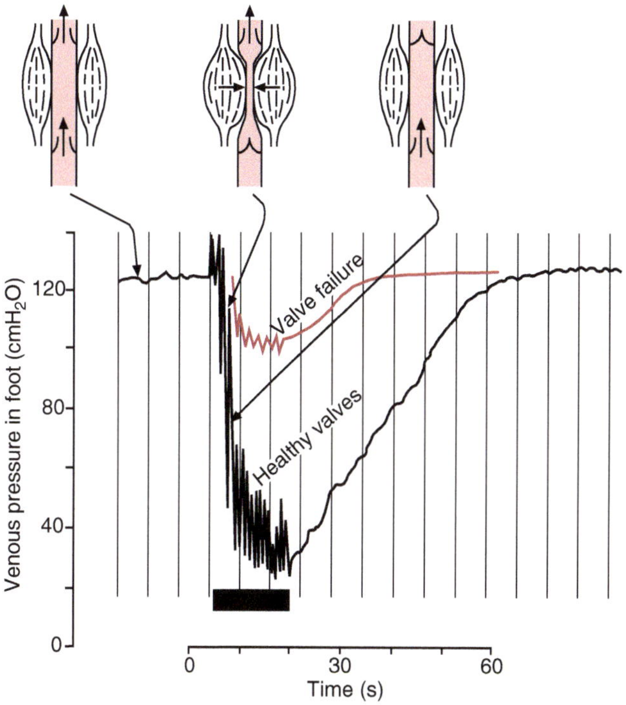

Figure 8.4 The skeletal muscle pump. Trace shows pressure in the dorsal vein of foot (solid line), initially standing still, then rhythmically contracting the calf muscles (black bar). Insets show how the muscle pump operates. Red line shows effect of failure of venous valves, as in varicose veins.

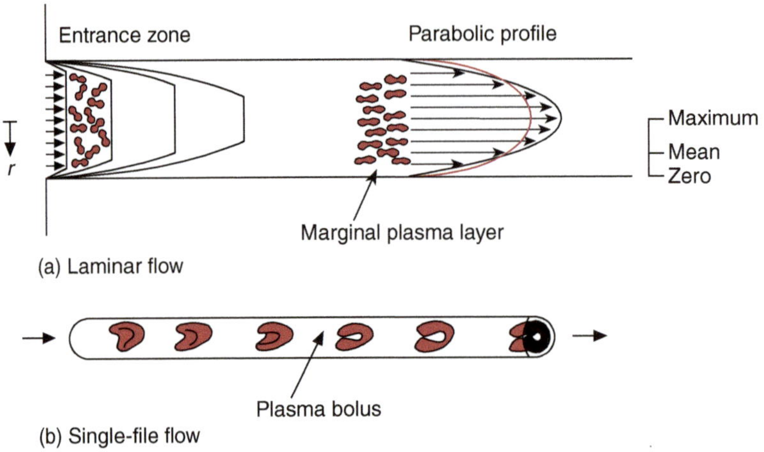

Figure 8.5 Blood flow patterns: (a) large vessels; arrow length represents velocity of each lamina. For a Newtonian fluid in fully developed laminar flow, velocity is a parabolic function of radial position. For non-Newtonian blood, the velocity profile is blunter (red line). The gradient of the velocity curve, the shear rate, is greatest at the edge. (b) In capillaries, the red cells must deform to traverse the vessel.

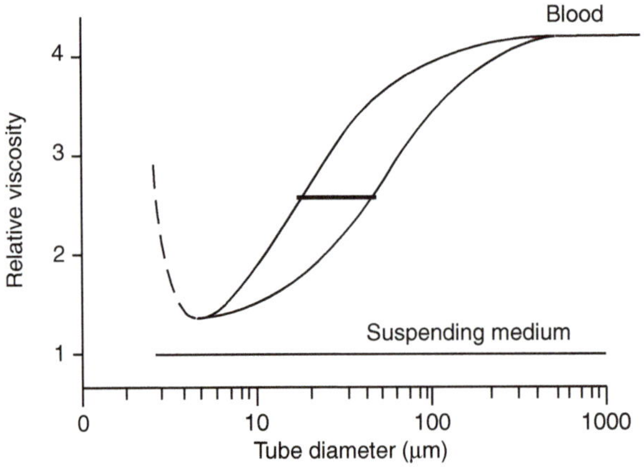

Figure 8.6 Anomalous viscosity of blood. Viscosity falls as tube diameter is reduced (Fåhraeus–Lindqvist effect), but water viscosity is unchanged. The effective viscosity of blood in the circulation is ~2.5 (black bar), implying that the functional diameter of the resistance vessels is ~30 μm (arterioles).

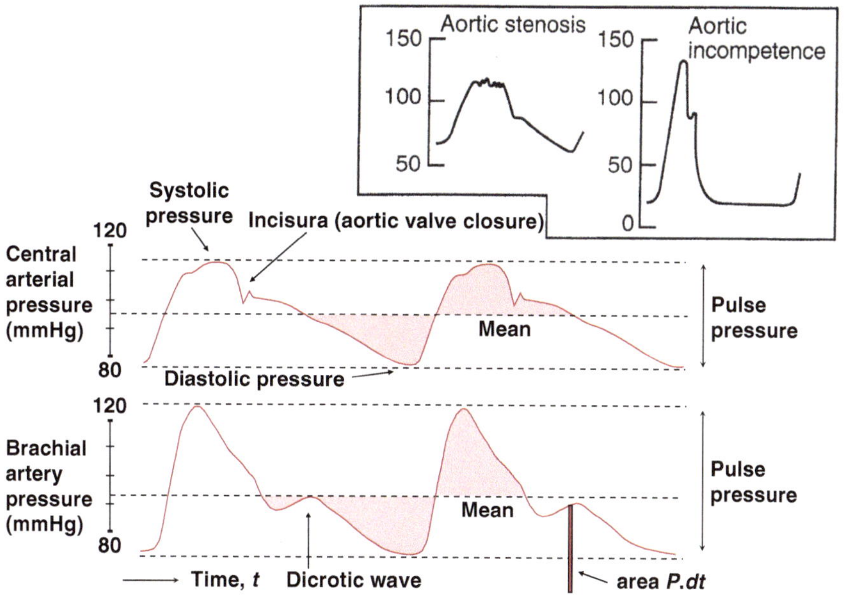

Figure 8.7 Pressure wave in aorta and brachial artery. Mean pressure is the sum of the thousands of thin rectangular strips of individual area *P.dt*, divided by time t (bottom right). The pressure-time product above mean pressure (pink area above central dashed line) equals that below the mean. In central arteries, mean pressure is halfway between systolic and diastolic pressures. In the brachial artery, the mean is diastolic + one-third pulse pressure, due to the altered wave shape. (*Insets*) Abnormal waveform in aortic valve stenosis (slow rise, prolonged plateau) and aortic incompetence (excessive pulse pressure, low diastolic pressure).

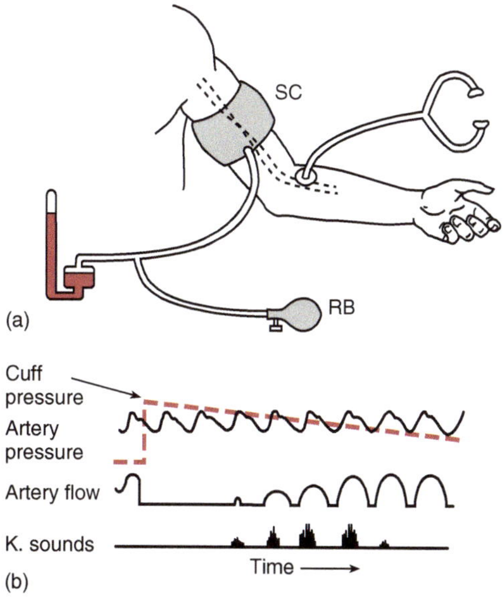

Figure 8.8 Measurement of human blood pressure. (a) Brachial artery is compressed by inflated sphygmomanometer cuff SC. Cuff pressure is controlled by the rubber bulb (RB). Cuff pressure has been measured for generations by a mercury column, but recent instruments use a dial gauge. (b) Korotkoff sounds begin when cuff pressure is reduced to just below systolic pressure. They cease when cuff pressure is below diastolic pressure.

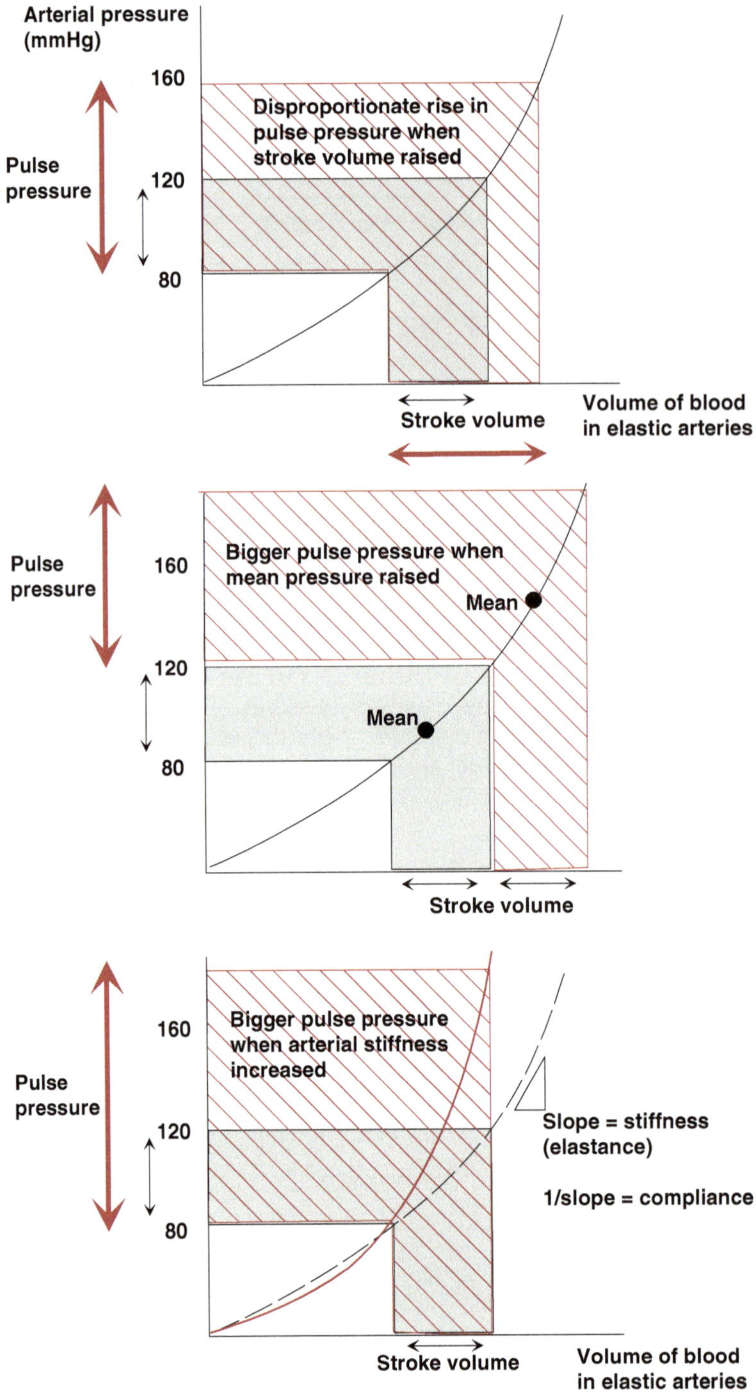

Figure 8.9 Non-linear pressure–volume relation of elastic arteries and effect on pulse pressure. (*Top*) A moderate increase in stroke volume increases pulse pressure disproportionately, because the artery gets stiffer with stretch, i.e. the curve gets steeper. (*Middle*) The same stroke volume ejected at a higher mean pressure (filled circles) causes a bigger pulse pressure, because distension increases the arterial stiffness (elastance). (*Bottom*) An increase in stiffness (e.g. arteriosclerosis of ageing) markedly increases the pulse pressure.

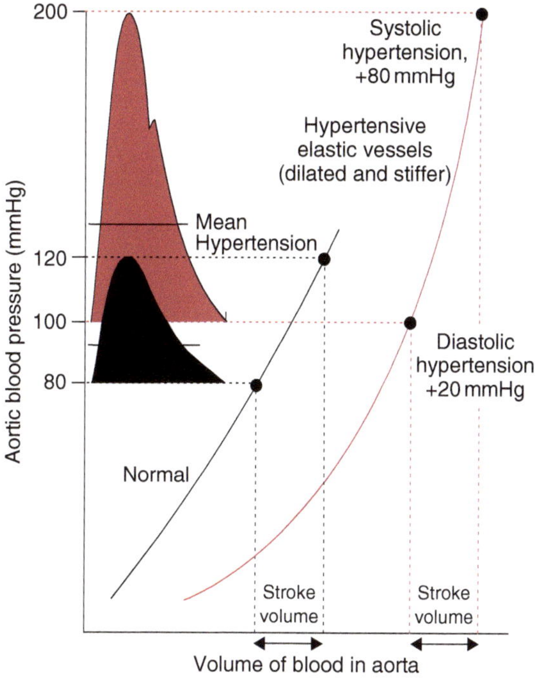

Figure 8.10 Increased stiffness of elastic arteries contributes to systolic hypertension. The central arteries are dilated, because elastin fragments with age and in hypertension. The arteries are stiffer (steeper slope. elastance) because dilatation stresses the collagen, and increases its deposition. The same stroke volume causes a bigger pulse pressure and systolic pressure. Diastolic pressure was raised 20 mmHg by increased peripheral resistance, but systolic pressure increased by 80 mmHg due to the stiffening of the dilated central arteries (reduced compliance).

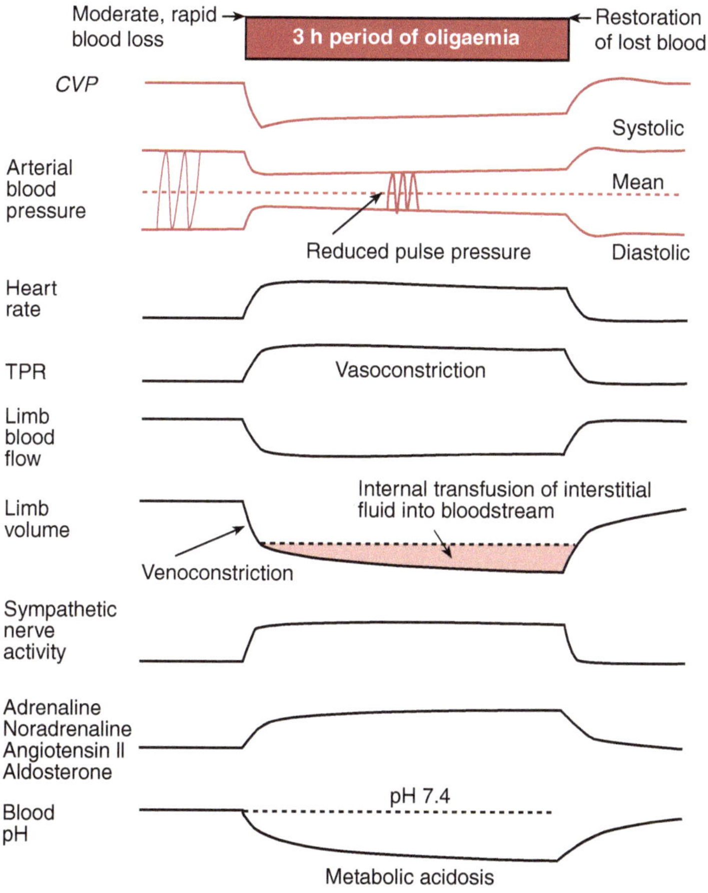

Figure 8.11 Cardiovascular changes following a haemorrhage of 20%. Reflex tachycardia and peripheral vasoconstriction maintain mean blood pressure, but the reduced CVP lowers the pulse pressure (Starling's law).

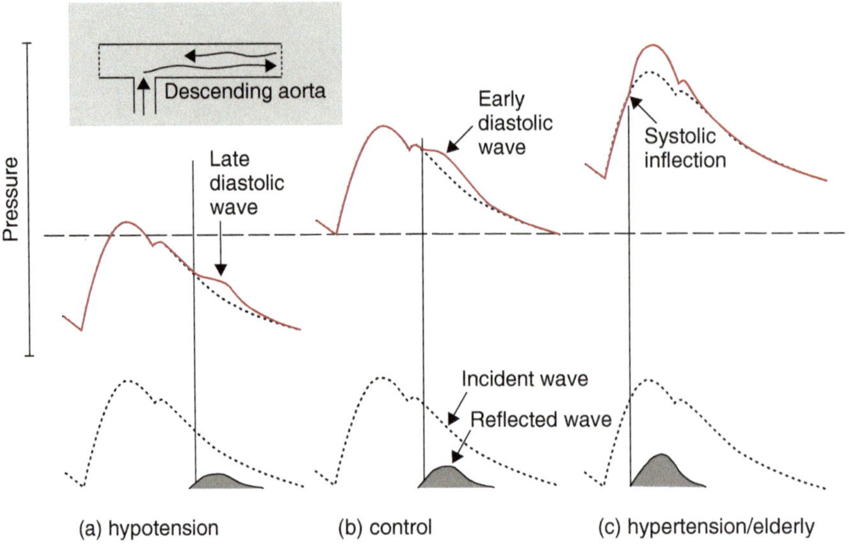

Figure 8.12 Effect of wave reflection on aortic pulse. (*Top*) Arterial system represented as an asymmetric T-tube; ends represent the average of all the reflection sites. The observed pulse (red) is composed of a basic 'incident' wave and a reflected wave. Time of return of reflected wave depends on pulse transmission velocity. (a) In hypotension, the low pressure reduces arterial stiffness (Figure 8.9). This slows pulse transmission velocity, so the reflected wave arrives back in late diastole. (b) At normal pressures in a young human, faster pulse transmission results in an early diastolic reflected wave. (c) In hypertensive or elderly humans, the increased arterial stiffness and transmission velocity result in a systolic reflected wave, seen as a systolic inflection.

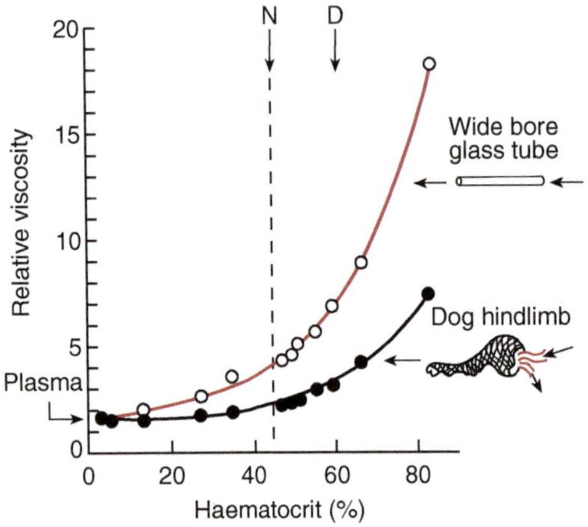

Figure 8.13 Effect of haematocrit on the viscosity of blood relative to water. Open circles: viscosity in a high-velocity, wide-bore glass viscometer. Closed circles: lower effective viscosity in an isolated, perfused dog hindlimb, due to the Fåhraeus–Lindqvist effect. N, normal haematocrit; D, haematocrit at which cells are packed so tightly that they deform even at rest.

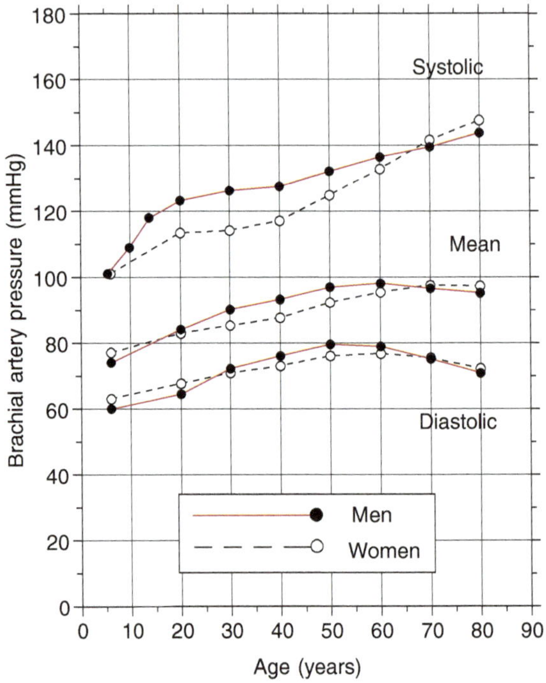

Figure 8.14 Change in arterial blood pressure with age in UK population.

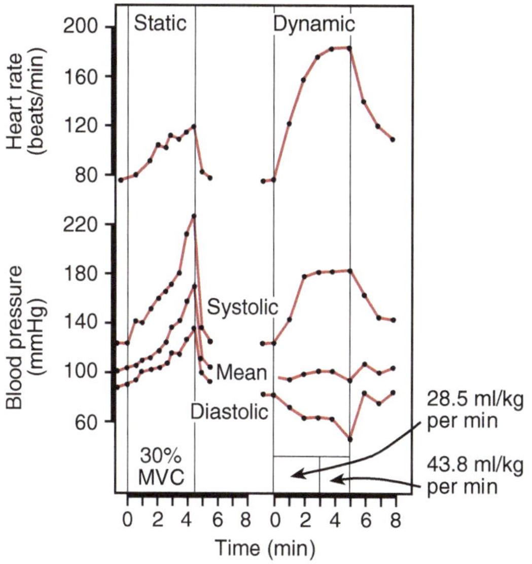

Figure 8.15 Exercise raises systolic blood pressure – static exercise (e.g. weight lifting) more so than dynamic exercise. MVC, maximum voluntary contraction. Arrow values are oxygen consumption.

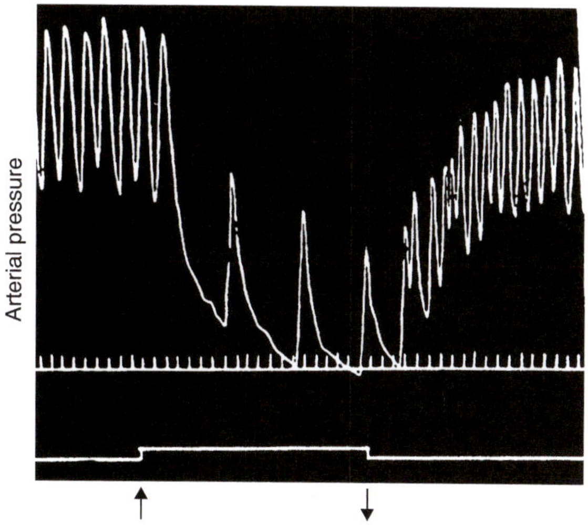

Figure 8.16 Arterial pressure trace, showing a reflex fall in pressure and a bradycardia in response to stimulation of carotid sinus baroreceptor fibres.

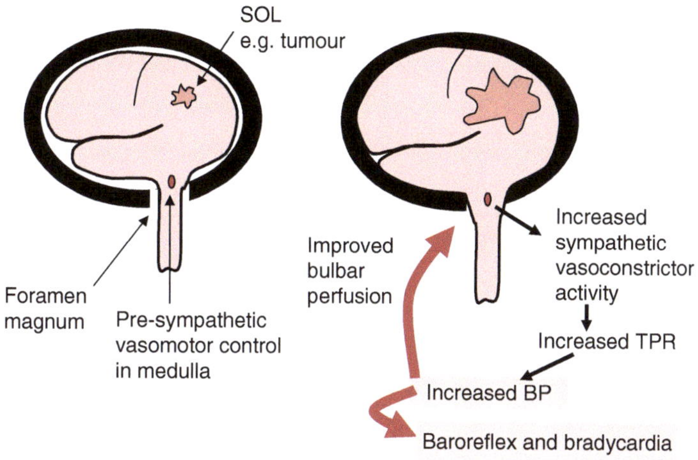

Figure 8.17 Bulbar ischaemia can result from herniation of the brainstem through the foramen magnum as a space-occupying lesion (SOL) expands within the cranium. This triggers increased sympathetic outflow, raising blood pressure to preserve brainstem perfusion. The hypertension elicits a baroreflex bradycardia (Cushing's reflex).

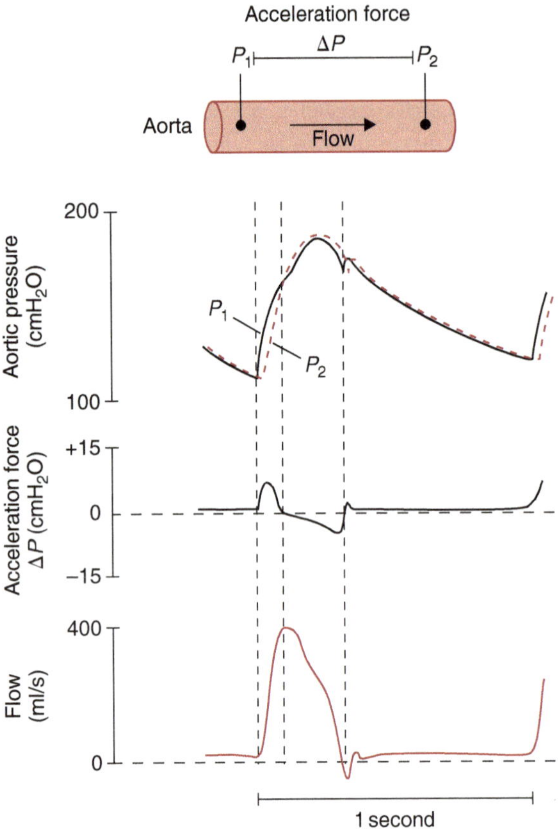

Figure 8.18 Flow, acceleration and pressure gradients in the human ascending aorta. The pressure difference ΔP at first accelerates flow along the aorta, then reverses and decelerates flow until a brief backflow closes the aortic valve. Proximal aortic flow is almost zero during diastole.

Poiseuille's law – what governs resistance?

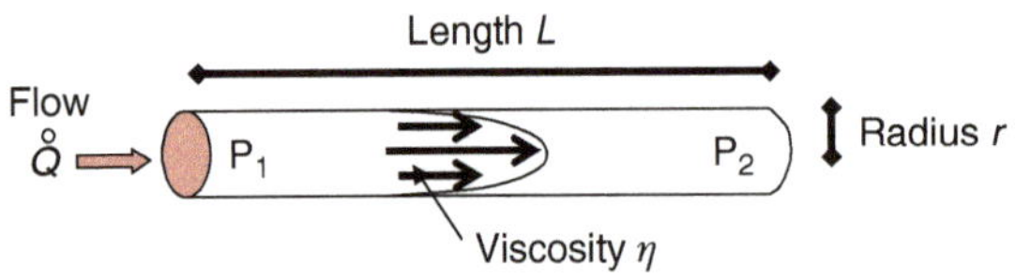

For laminar flow down a tube of radius r,

$$\mathring{Q} = (P_1 - P_2)\,\frac{\pi r^4}{8\eta L}$$

Since flow equal pressure drop $(P_1 - P_2)$ divided by resistance,

$$\text{Resistance } R = \frac{8\eta L}{\pi r^4}$$

Resistance depends on-

- radius r^4
- viscosity η
- length L

Figure 8.19 Poiseuille's law describes laminar flow along a cylindrical tube, and the factors that govern the resistance to flow.

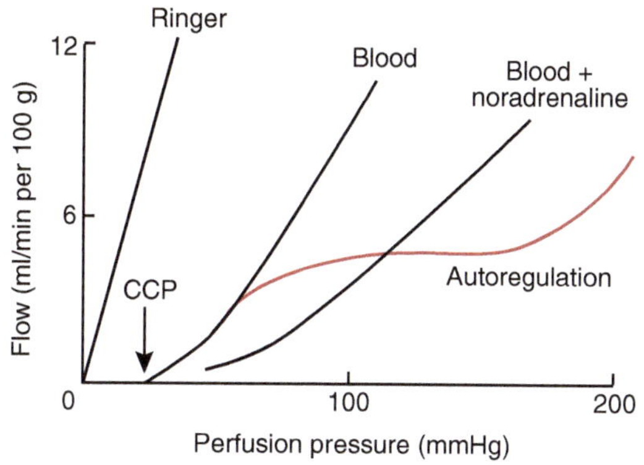

Figure 8.20 Pressure–flow curves in perfused muscle. 'Autoregulation' curve applies under physiological conditions, because arterioles respond myogenically to pressure changes. 'Blood' curve is observed if autoregulation is abolished. 'Blood + noradrenaline' curve is less steep (lower conductance), because noradrenaline causes vasoconstriction, which raises vascular resistance. 'Ringer' line; perfusion with a saline solution; relation is steeper, because low viscosity reduces resistance to flow (Poiseuille's law).

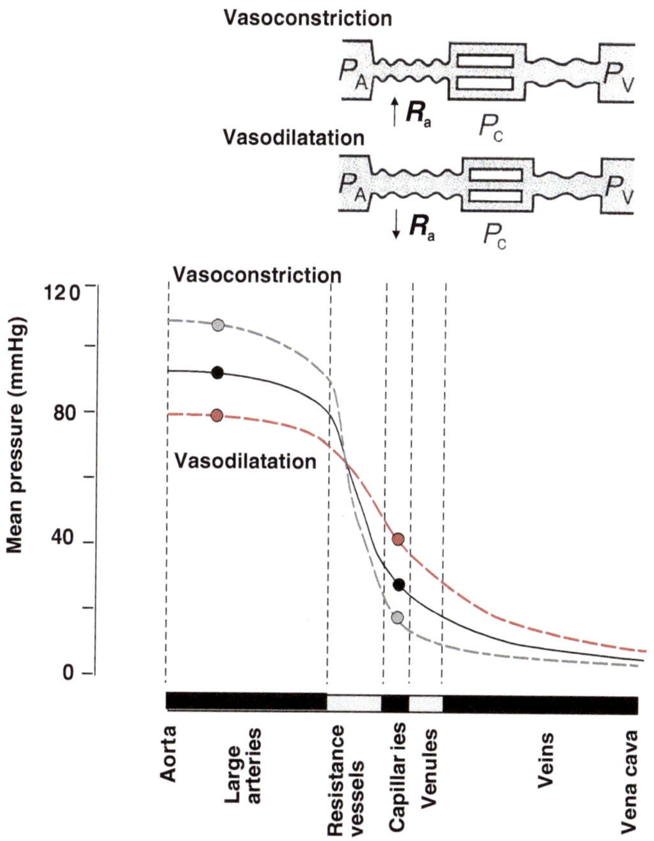

Figure 8.21 Changes in pressure distribution across the circulation caused by widespread vasoconstriction/vasodilatation of resistance vessels (terminal arteries and arterioles, resistance R_a). Vasoconstriction raises arterial pressure (P_A), at a given cardiac output, because blood escapes less easily from the upstream arteries through the raised downstream resistance. Vasoconstriction also reduces capillary pressure P_C, because more pressure is lost as blood traverses the raised precapillary resistance R_a; less pressure 'gets through'. Conversely, a widespread vasodilatation tends to lower arterial pressure and raise capillary pressure.

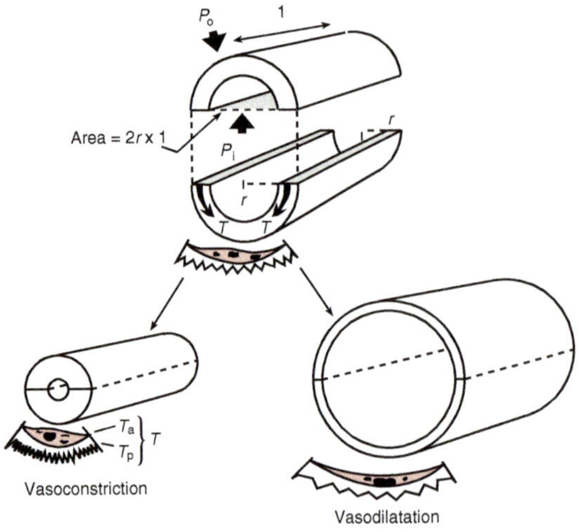

Figure 8.22 Laplace wall mechanics in a tube. (*Upper panel*) The distending pressure (internal pressure P_i minus external pressure P_o) is countered by the wall tension T on each side of the cylinder. $T = (P_i - P_o)r$ (Laplace's law). (*Lower panels*) Tension T is the sum of active tension in smooth muscle, T_a, and passive tension in elastin/collagen fibres, T_p, shown as a spring. The spring on the left is in its relaxed state and that on the right is stretched and tense. T_a and T_p change in opposite directions during vasoconstriction to achieve mechanical stability.

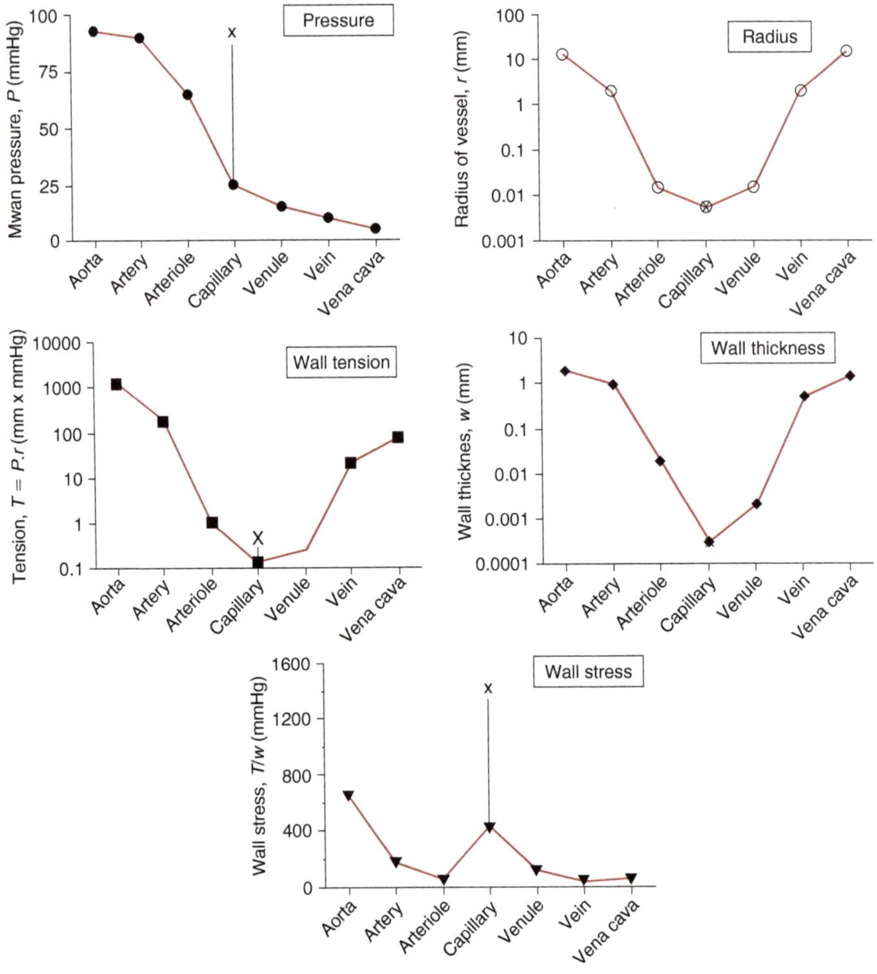

Figure 8.23 Pressure, radius, wall tension and stress in different categories of blood vessel at heart level (Laplace's law). Vessel wall thickness affects stress, which is tension/thickness. Crosses represent capillaries in foot during quiet standing, when gravity raises capillary pressure to ~90 mmHg.

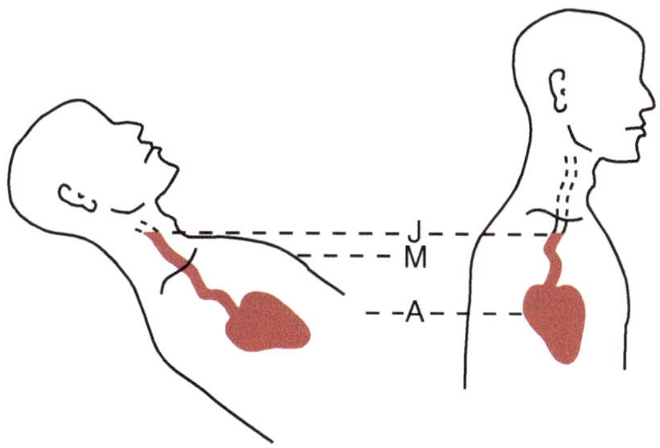

Figure 8.24 Central venous pressure (CVP) is vena cava blood pressure at junction with the right atrium. It equals the vertical distance J–A, between the point of collapse of the jugular vein (J, venous blood at atmospheric pressure) and right atrium (A). Since A is not visible, the vertical height of J above the manubriosternal angle (M) is measured in cm, and an average vertical distance M − A (~5 cm) is added on. Thus CVP = (J − M) cm + 5 cm, in cm blood (almost same as cmH_2O). In the upright position, the entire jugular vein is normally collapsed, so is not visible.

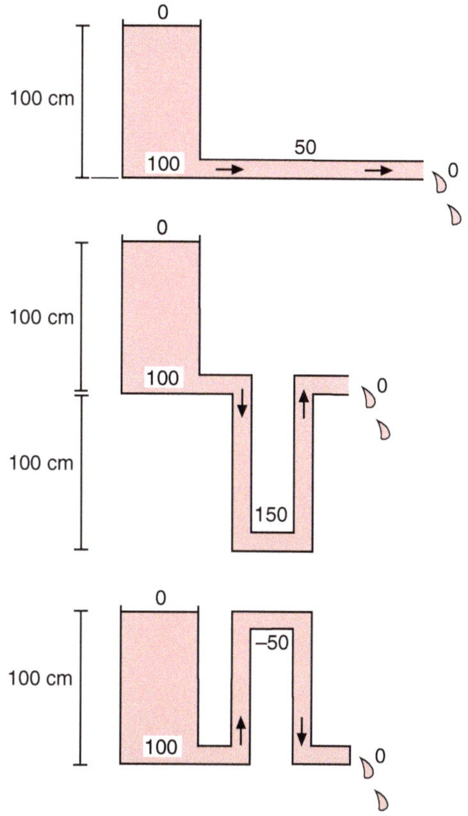

Figure 8.25 The siphon principle. The pressure head in the feed-tank, 100 cmH_2O, drives the flow. Pressure is 50 cmH_2O halfway along the tube when horizontal. If the tube is bent into a U shape, the pressure difference driving flow from tank to outlet is the same, so the flow is identical – irrespective of which way up the U tube is. Only the intermediate pressures are changed (numbers, cmH_2O). The middle sketch is equivalent to the situation in the leg vasculature during standing.

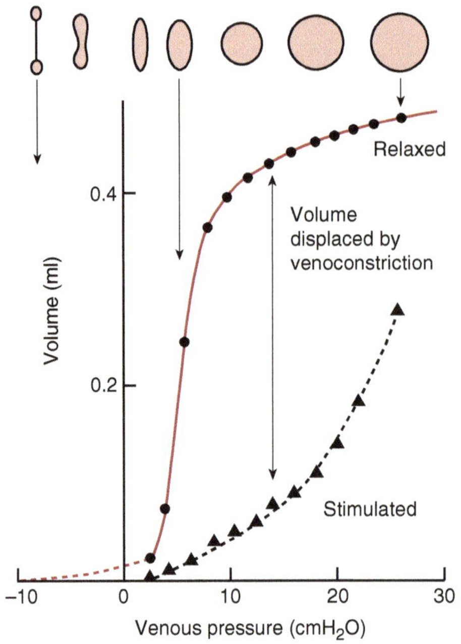

Figure 8.26 Venous pressure–volume curves, when veins are relaxed (circles) or maximally venoconstricted (triangles). Change in venous cross section with pressure in relaxed state shown above.

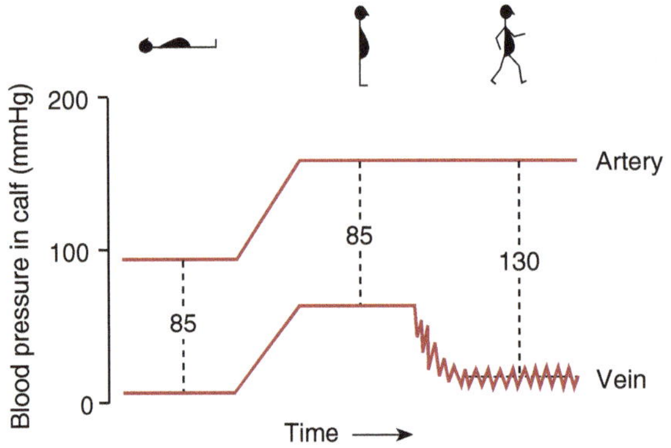

Figure 8.27 Effect of standing and walking (calf muscle pump) on the pressure gradient driving blood through the lower leg.

CHAPTER 9

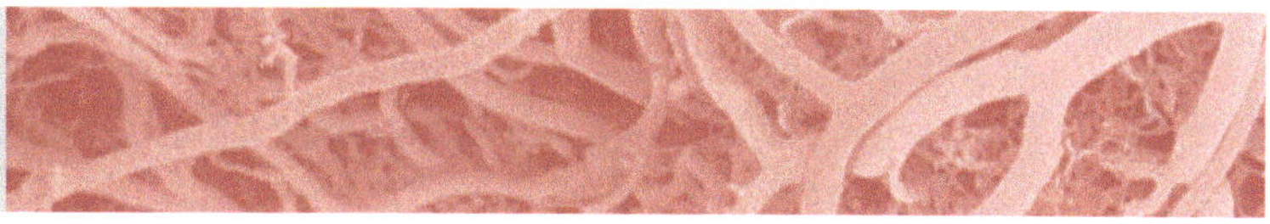

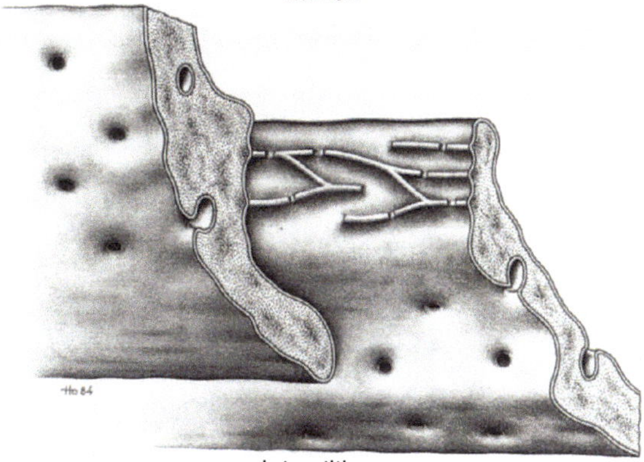

Figure 9.1 Three-dimensional structure of capillary intercellular cleft. Water and small lipophobic solutes follow the tortuous pathway through the breaks in the junctional strands.

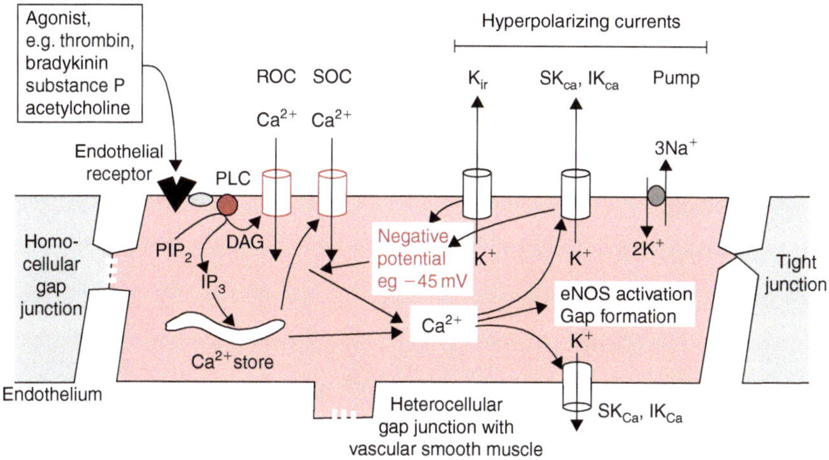

Figure 9.2 Endothelial electrophysiology and Ca^{2+} regulation. eNOS, endothelial nitric oxide synthase; IK_{Ca}, SK_{Ca} intermediate and small conductance calcium-activated potassium channels; K_{ir}, inward rectifying K^+ channel; PIP_2, phosphatidyl inositol bisphosphate (an inner membrane phospholipid); PLC, phospholipase in membrane, linked by G protein (grey) to agonist receptor; ROC, receptor operated Ca^{2+} channel; SOC, store operated Ca^{2+} channels.

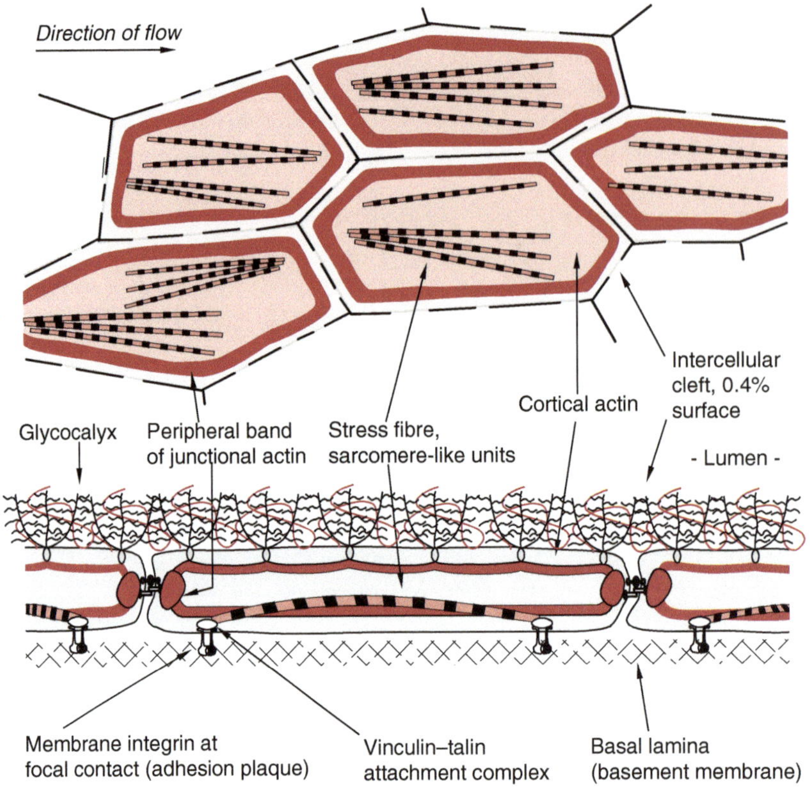

Figure 9.3 Organization of endothelial cytoskeleton and intercellular junctions, viewed *en face* (*top*) and in cross section (*bottom*). Black intercellular lines *en face* represent sealed section of cleft (~90%); the grey lines are the open, permeable parts of the cleft, at breaks in the junctional strands. Glycocalyx molecules form hairy tufts attached to cell membrane and linked to the cortical actin cytoskeleton at ~100 nm intervals.

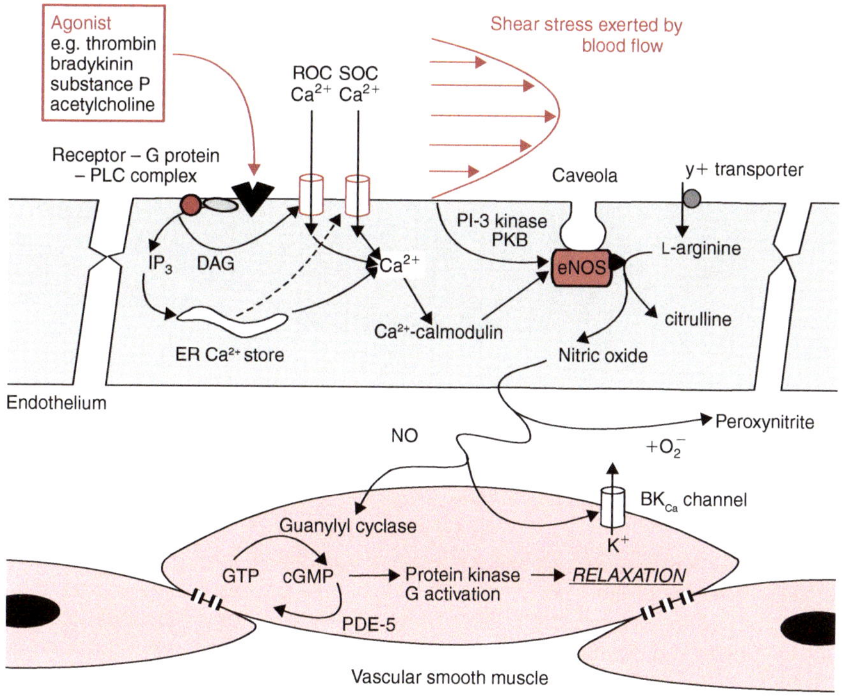

Figure 9.4 Regulation of NO production and its effect on neighbouring vascular smooth muscle. *Key* as for Figure 9.2; eNOS endothelial nitric oxide synthase; ER endoplasmic reticulum; PDE-5 phosphodiesterase 5 (inhibited by sildenafil, Viagra); PI-3 kinase, phosphatidyl inositol-3 kinase; PKB protein kinase B (akt).

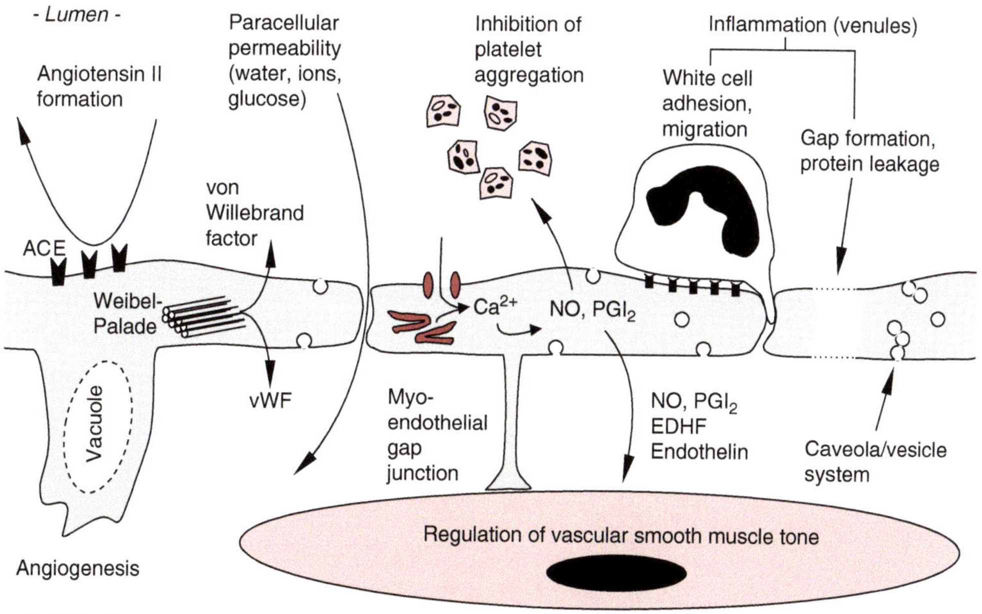

Figure 9.5 Multiple functions of endothelial cell; lumen is at top. NO, nitric oxide; PGI_2, prostacyclin; EDHF, endothelium-derived hyperpolarizing factor; ACE, angiotensin I-converting enzyme; vWF, von Willebrand haemostatic factor.

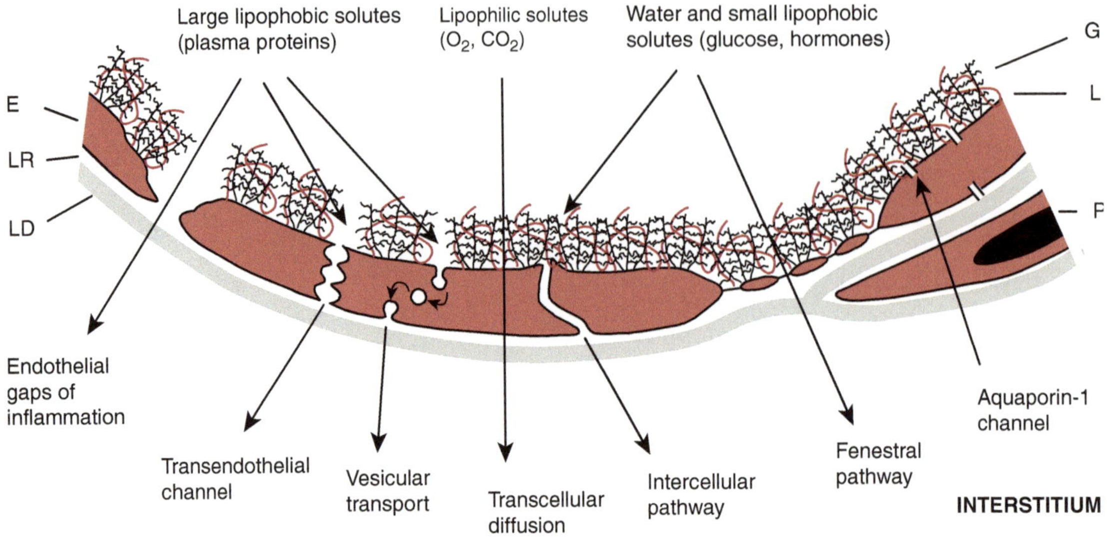

Figure 9.6 Transport pathways across a capillary. Water flows mainly through the small pore system, i.e. glycocalyx overlying intercellular clefts and fenestrae. Only a little passes through membrane aquaporin-1 channels or the scanty large pore system. Note large gap and break in glycocalyx in inflammation. E, endothelium; G, glycocalyx; L, lipid plasma membrane; LR and LD, lamina rara and lamina densa of basement membrane, respectively; P, pericyte.

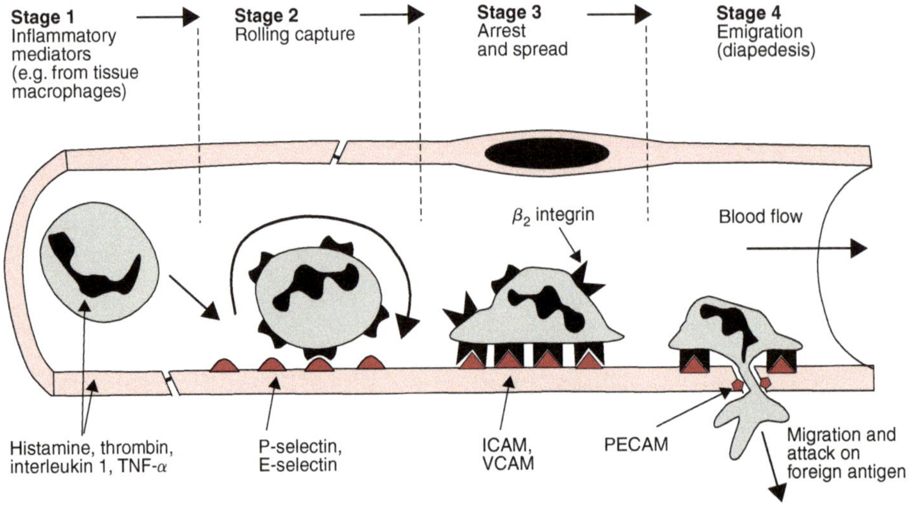

Figure 9.7 Rolling capture, arrest and extravasation of leukocyte during the inflammatory response. TNF-α, tumour necrosis factor α.

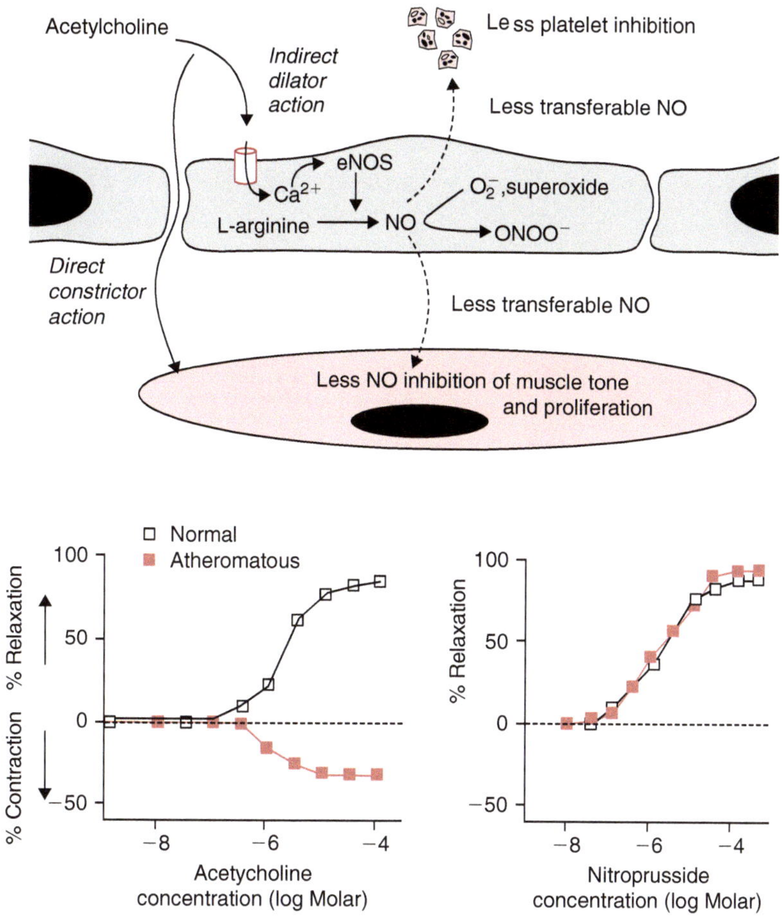

Figure 9.8 Reduced NO availability in atheromatous arteries. Response of normal (open circles) and atheromatous iliac artery (filled circles) of monkey to acetylcholine (*bottom left*) or the NO donor nitroprusside (*bottom right*). The NO-dependent vasodilator response to acetylcholine becomes a constrictor response in atheromatous arteries. Sketch shows explanation – a fall in transferable NO due to high levels of endothelial superoxide radicals in atheromatous vessels.

CHAPTER 10

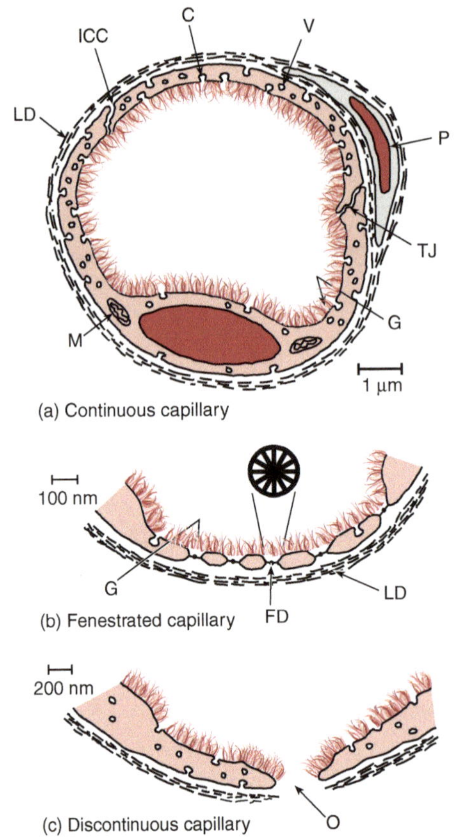

Figure 10.1 Capillary wall in transverse section. C, caveola (open surface vesicle); FD, fenestral diaphragm; inset shows diaphragm *en face*; G, glycocalyx; ICC, intercellular cleft; LD, lamina densa of basal lamina; M, mitochondrion; O, open gap; P, pericyte; TJ, tight part of intercellular junction; V, vesicle.

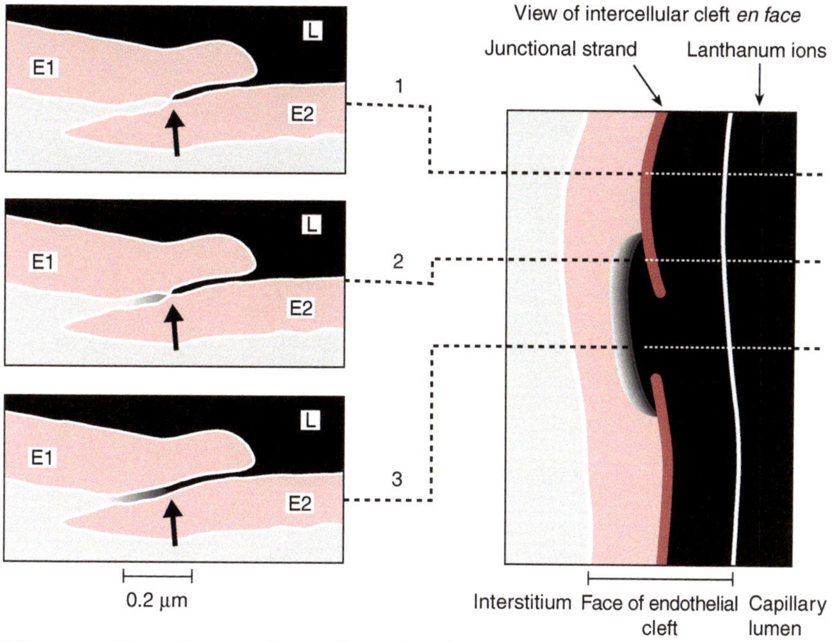

Figure 10.2 Three sections along an intercellular cleft (left). The capillary was perfused with a solution of lanthanum ions (black). The cleft is viewed *en face* on the right. The tight junction (red lines on right, arrows on left) blocks the cleft in Section 1, but a break in the junctional strands creates an open pathway in Section 3. L, lumen; E1 and E2, endothelial cells.

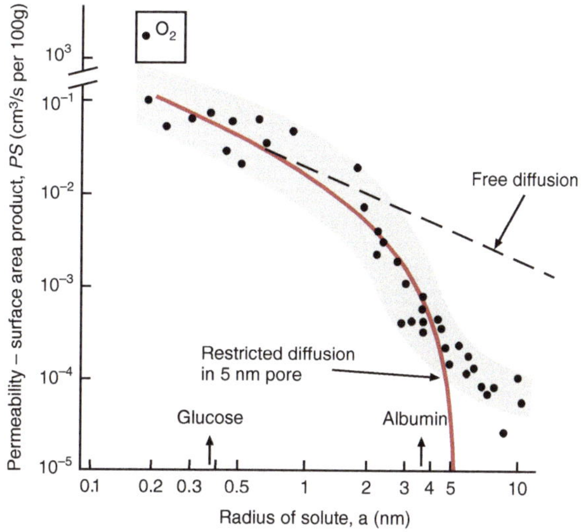

Figure 10.3 Effect of solute radius on capillary permeability. Except for O_2, the points denote lipophobic solutes. Dashed line of slope −1 shows effect of fall in free diffusion coefficient with increasing molecular size. Red line shows predicted fall in permeability for cylindrical pores of radius 5 nm. The low, persistent permeability to solutes larger than albumin is due to a small number of larger pores or vesicular transport.

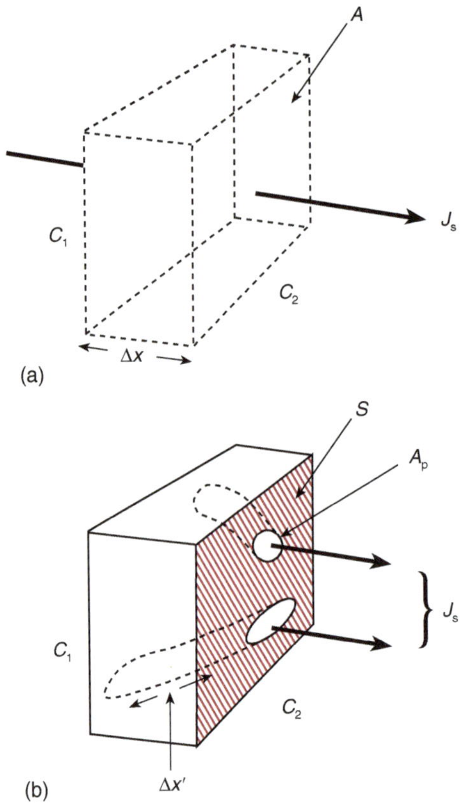

Figure 10.4 (a) Free diffusion in bulk solution. The solute diffuses through an unimpeded layer of fluid of thickness Δx and surface area A, driven by concentration difference ($C_1 - C_2$). J_s is the diffusion rate (mole/s). (b) A porous membrane reduces J_s by confining the solute to pores of total area A_p. The pore pathlength $\Delta x'$ is usually greater than the membrane thickness Δx.

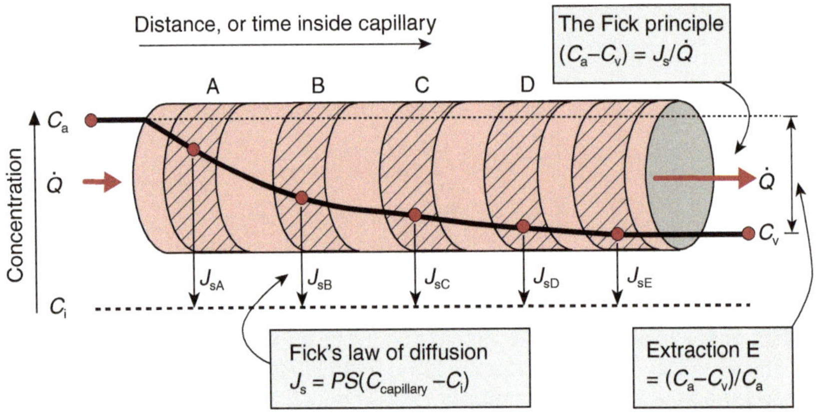

Figure 10.5 Concentration of a rapidly diffusing solute falls non-linearly along a capillary, from arterial concentration C_a to venous concentration C_V. Black arrows indicate size of diffusional fluxes J_s. PS, permeability–surface area product; $\dot{Q}$, blood flow. The concentration profile is exponential, if the interstitial concentration C_i is zero or uniform. The mean intracapillary concentration is less than (arterial + venous)/2.

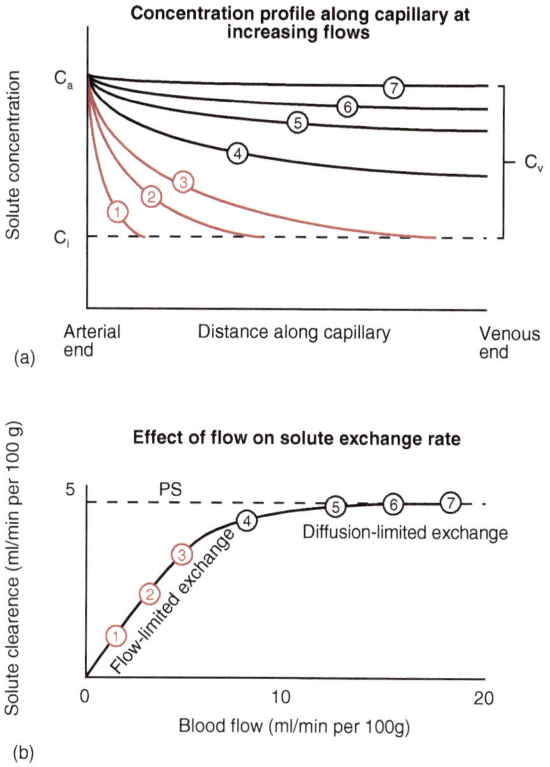

Figure 10.6 Effect of blood flow on diffusive transport across capillary wall. (a) Decay of plasma concentration along capillary at low to high blood flows (curves 1–7), for a constant or zero pericapillary concentration C_i. C_a, C_v, arterial and venous concentrations. Slow transits allow time for equilibration ($C_v = C_i$) before the end of the capillary (curves 1–3). This is flow-limited exchange. With fast transits, there is not enough time for equilibration, so C_v is $>C_i$ (curves 5–7). This is diffusion-limited exchange. (b) Resulting effect of blood flow on transcapillary exchange, expressed as plasma clearance (solute flux/C_a). Plateau clearance value equals the capillary diffusion capacity, *PS*.

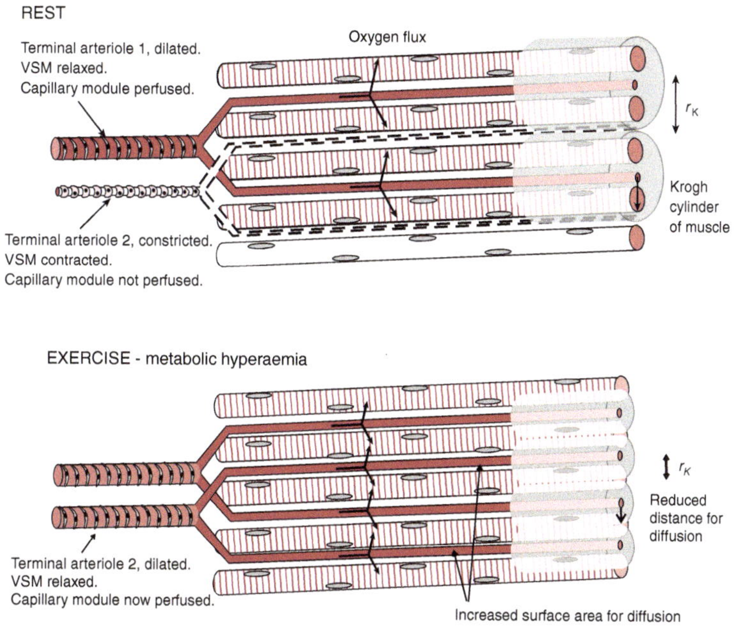

Figure 10.7 The Krogh muscle cylinder and capillary recruitment. In resting skeletal muscle, contraction of terminal arteriole 2 arrests the perfusion of some capillaries (dashed lines). Each perfused capillary therefore has to supply a broad cylinder of muscle (Krogh cylinder). The radius of the Krogh cylinder, r_K, is the maximum diffusion distance. During exercise, metabolic vasodilatation dilates terminal arteriole 2, so the previously closed-off capillaries are now perfused. This improves the homogeneity of O_2 supply, increases the perfused capillary surface area, reduces the radius of each Krogh cylinder, and thus reduces the maximum diffusion distance r_K.

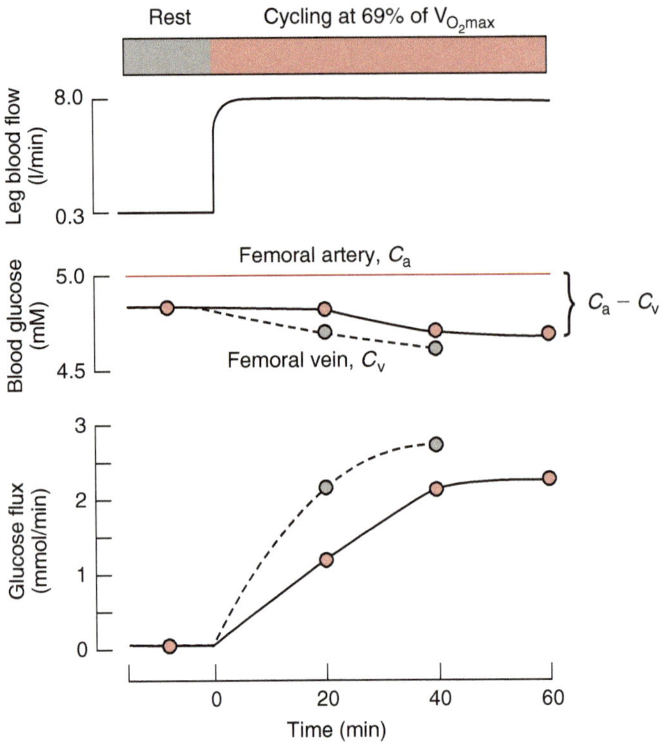

Figure 10.8 Increase in glucose flux from blood to leg muscles during cycling. At first the muscle utilizes both stored glycogen and extracted glucose. As the glycogen store is depleted, blood glucose extraction $(C_a - C_v)/C_a$ increases. When muscle glycogen was depleted prior to exercise, glucose extraction is increased (dashed lines with grey circles).

CHAPTER 11

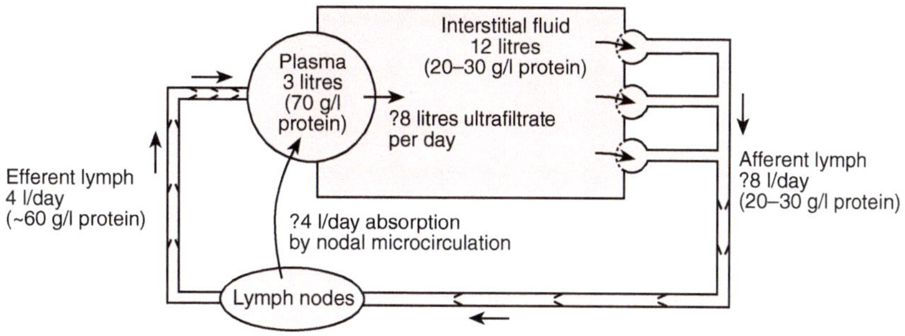

Figure 11.1 Estimated circulation of fluid between plasma, interstitial compartment and lymph in a 65 kg human.

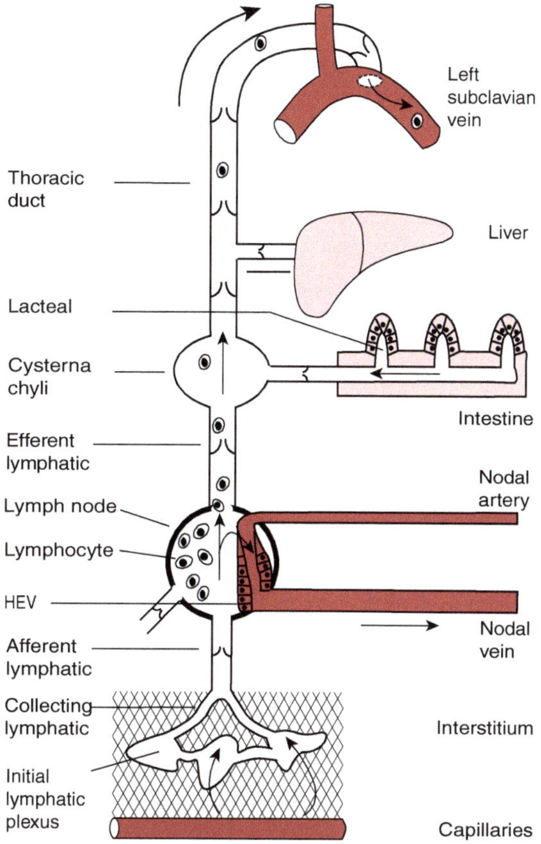

Figure 11.2 The lymphatic system. Curved arrow within node indicates absorption of some of the fluid by nodal capillaries. HEV, high endothelial venule, where circulating lymphocytes re-enter the node.

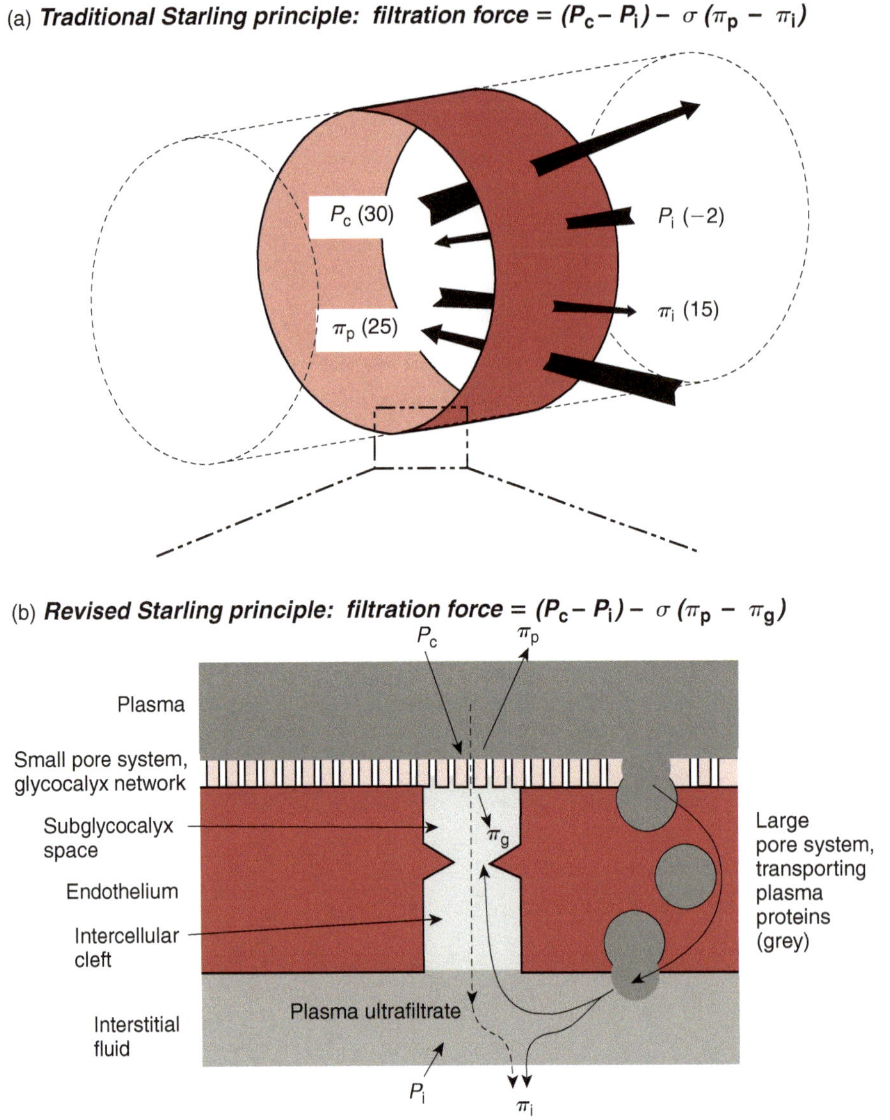

Figure 11.3 (a) Four classic Starling pressures influencing fluid exchange (mmHg, human skin, heart level). P_c, capillary blood pressure P_i, interstitial fluid pressure. π_p, plasma colloid osmotic pressure (COP). π_i, interstitial fluid COP. Pressures are relative to atmospheric pressure (760 mmHg), so $P_i = -2$ mmHg means an absolute pressure of 758 mmHg – hence arrow direction. (b) Cross section of intercellular cleft to show gradient of extravascular plasma protein extending into subglycocalyx space (COP is π_g); concentration indicated by shade of grey. Gradient is result of battle between upstream diffusion of extravascular plasma protein (solid curves) and its washout by plasma ultrafiltrate emerging from the glycocalyx small pore system (dashed line).

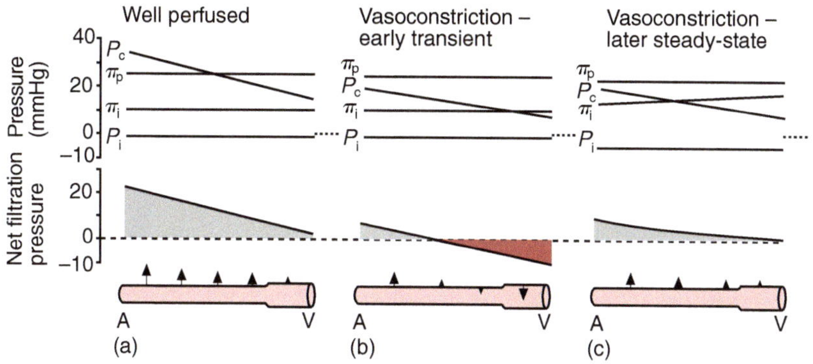

Figure 11.4 Capillary pressure gradients from arterial end of capillary (A) to venule (V). Shaded region shows sum of four classic Starling pressures, $(P_c - P_i) - \sigma(\pi_p - \pi_i)$, as measured in skin, muscle and mesentery at heart level. Arrows show fluid flux inferred from Starling forces. A broadly similar pattern is predicted when differences between π_i and π_g are taken into account. (a) Net filtration along entire length of a well-perfused capillary. Note that neglect of measured π_i and P_i would lead to the spurious prediction of absorption in downstream half of capillary. (b) Transient absorptive force immediately after a haemorrhage and/or arteriolar constriction, which lower P_c. (c) Disappearance of absorptive force with time, due to progressive rise in π_i and π_g and fall in P_i.

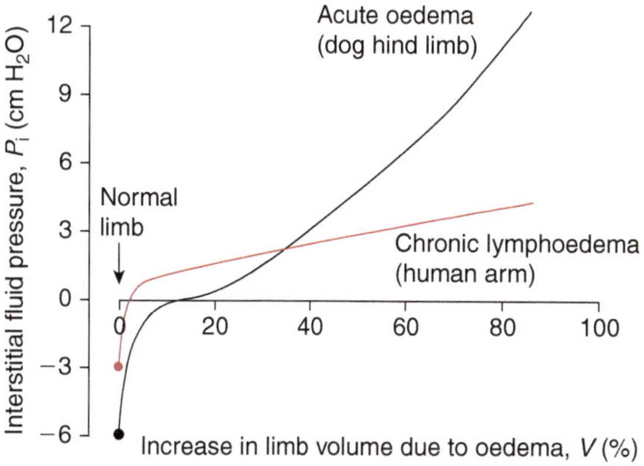

Figure 11.5 The interstitial compliance curve of limb subcutis. The steeper relation occurred in dog hind limbs made acutely oedematous by intravenous saline infusion. Pressure gradually declines with time, for a given degree of swelling ('creep'). Consequently, in the chronically swollen human arm (lymphoedema caused by breast cancer surgery) the interstitial compliance curve is flatter.

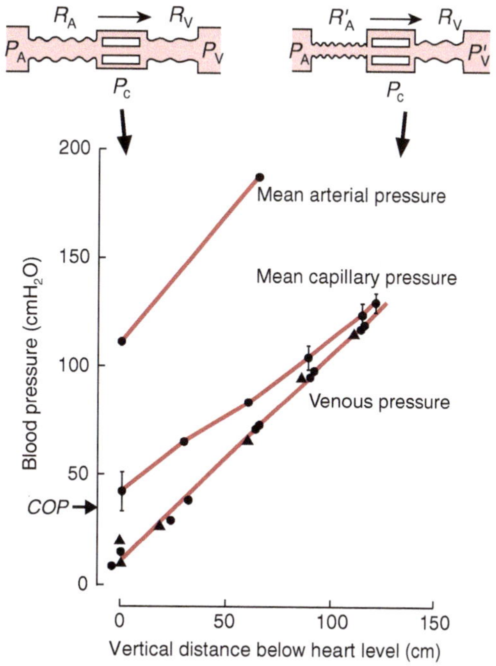

Figure 11.6 Capillary blood pressure in skin of human foot at various distances below heart level. Popliteal artery pressure and dorsal foot vein pressure increase with distance below heart level due to gravity. Capillary pressure increases less than expected. *Top insets* show how the rise in capillary pressure is attenuated by the vasoconstrictor 'veni-arteriolar response', which raises the pre- to postcapillary resistance ratio R_A/R_V.

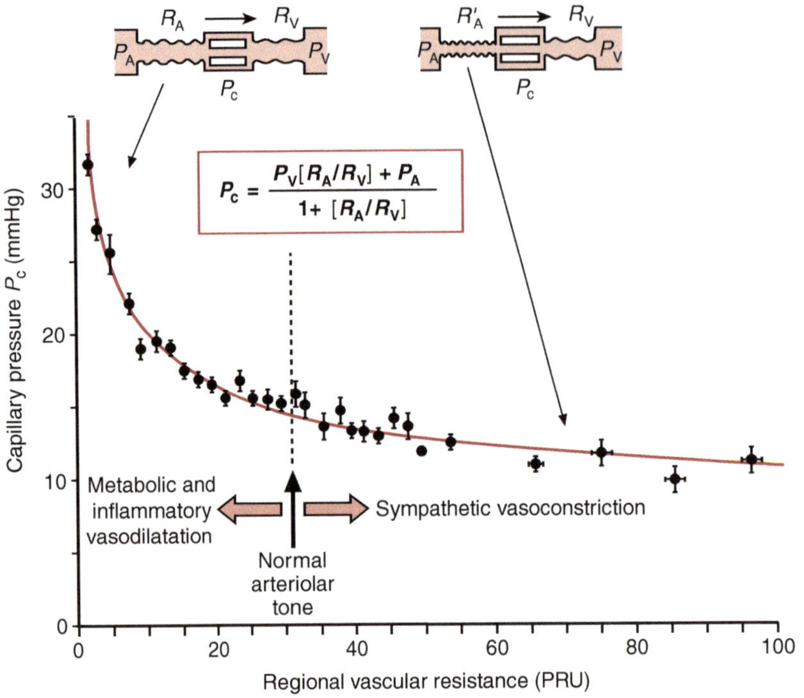

Figure 11.7 Control of capillary pressure P_c by precapillary resistance R_A, relative to postcapillary resistance R_V.

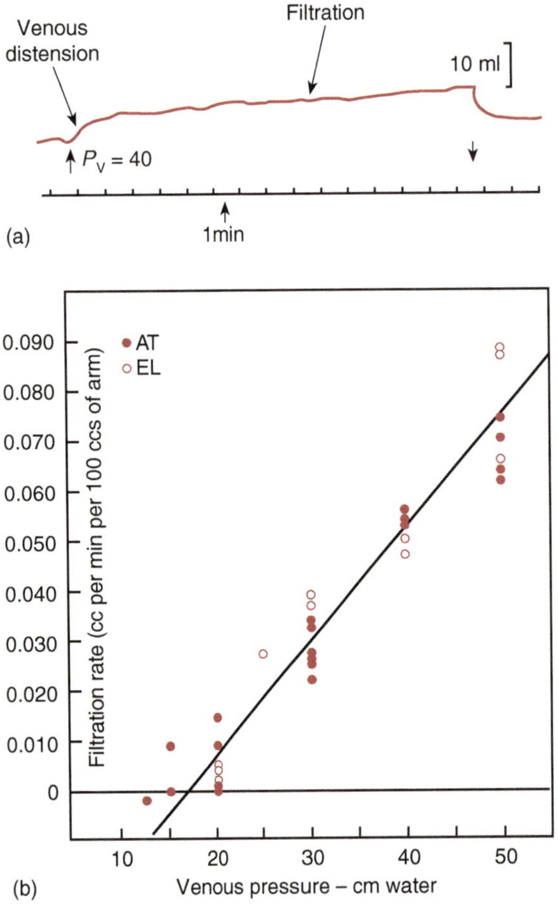

Figure 11.8 Effect of venous pressure on capillary filtration into the human forearm. (a) Inflation of venous congesting cuff around upper arm raises forearm volume (*top trace*). After the initial phase of venous distension (~2 min), the slow swelling is caused by capillary filtration. (b) Capillary filtration rate as a function of venous pressure.

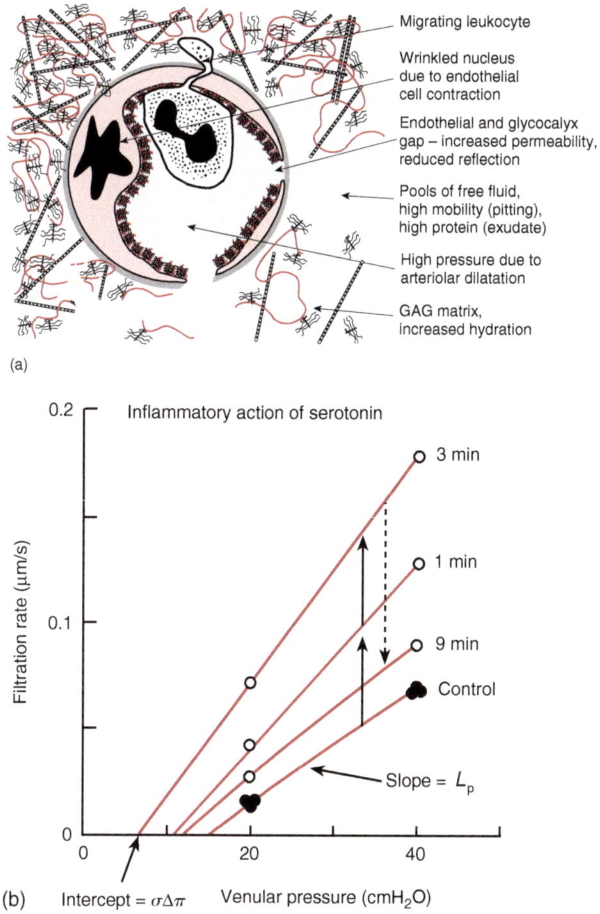

Figure 11.9 (a) Gap formation, oedema and leukocyte migration in acutely inflamed, postcapillary venule. (b) Effect of an inflammatory agonist, serotonin, on permeability of a single venule (rat). Hydraulic permeability increases (slope, *L*p) and osmotic reflection coefficient decreases (intercept at zero filtration, $\sigma\Delta\pi$).

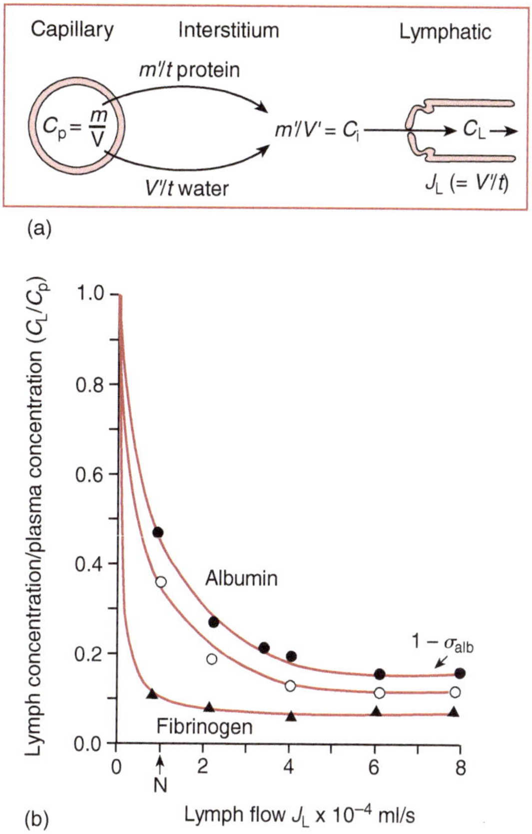

Figure 11.10 Effect of capillary filtration on interstitial plasma protein concentration. *(a)* Mass of protein entering the interstitium in a given time (m'/t or J_s) is diluted by the volume of filtrate produced over the same time interval (V'/t or J_v); so interstitial protein concentration $C_i = J_s/J_v$. Prenodal lymph protein concentration is same as interstitial protein concentration. *(b)* Effect of filtration rate (recorded as lymph flow J_L) on lymph/plasma concentration ratio, C_L/C_p. *N* is normal value (dog paw). At high flows C_L/C_p reaches its lowest possible value, the transmitted fraction 1-σ (σ is the capillary reflection coefficient).

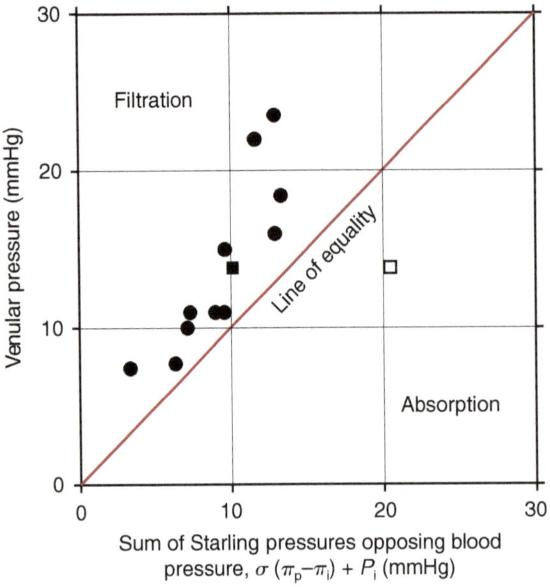

Figure 11.11 Comparison of venular blood pressure and the net pro-absorption Starling pressures in 12 tissues, showing a small net filtration force even in the venules. When differences between π_i and π_g are taken into account, the net filtration force is even smaller. Tissues range from lung (lowest left point) to mesentery (highest right point). Unfilled square is absorbing intestinal mucosal capillaries after drinking water.

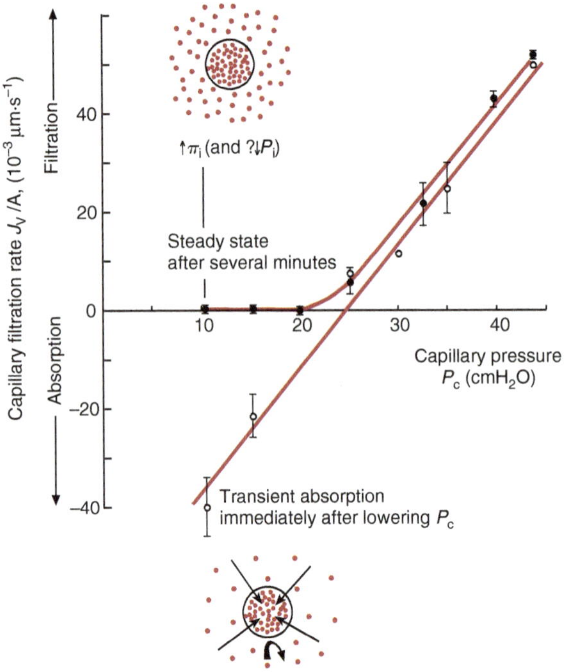

Figure 11.12 Experiment showing that lowering capillary pressure below plasma COP (32 cmH_2O here) causes a transient but not sustained fluid absorption. *Lower inset* shows extravascular plasma protein (dots) reflected by capillary wall during transient phase of water absorption (long arrows). This raises extravascular protein concentration (*upper sketch*).

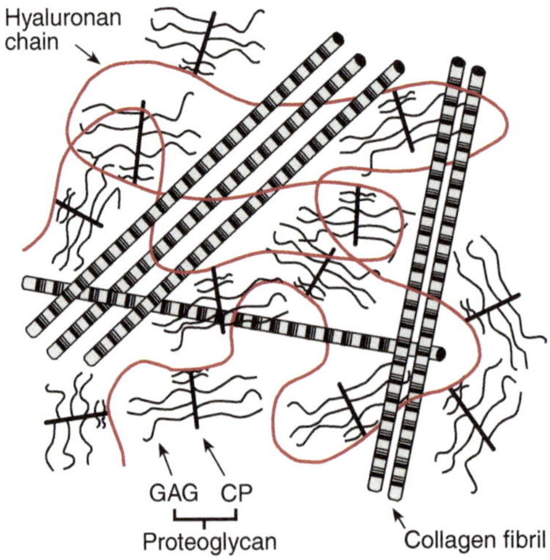

Figure 11.13 Interstitial matrix is a network of fibrous biopolymers; interstitial fluid occupies the tiny spaces between the chains. GAG, sulphated glycosaminoglycan chains, namely chondroitin sulphate and keratan sulphate; CP, core protein of proteoglycan.

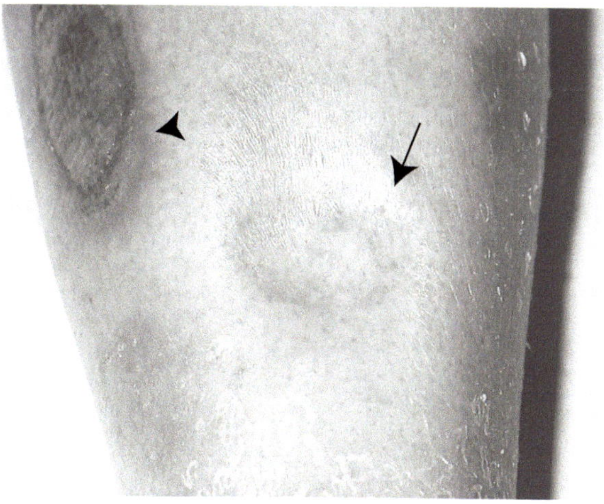

Figure 11.14 Human calf showing pitting oedema (arrow) in a patient with cardiac failure. The skin damage (arrowhead, top left) was caused by an oedema blister.

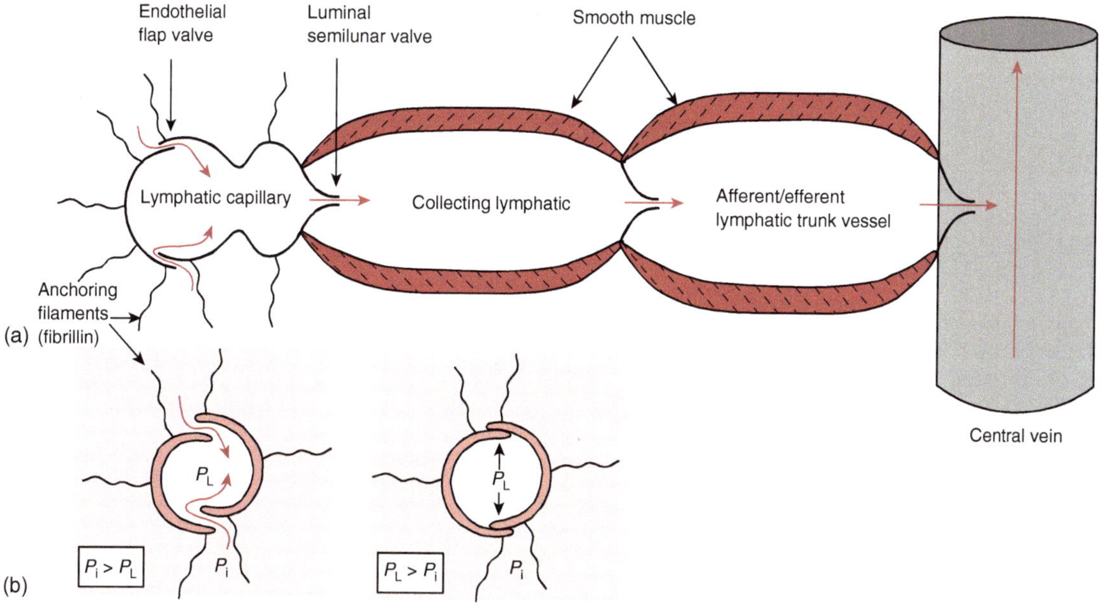

Figure 11.15 Lymphatic transport mechanisms. (a) Interstitial fluid enters the initial lymphatic through the intercellular cleft flap valves down a pressure gradient. Each muscular segment then pumps lymph into the next segment and ultimately into the venous system. (b) Proposed operation of initial lymphatic endothelial junctions as flap valves. P_i, interstitial pressure; P_L, lymph pressure.

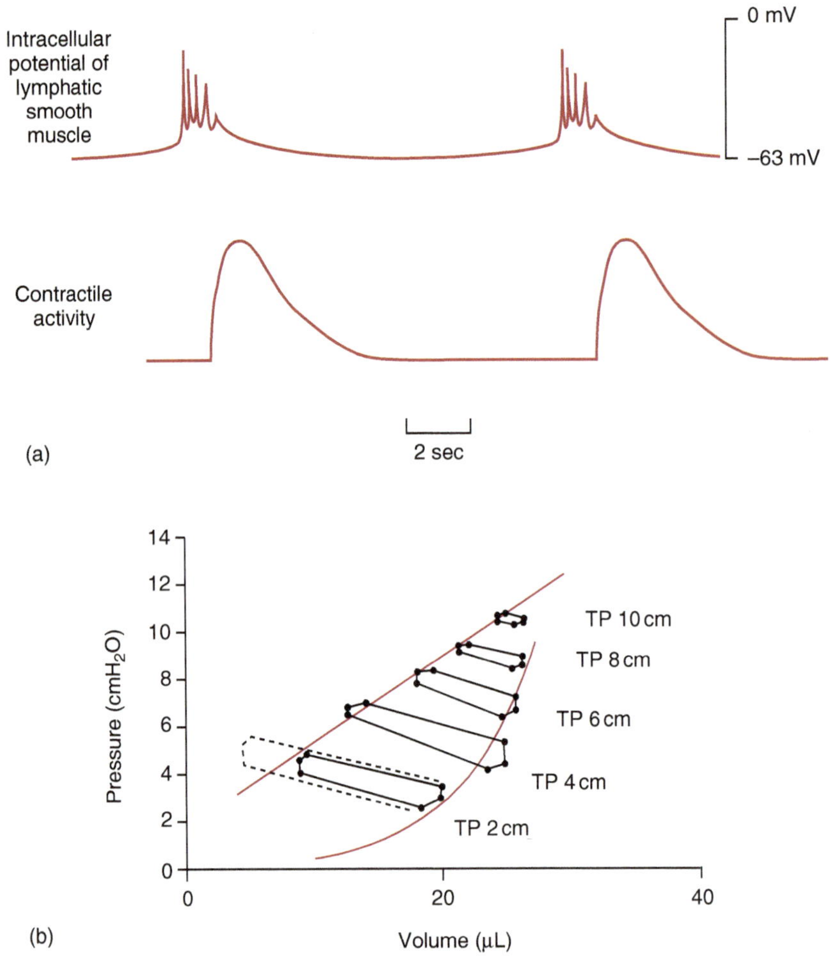

Figure 11.16 Electrical and contractile properties of lymphatic smooth muscle. (a) Periodic depolarization triggers action potentials and contraction in a bovine lymphatic. (b) Pressure–volume cycle of contracting sheep mesenteric lymphatic vessels at various diastolic distensions (TP, transmural pressure). Dashed loop shows increased contractility and ejection fraction after a haemorrhage.

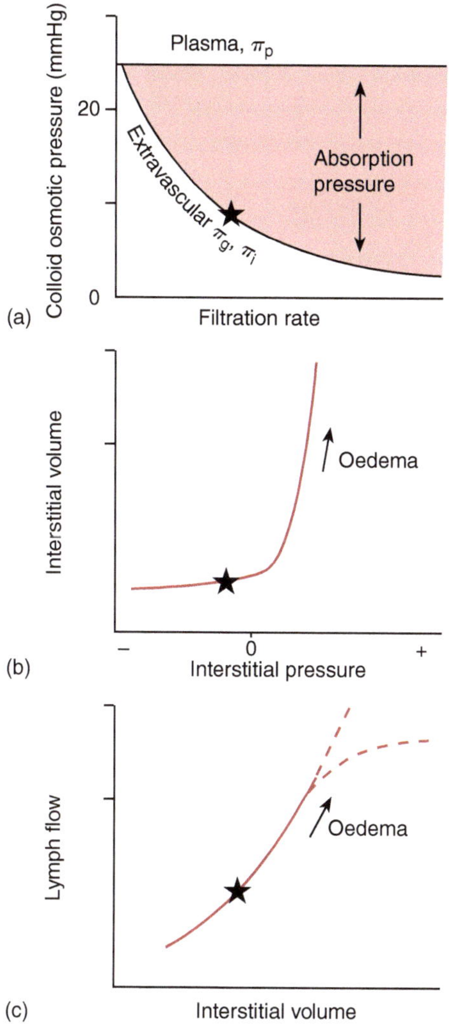

Figure 11.17 Three safety factors against oedema. Stars indicate normal state. (a) When capillary filtration rate increases, the COP difference opposing filtration ($\pi_p - \pi_g$) increases, because extravascular plasma protein concentration falls in the interstitial and subglycocalyx compartments. (b) Interstitial fluid pressure changes markedly with hydration in normal subcutis; this is Figure 11.5 turned on its side. Once oedema develops, however, interstitial compliance becomes very large, so there is little further rise in pressure to prevent fluid accumulation. (c) Lymphatic drainage rate increases with increasing interstitial hydration, thereby opposing oedema formation.

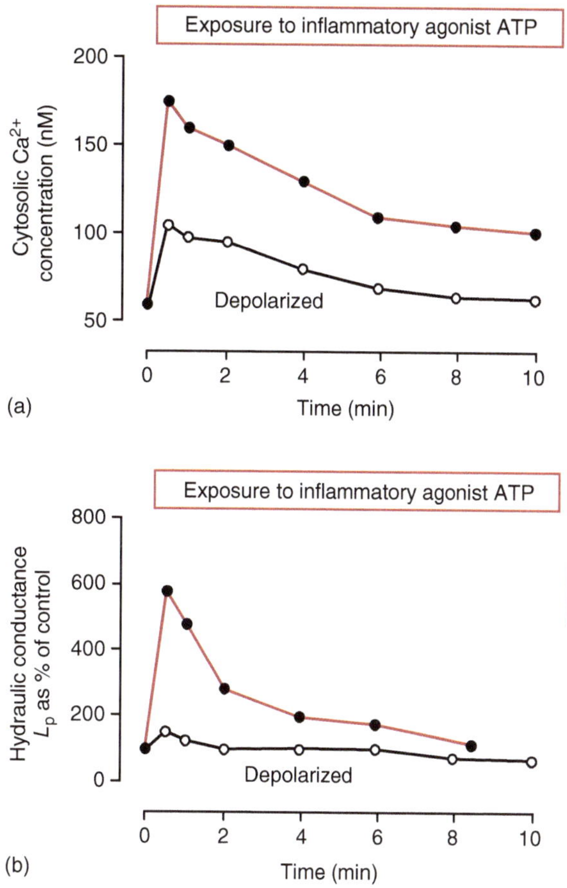

Figure 11.18 Parallel changes in free cytosolic Ca^{2+} (a) and hydraulic permeability (b) during the inflammatory response of frog venule to inflammatory agonist ATP. ATP was used because frogs do not respond to mammalian agonists such as histamine. Endothelial depolarization by a high K^+ solution (open symbols) reduced the Ca^{2+} transient and hence the hydraulic conductance change.

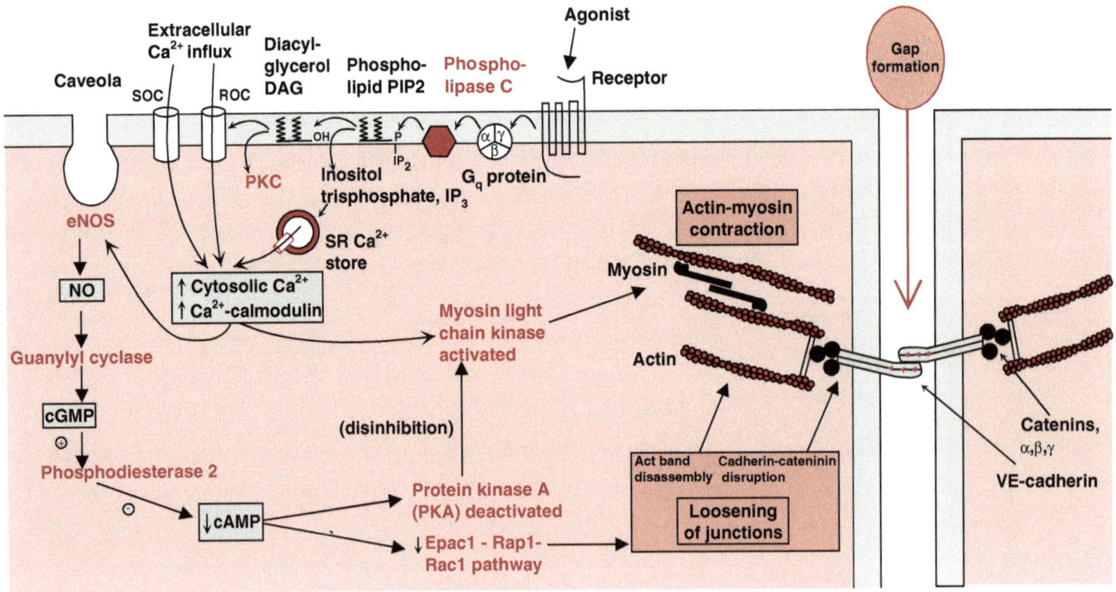

Figure 11.19 Signal transduction cascade implicated in endothelial gap formation during inflammation. Major second messengers are in grey boxes, enzymes in red. PIP_2, phosphatidyl inositol bisphosphate. PKC, protein kinase C – this activates a MAP kinase cascade implicated in some inflammatory responses. Epac, exchange protein activated by cAMP.

CHAPTER 12

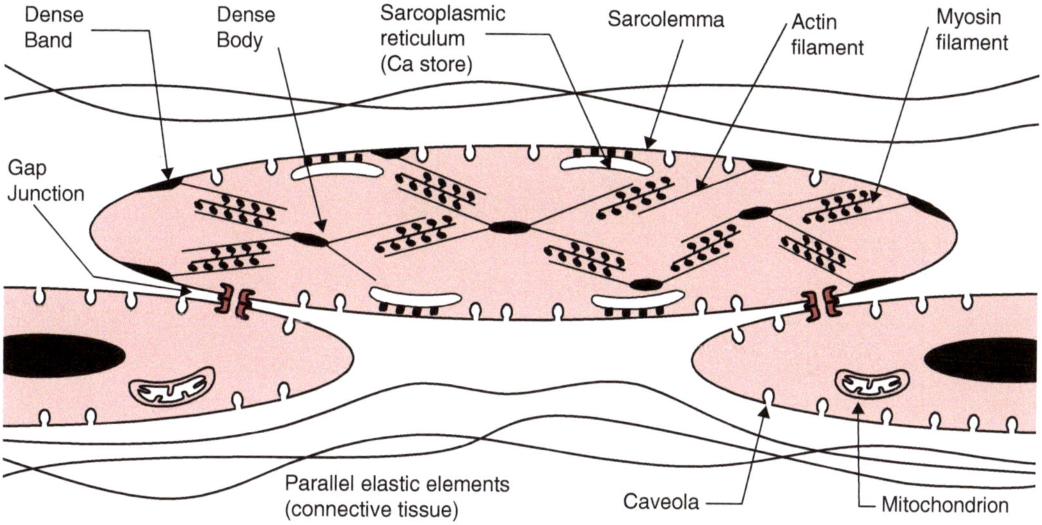

Figure 12.1 Vascular myocyte structure.

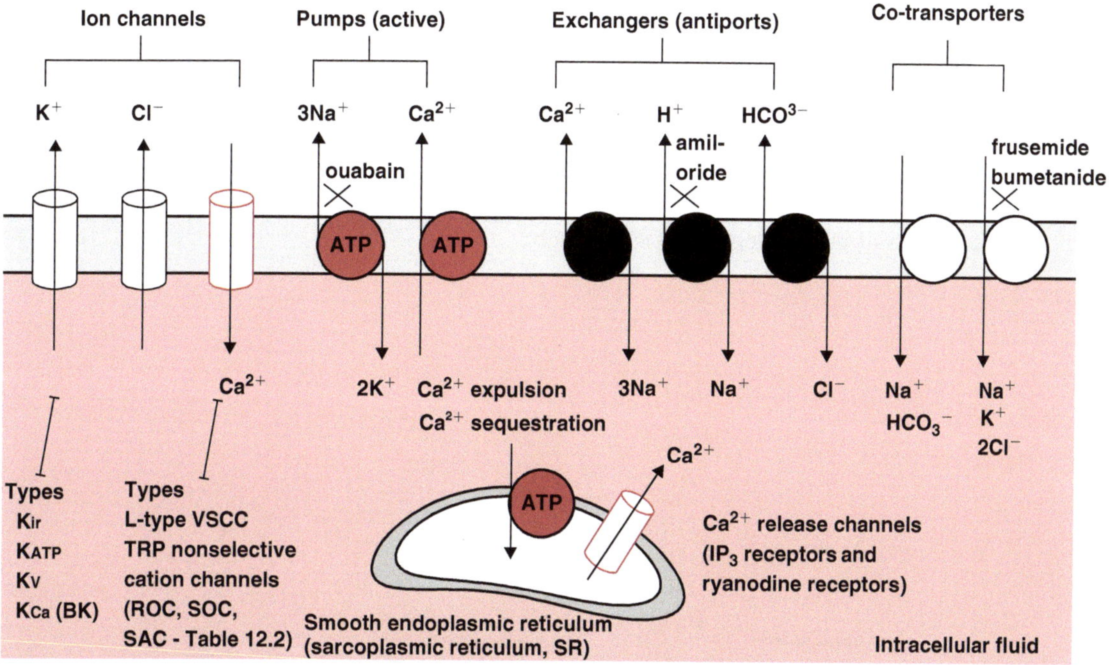

Figure 12.2 Ion channels and transporters in sarcolemma of vascular myocyte. The $Na^+K^+2Cl^-$ co-transporter and HCO_3^-–Cl^- exchanger generate a high intracellular chloride concentration.

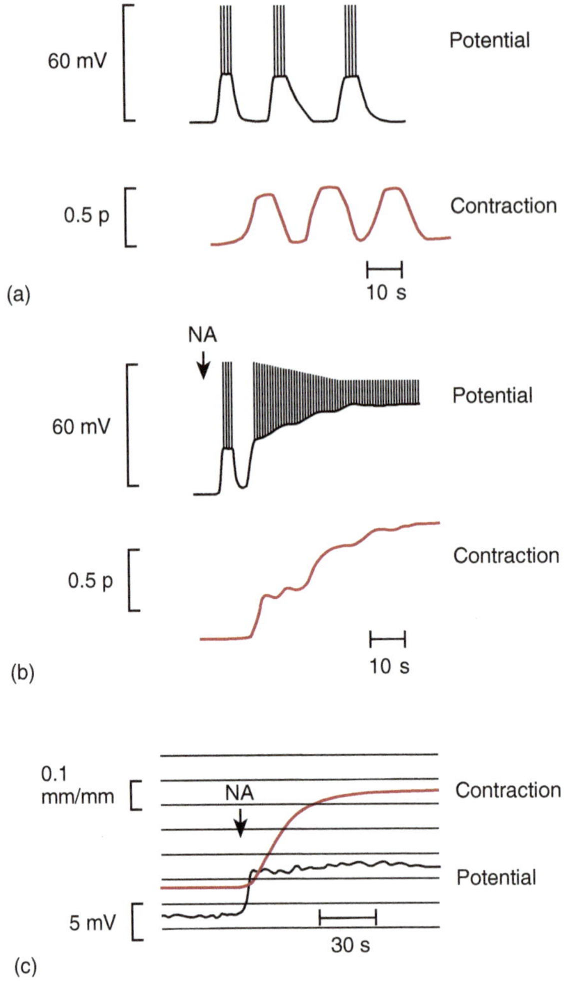

Figure 12.3 Diverse characteristics of vascular smooth muscle. (a) Spontaneously active portal vein; action potentials trigger contraction. (b) Response of portal vein to noradrenaline (NA) showing further depolarization-dependent contraction. (c) Contrasting response of sheep carotid artery to noradrenaline – no action potentials, but a sustained contraction. The latter is not dependent on the slight accompanying depolarization (depolarization-independent contraction).

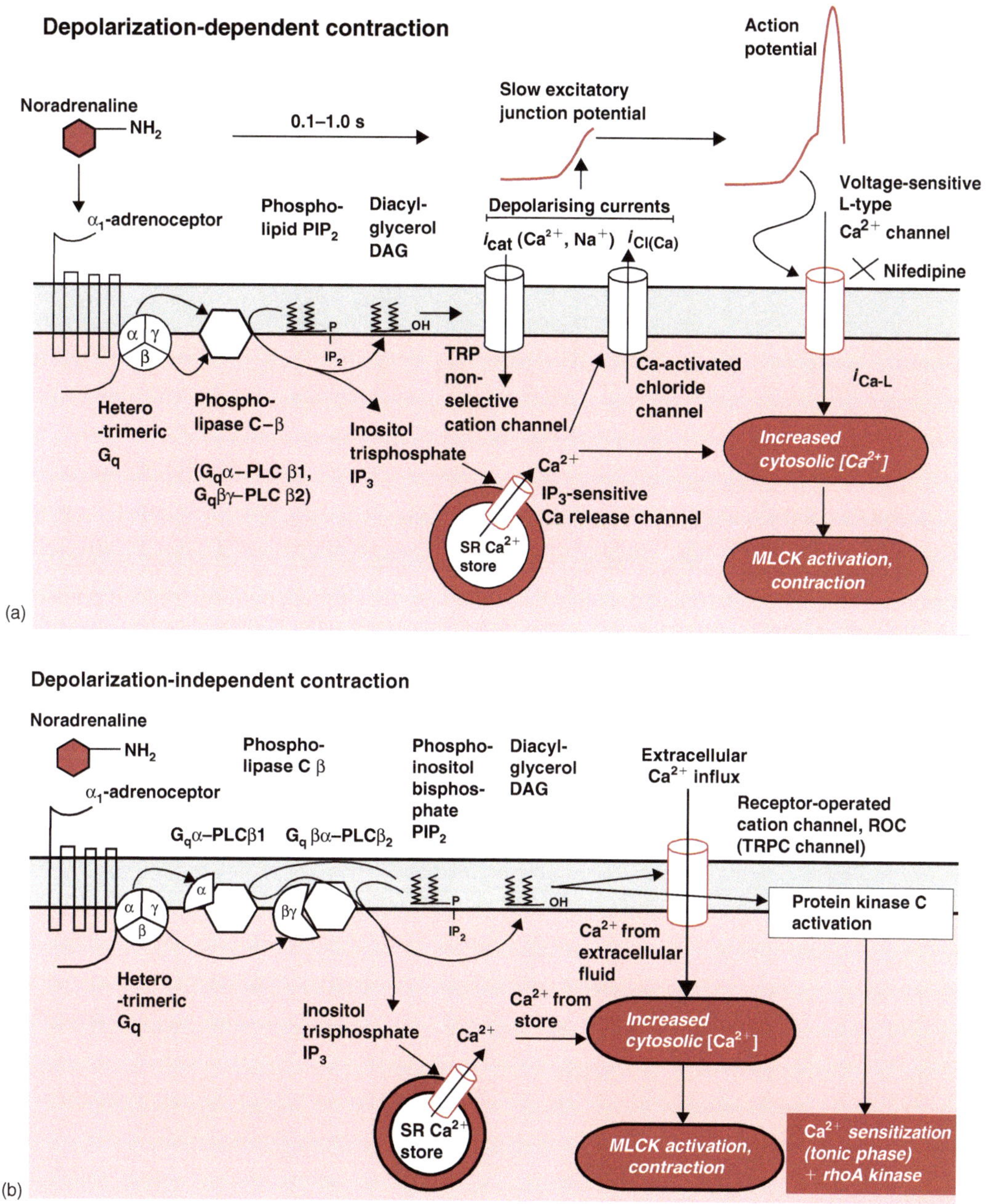

Figure 12.4 Pathways by which noradrenaline α_1 receptors evoke depolarization-dependent contraction (a) and depolarization-independent contraction (b). PIP_2, phosphatidyl inositol bisphosphate; *i*, current; MLCK, myosin light chain kinase.

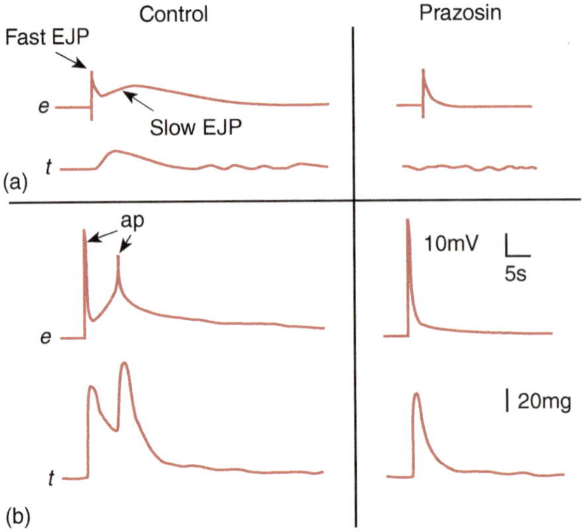

Figure 12.5 Contractile tension (*t*) and membrane potential (*e*) in an artery. Sympathetic nerves were stimulated by a single external pulse in each frame in the absence (*left*) or presence (*right*) of an α-adrenoceptor blocker, prazosin. (a) Medium intensity stimulation produced a fast excitatory junction potential (fast EJP, ATP-mediated) and a slow EJP (noradrenaline-mediated). Contraction *preceded* the slow EJP, yet was blocked by prazosin, so it was a depolarization-independent contraction. (b) Stimulation at higher intensity evoked larger fast and slow EJPs, each of which triggered an action potential (ap), with associated twitch contractions (depolarization-dependent contractions).

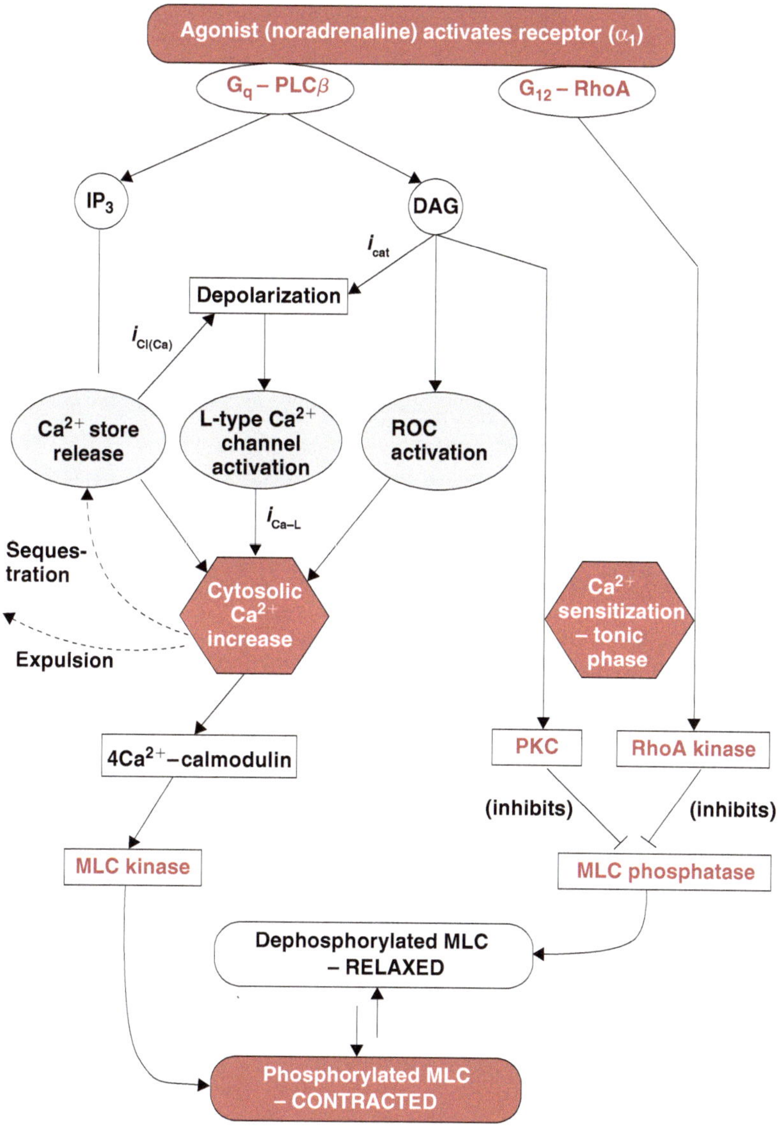

Figure 12.6 Pathways mediating noradrenaline-induced vasoconstriction. Relative importance of various pathways varies with vessel type, tissue and agonist.

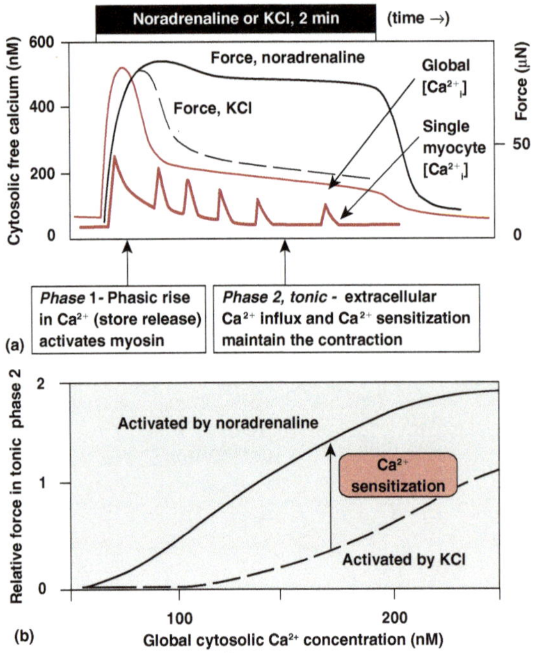

Figure 12.7 Contraction and cytosolic free Ca^{2+} concentration in an artery. (a) Noradrenaline evokes a well sustained contraction (upper black line). Depolarizing by extracellular KCl had a less sustained effect (lower, dashed line). 'Global' cytosolic Ca^{2+} concentration over the whole tunica media (upper red line) is average of hundreds of asynchronous Ca^{2+} waves in individual myocytes (lower red line). Noradrenaline-induced contraction is maintained despite a fall in [Ca^{2+}] during the tonic phase, showing that the sensitivity to Ca^{2+} has increased. (b) Dependence of contractile force on mean cytosolic free [Ca^{2+}] in the tonic phase. Noradrenaline steepens the relation, demonstrating Ca^{2+} sensitization.

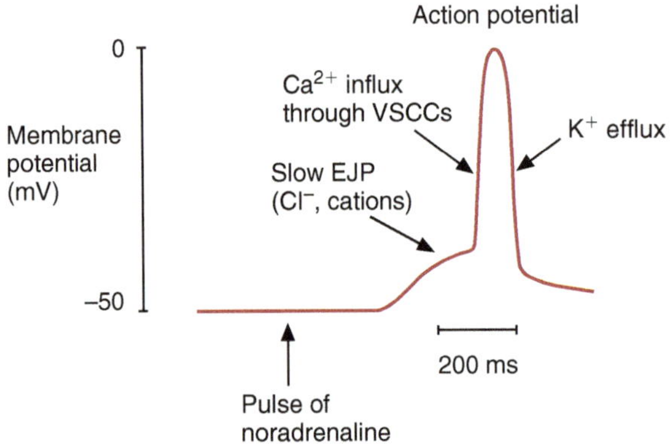

Figure 12.8 Response of an action potential-generating vascular myocyte to a pulse of noradrenaline. VSCC, voltage-sensitive channel permeable to Ca^{2+}.

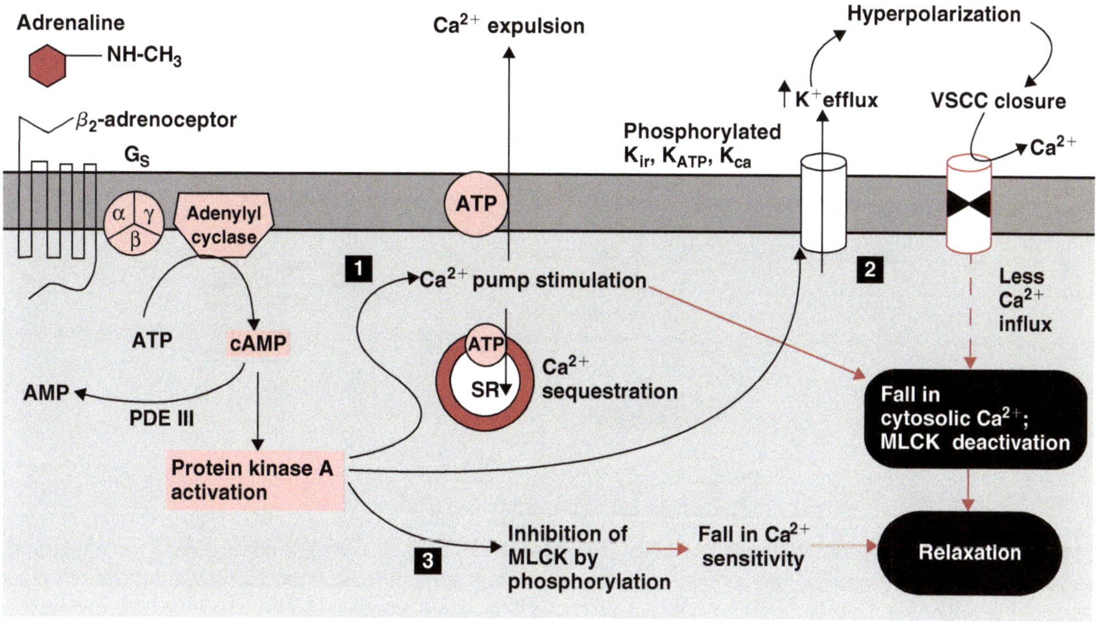

Figure 12.9 Vasodilatation evoked by adrenaline-activated β_2-adrenoceptors. AMP, adenosine monophosphate. PDE III, phosphodiesterase III.

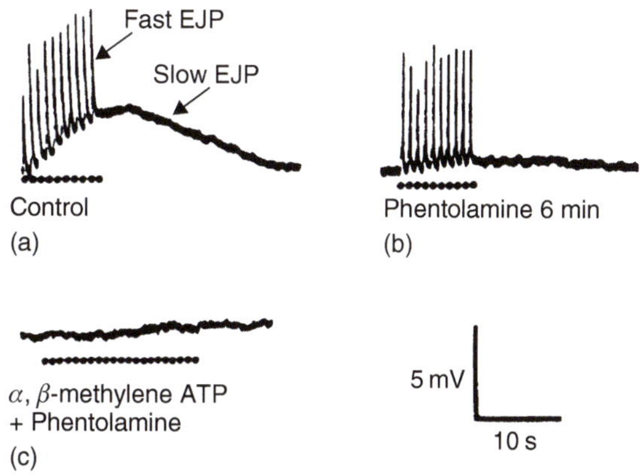

Figure 12.10 Sympathetic transmission by both noradrenaline and ATP in an artery. Sympathetic stimulation (dots) caused fast excitatory junction potentials (fast EJP, spikes, not action potentials,) on top of a slower depolarization (slow EJP, baseline under spikes). (b) Phentolamine, an α-adrenoceptor blocker, abolishes the slow EJP. (c) Desensitization of purinergic receptors by α,β-methylene ATP abolishes the fast EJPs.

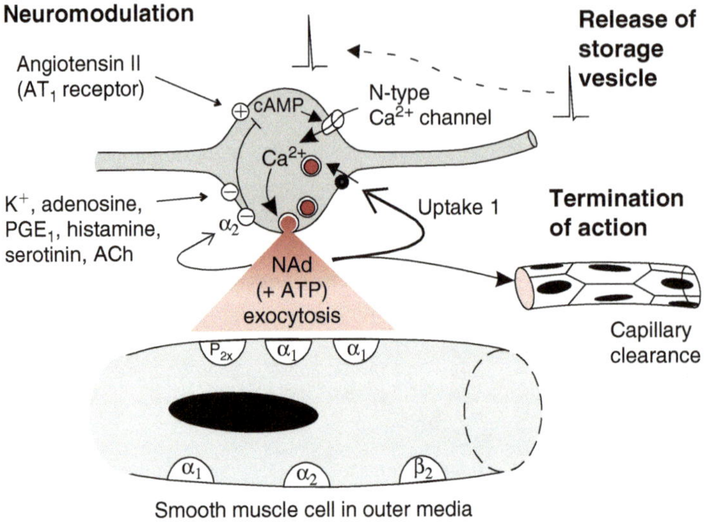

Figure 12.11 Sympathetic transmission by release of vesicles of noradrenaline (NAd) from terminal varicosities. Prejunctional α_2 receptors, and receptors for many intrinsic vasodilators, attenuate vesicle release (negative sign). Angiotensin receptors promote it (positive sign).

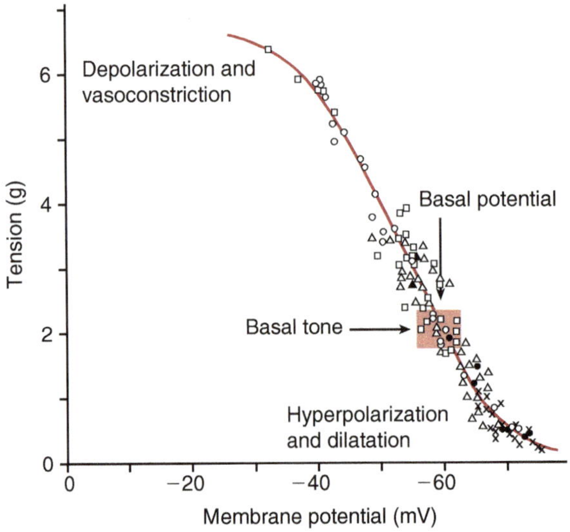

Figure 12.12 Dependence of vascular tone on membrane potential. Membrane potential was altered by extracellular H^+ (△), extracellular K^+ (□), extracellular Ca^{2+} (●), noradrenaline (○) and hypoxia (×).

CHAPTER 13

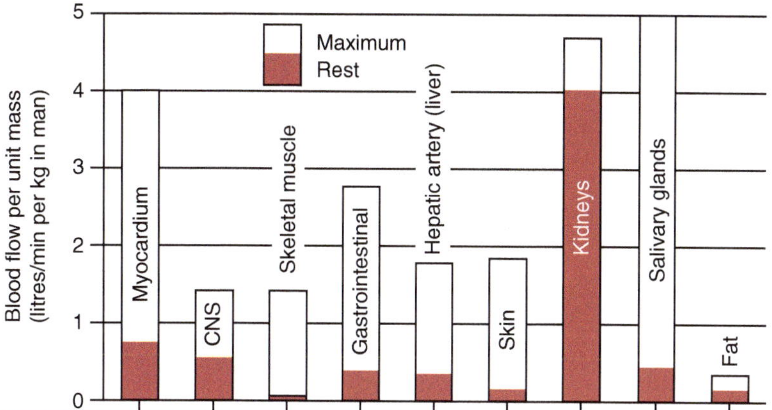

Rest (l/min)	0.21	+	0.75	+	0.75	+	0.7	+	0.5	+	0.2	+	1.2	+	0.02	+	0.8	= 5.1
Maximum	1.2		2.1		18.0		5.5		3.0		3.8		1.4		0.25		3.0	(= 38!)
Weight (kg)	0.3		1.5		30		2		1.7		2.1		0.3		0.05		10	= 48

Figure 13.1 Regulated range of human blood flow, from rest to maximal.

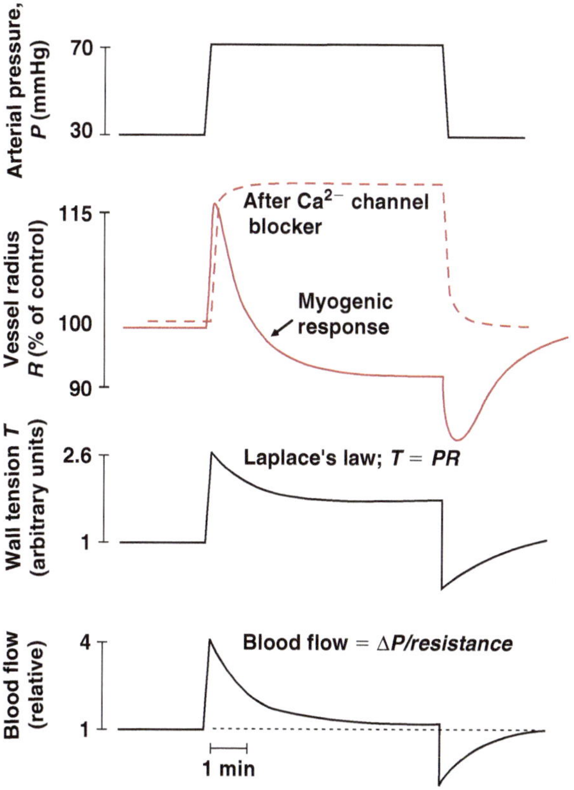

Figure 13.2 Change in diameter of isolated rat cerebral artery upon raising luminal pressure P. Initial passive stretch is followed by active contraction – the Bayliss myogenic response. This is abolished by the L-type Ca^{2+} channel blocker, nimodipine. The rise in wall tension T provides a maintained stimulus.

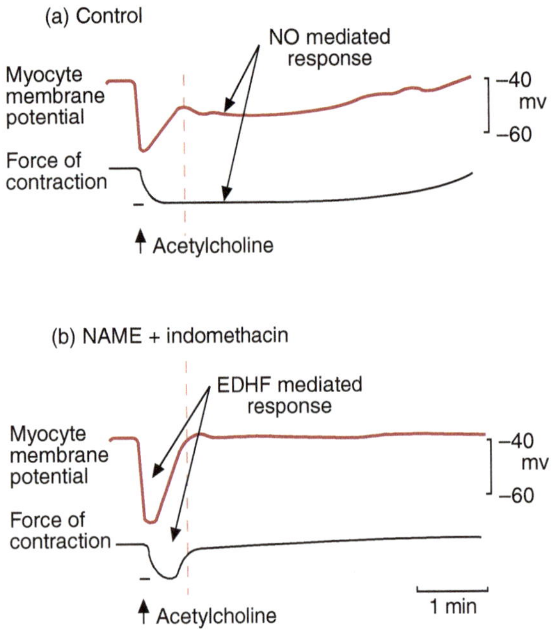

Figure 13.3 (a) Endothelium-dependent relaxation of coronary artery (black line) in response to acetylcholine (bar). The relaxation is mediated partly by hyperpolarization of the vascular smooth muscle (red line). (b) Blockage of NO production (by nitroarginine methyl ester, NAME) and prostacyclin production (by indomethacin) abolishes late part of the response. The early hyperpolarization and relaxation is mediated by EDHF and persists.

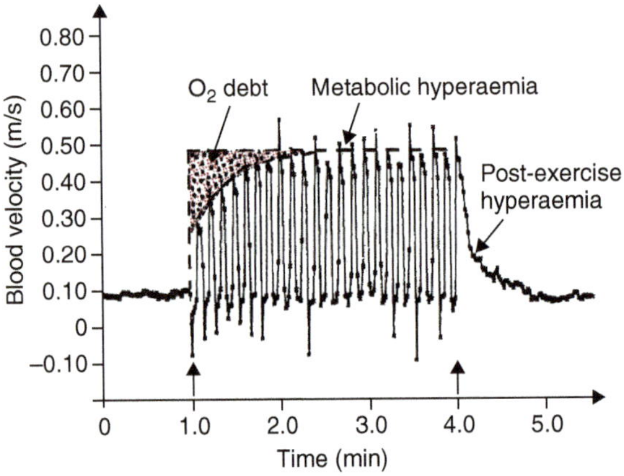

Figure 13.4 Oscillating increase in blood flow (metabolic hyperaemia) in human femoral artery during rhythmic quadriceps exercise. The relatively slow onset of the hyperaemia creates an oxygen debt. Post-exercise hyperaemia repays the nutritional debt.

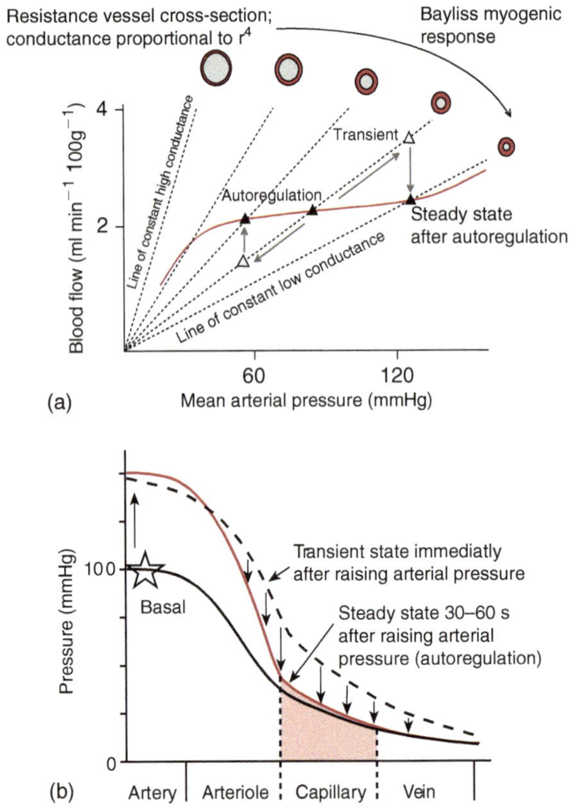

Figure 13.5 Autoregulation of (a) blood flow and (b) capillary pressure in isolated, perfused skeletal muscle. (a) Raising or lowering blood pressure transiently raises or lowers blood flow as dictated by Poisueuille's law (dashed lines of constant conductance). The myogenic response then actively changes the resistance vessel radius, producing a new isoconductance line and restoring flow to close to its former level in the steady state (vertical grey arrows). (b) Dashed lines show the transient state immediately after changing perfusion pressure from a control level of 100 mmHg (star), before autoregulation has had time to kick in. Over the next 30–60 s arteriolar contraction/dilatation (arrows) readjusts the flow and capillary pressure to a steady-state value similar to before (solid red curve).

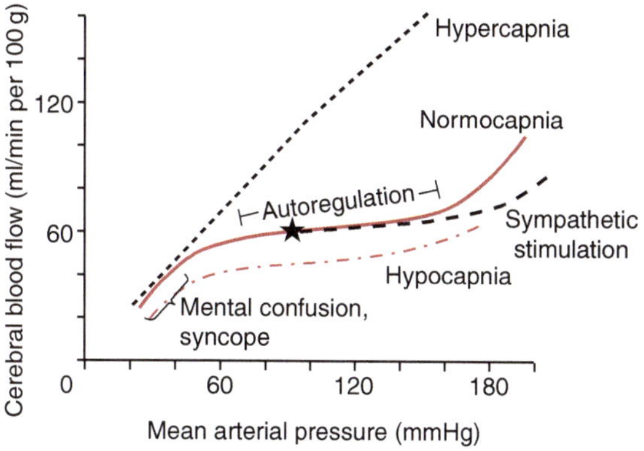

Figure 13.6 Autoregulation of cerebral perfusion at normal arterial P_{CO_2} (solid line); flow changes by only 6% per 10 mmHg pressure change. A raised arterial CO_2 causes cerebral vasodilatation (upper dashed line); a low CO_2, usually due to hyperventilation, cause vasoconstriction, leading to dizziness. Local sympathetic stimulation affects flow significantly only when arterial pressure is high.

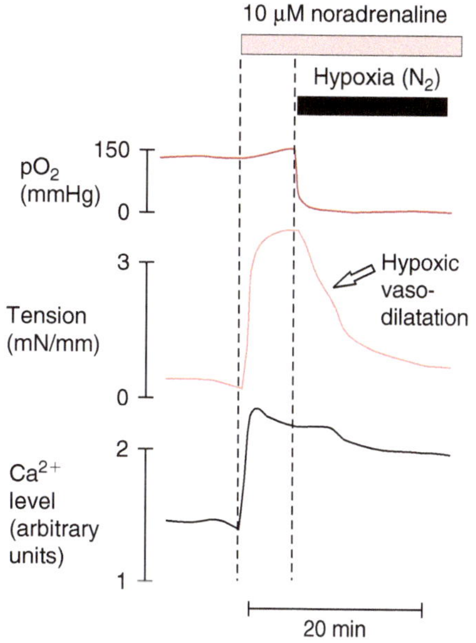

Figure 13.7 Noradrenaline causes vasoconstriction. Acute hypoxia causes small artery vasodilatation. The hypoxic vasodilatation involved little to no fall in Ca^{2+}, and was brought about by a fall in sensitivity to Ca^{2+}. In some arteries, hypoxia reduces intracellular free Ca^{2+} via hyperpolarization-mediated closure of L-type Ca^{2+} channels.

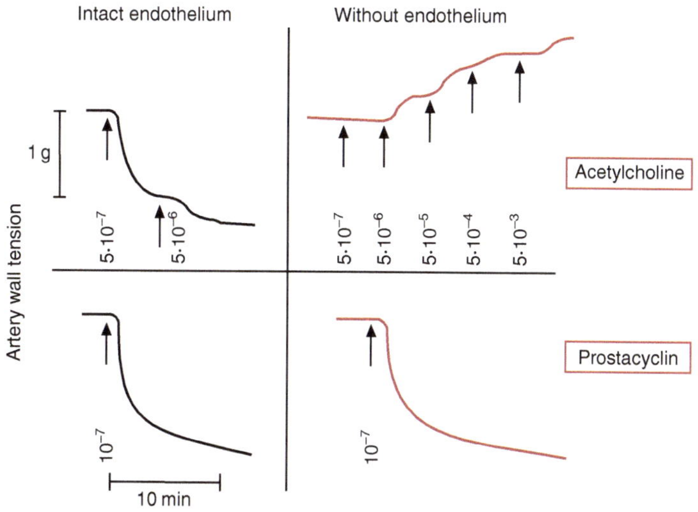

Figure 13.8 Arterial dilatation is evoked by acetylcholine and prostacyclin (*left panels*). In the case of acetylcholine, dilatation is endothelium-dependent (NO secretion); the direct action of acetylcholine on smooth muscle is contraction (*top right*). Prostacyclin has a direct vasodilator action on the smooth muscle (*bottom right*).

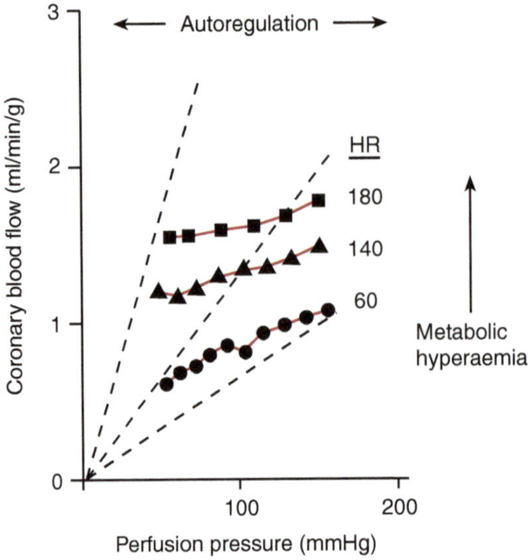

Figure 13.9 At any given perfusion pressure, coronary blood flow increases with metabolic rate (heart rate HR). This is *metabolic hyperaemia*. But at any given metabolic rate, coronary flow increases relatively little with perfusion pressure. This is *autoregulation*. Dashed lines are pressure–flow lines at constant conductance.

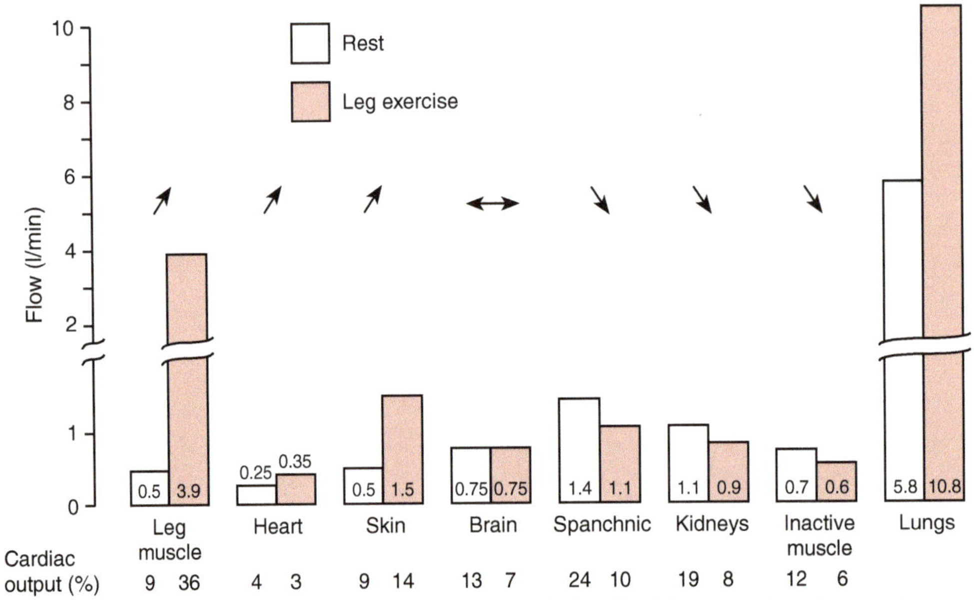

Figure 13.10 Redistribution of human cardiac output during light leg exercise at room temperature. Number at base of each column is blood flow in litre/min. Most of increased flow to legs derives from the increase in cardiac output; flow 'diverted' from other tissues by vasoconstriction makes only a minor contribution.

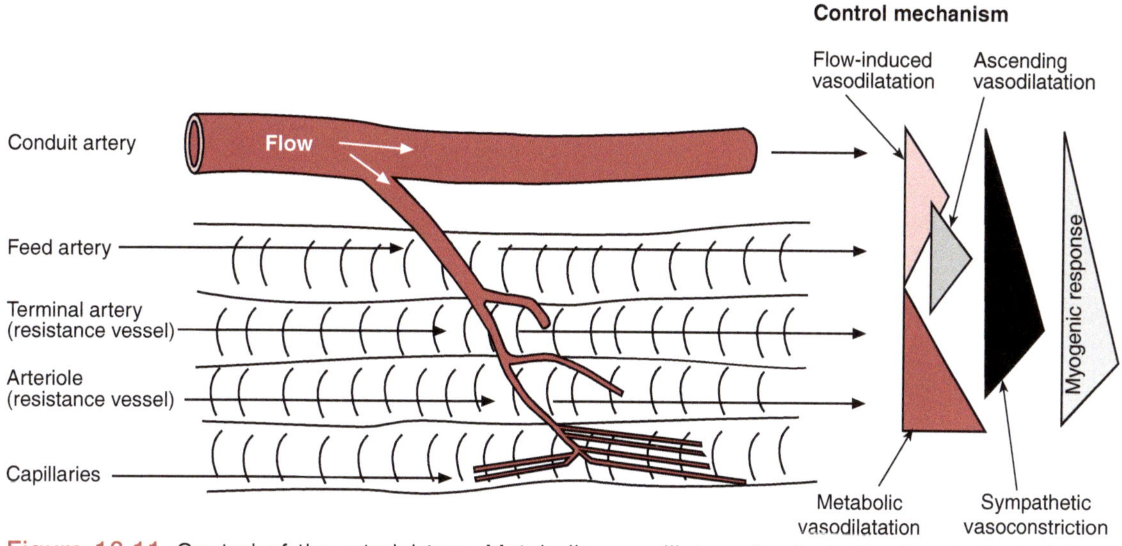

Figure 13.11 Control of the arterial tree. Metabolic vasodilators dominate the *terminal arterioles*. Sympathetic vasoconstrictor nerves dominate the more *proximal resistance vessels*. Ascending (conducted) vasodilatation regulates *feed arteries*. Flow-induced vasodilatation, mediated by nitric oxide, is important in the *conduit* and proximal feed arteries.

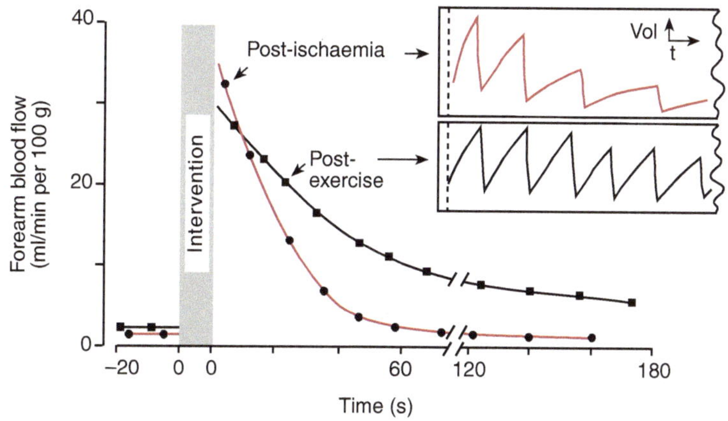

Figure 13.12 Post-ischaemic hyperaemia (red line) in human forearm, following arrest of arterial flow by a brachial artery occlusion for 120 s. Black line show post-exercise hyperaemia, following 30 s strenuous forearm exercise. Insets are venous occlusion plethysmography recordings; slopes represent blood flow.

CHAPTER 14

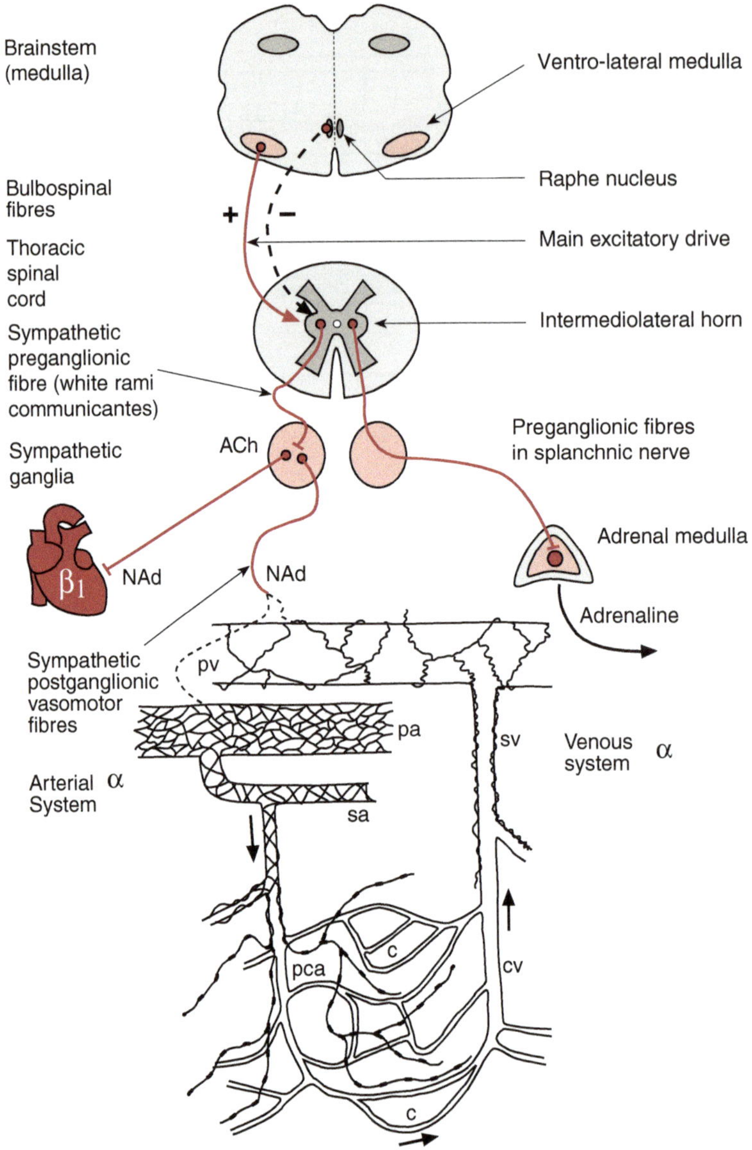

Figure 14.1 Cardiovascular sympathetic innervation. Alpha and β refer to predominant adrenoceptor. NAd, noradrenaline; ACh, acetylcholine. One descending tract (bulbospinal tract) excites the sympathetic IML cells; other bulbospinal fibres inhibit the cell. pa and pv, primary, conduit artery and vein to an organ; sa and sv, small artery and vein; pca, precapillary arteriole; c, capillary; cv, collecting venule.

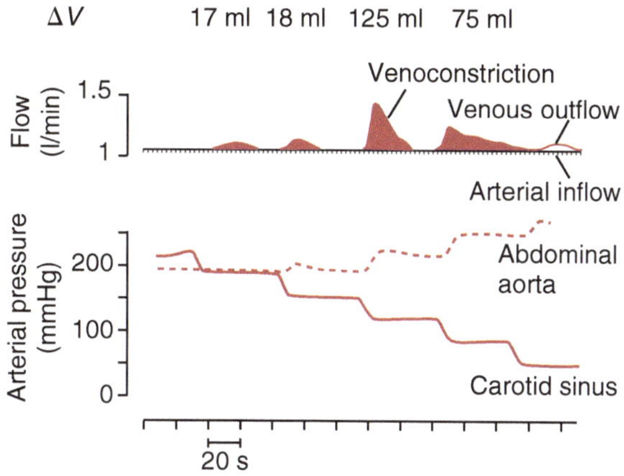

Figure 14.2 Active splanchnic venoconstriction and increase in blood pressure (abdominal aorta trace) mediated by increased sympathetic activity. Latter was evoked by the baroreflex when pressure was lowered in an isolated carotid sinus. Each transient excess of splanchnic venous outflow over arterial inflow marks an episode of venoconstriction. ΔV, displaced blood volume.

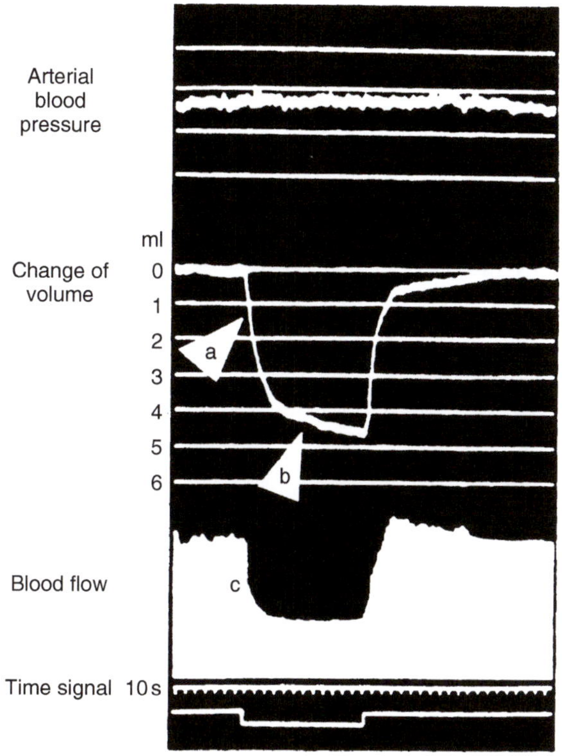

Figure 14.3 Effects of sympathetic stimulation (square signal) in cat hindquarters. Arrow *a* shows fall in venous volume of blood, caused by a fall in venous pressure as the resistance vessels contract (skeletal muscle veins have little direct innervation). Arrow *b* shows slow fall in tissue volume due to capillary absorption of interstitial fluid, as capillary pressure is reduced by resistance vessel contraction. Arrow *c* shows fall in blood flow caused by resistance vessel contraction.

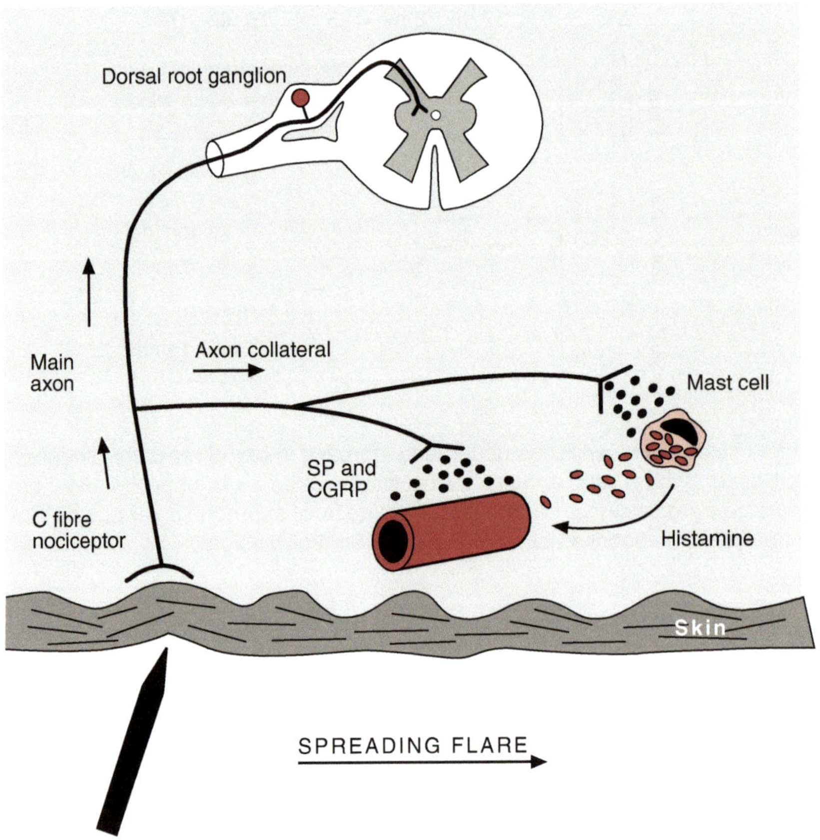

Figure 14.4 The sensory axon reflex and spreading flare response to a scratch. Vasodilatation is due to the release of substance P (SP) and CGRP from nociceptive C-fibre axon branches. In rat skin and possibly some human dermatological conditions, collateral endings near mast cells also trigger histamine granule release, which augments the flare.

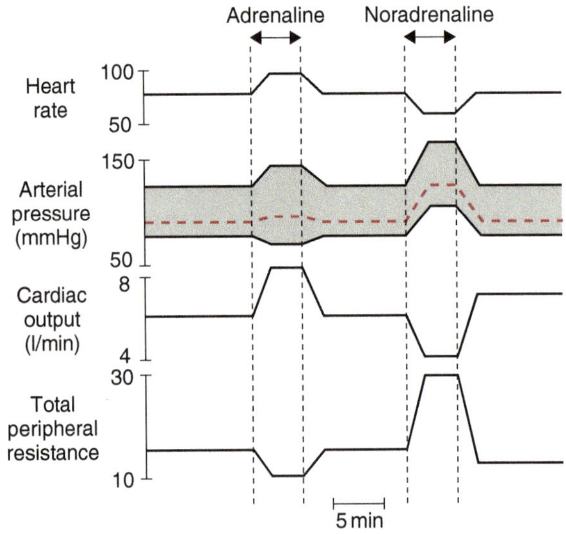

Figure 14.5 Contrasting effects of intravenous adrenaline and noradrenaline in man. Dashed red line is mean blood pressure.

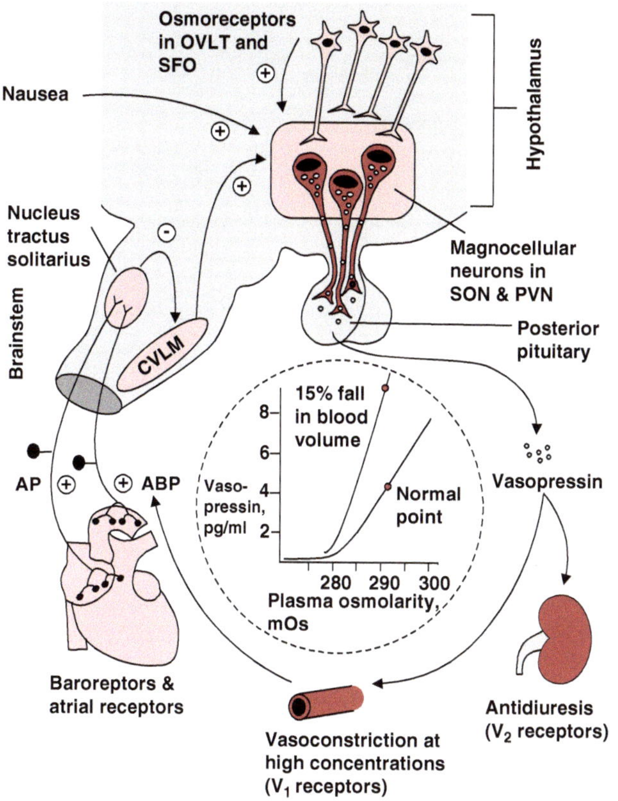

Figure 14.6 Regulation of vasopressin secretion. ABP, arterial blood pressure, regulated by resistance vessel tone; AP, atrial pressure, regulated by renal control of extracellular fluid volume; OVLT, organum vasculosus lamina terminalis; SFO, subfornicular organ; SON, supraoptic nucleus; PVN, paraventricular nucleus; CVLM, caudal ventrolateral medulla.

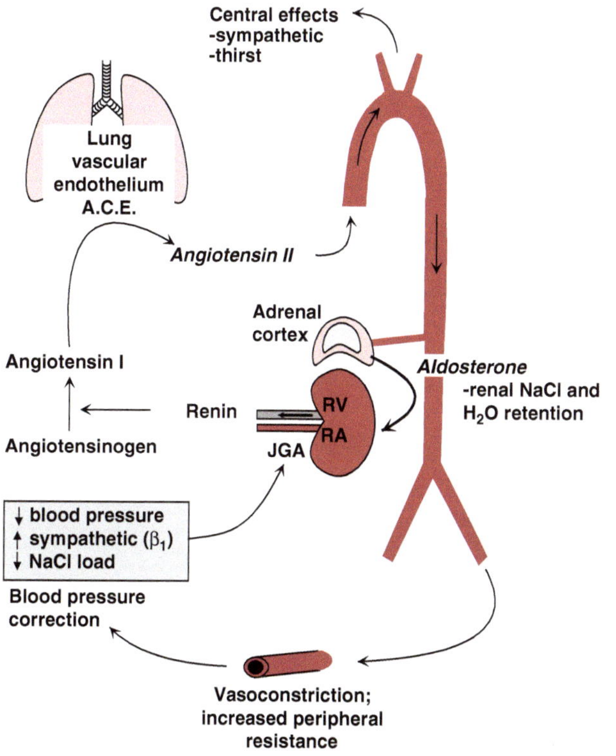

Figure 14.7 Renin–angiotensin–aldosterone system. JGA, juxtaglomerular apparatus, RA and RV, renal artery and vein. Central effects of angiotensin II are stimulation of sympathetic outflow, reduction in sensitivity of baroreceptor reflex and stimulation of thirst.

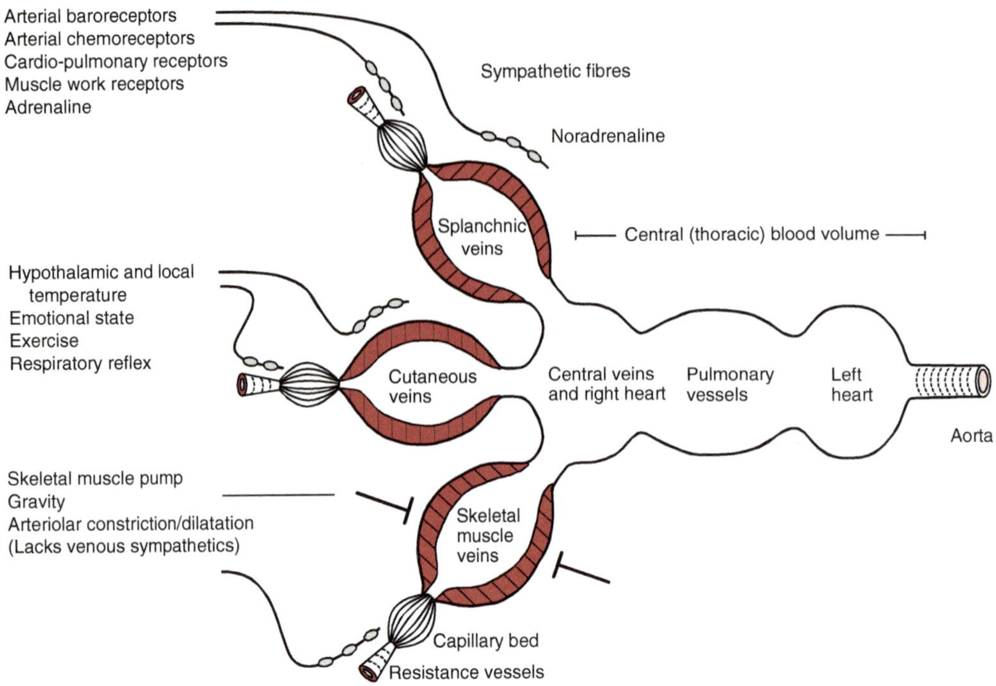

Figure 14.8 Differentiation within the venous system. Changes in central blood volume and cardiac filling pressure are brought about by contraction of peripheral veins, especially splanchnic veins. Factors regulating the different venous beds are listed on the left.

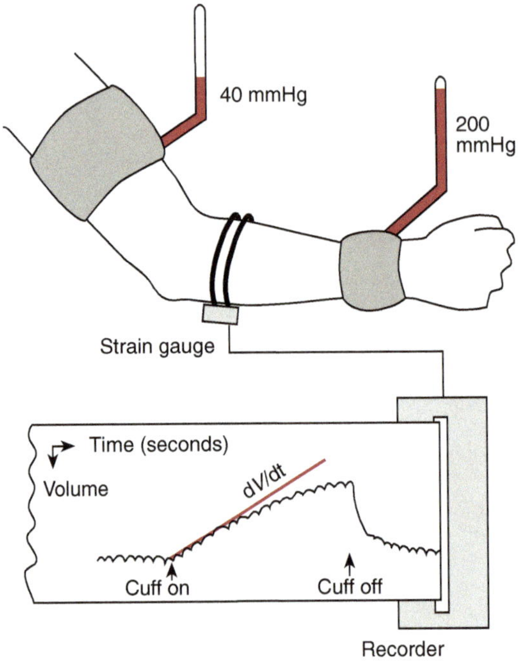

Figure 14.9 Venous occlusion plethysmography. The 'congesting cuff' (upper arm) occludes venous return; the wrist cuff eliminates hand blood flow from the measurement. The strain gauge measures the increase in forearm circumference due to the continuing arterial inflow (see the trace). The swelling rate dV/dt measures forearm blood flow.

CHAPTER 15

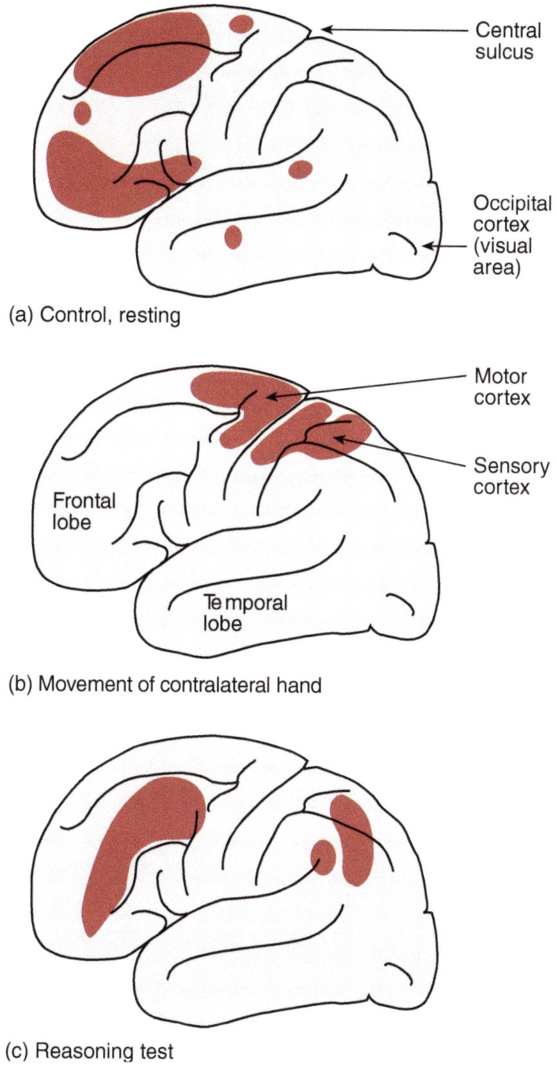

Figure 15.1 Xenon-133 imaging of cerebral perfusion, showing local functional/metabolic hyperaemia in human cortex. Red areas show raised flow. (a) Frontal lobe hyperaemia in resting, pensive subject. (b) Hyperaemia of the hand area of the upper motor, premotor and sensory cortex during voluntary movement of contralateral hand. (c) Hyperaemia in precentral and postcentral areas during a reasoning test.

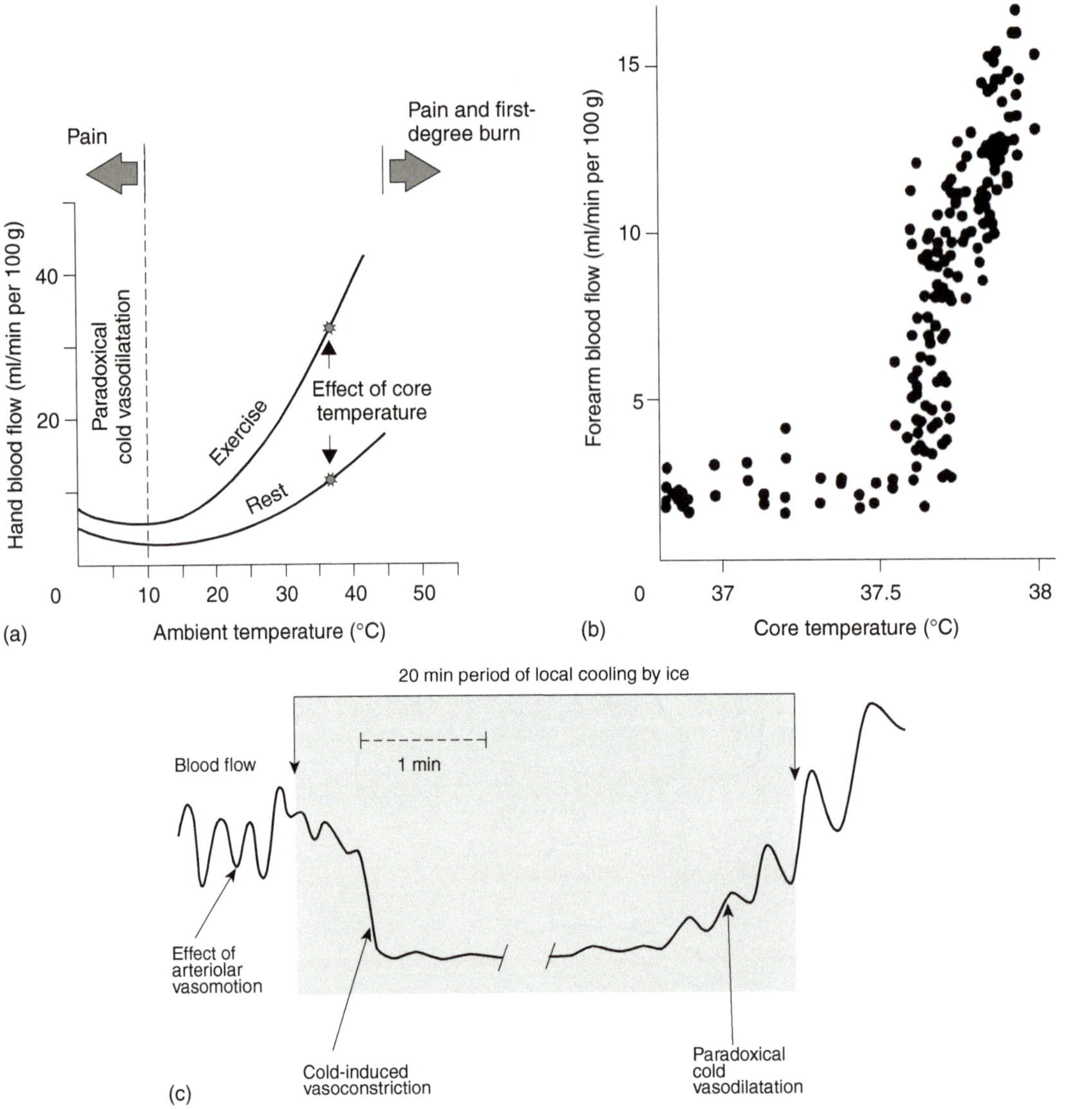

Figure 15.2 Effect of external (ambient) temperature and internal (core) temperature on skin blood flow. (a) Response of immersed hand to water temperature, when internal heat load is low (rest) or high (exercise). (b) Response of forearm skin blood flow to rise in core temperature induced by leg exercise. (c) Cold-induced vasoconstriction in human calf skin, changing to paradoxical cold vasodilatation after 10–20 min.

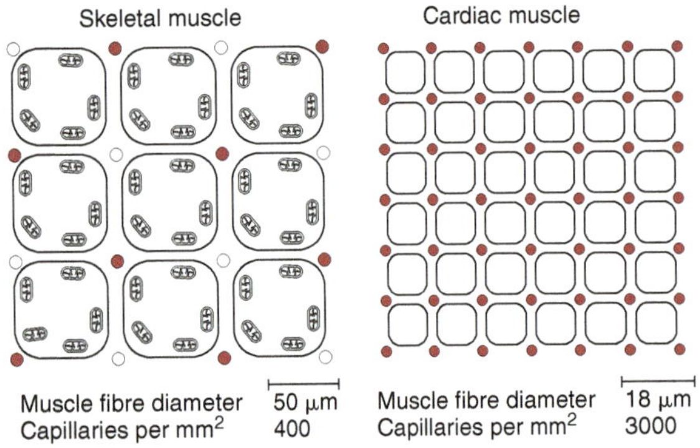

Figure 15.3 Capillaries density (number/area) in skeletal and cardiac muscle, on same scale. Each tissue has ~1 capillary (red circle) per muscle fibre; but myocardial fibres are smaller, so myocardial capillary density is greater and diffusion distance correspondingly shorter. Open circles in skeletal muscle are capillaries not perfused with blood at any given moment in resting muscle.

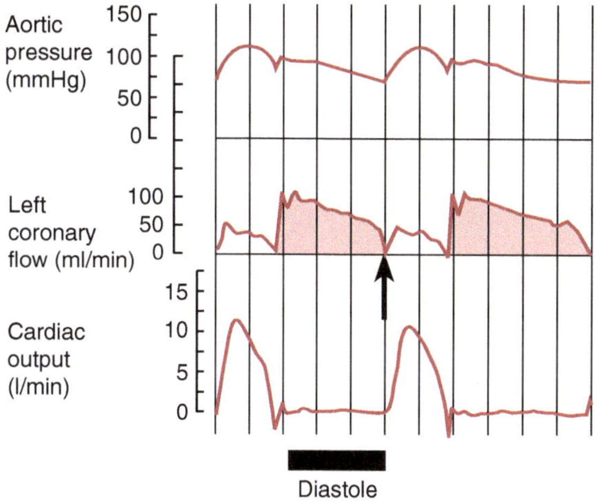

Figure 15.4 Blood flow in left coronary artery. Note the sharp curtailment of flow at the onset of systole (arrow). Most coronary flow occurs during diastole (shaded area).

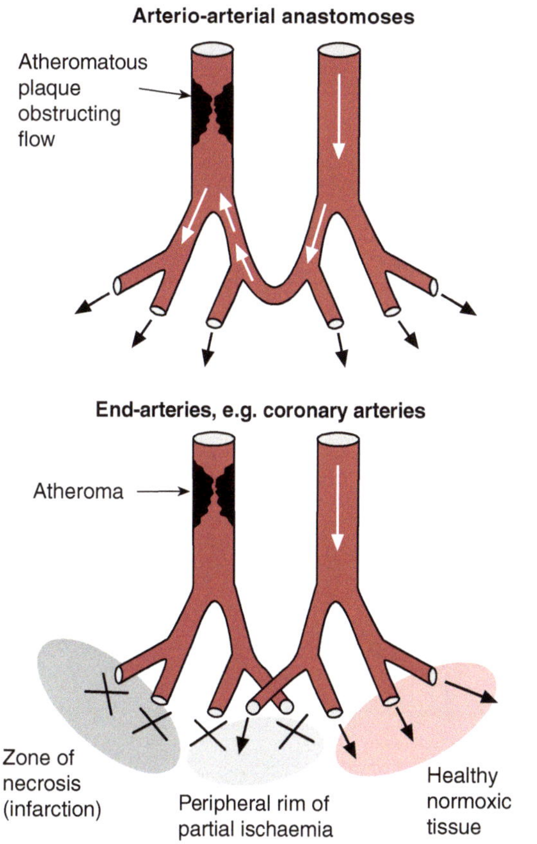

Figure 15.5 Arterio-arterial anastomoses affect susceptibility to infarction following arterial obstruction. (*Lower panel*) Human, baboon, rabbit and pig coronary arteries are functional end-arteries. Acute ligation of a major vessel in the pig heart reduces perfusion to 0.6% in the downstream territory. (*Upper panel*) Dog coronary circulation has better arterio-arterial anastomoses. Acute ligation of a major canine coronary artery reduces myocardial perfusion less severely, to ~16%.

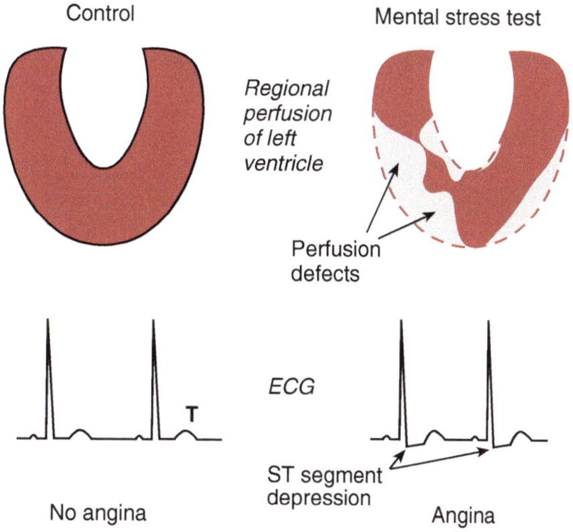

Figure 15.6 Nuclear imaging of human left ventricle myocardial perfusion, using intravascular rubidium. Control: Uniform perfusion and normal ECG with patient relaxed. Stress test (mental arithmetic) caused angina, areas of defective myocardial perfusion (cold spots) and ST segment depression (ischaemia), due to increased cardiac work and sympathetic coronary vasoconstriction. Exercise causes similar changes.

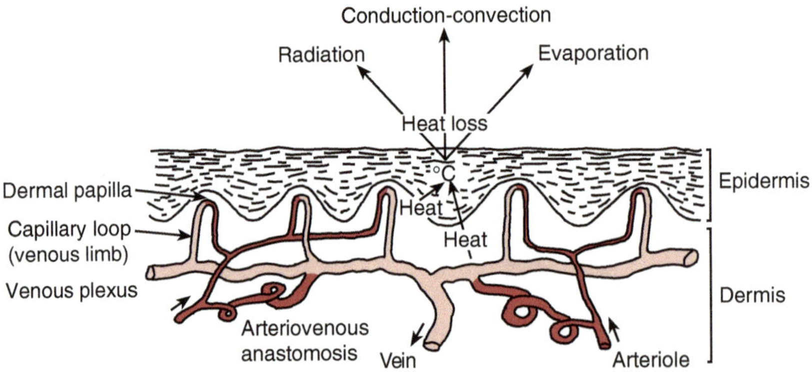

Figure 15.7 Skin circulation and heat flux in a human extremity, e.g. fingers, ear lobe (acral skin). Non-acral skin of limbs and trunk lacks arteriovenous anastomoses. Red cell volume and O_2 status in subpapillary venous plexus influence skin colour.

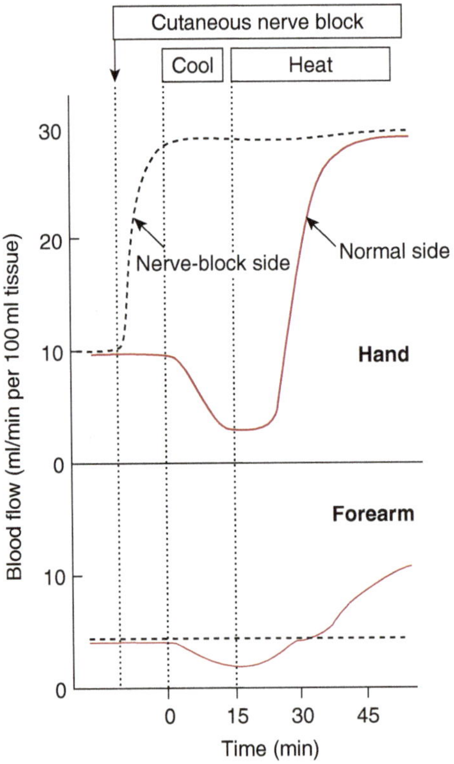

Figure 15.8 Contrast between cutaneous vascular control in hand and arm. Dashed line shows marked effect in hand, but not forearm, of sympathetic block by local anaesthetic. Core temperature was then cooled, followed by heating, by placing legs in cold/hot water (upper limbs at room temperature). In the hand, sympathetic restraint of arteriovenous flow is substantial at thermoneutrality, and heat-mediated dilatation is due chiefly to abolition of restraint. In more proximal skin (arm) sympathetic-induced tone is slight and vasodilatation depends on increased sympathetic cholinergic fibre activity.

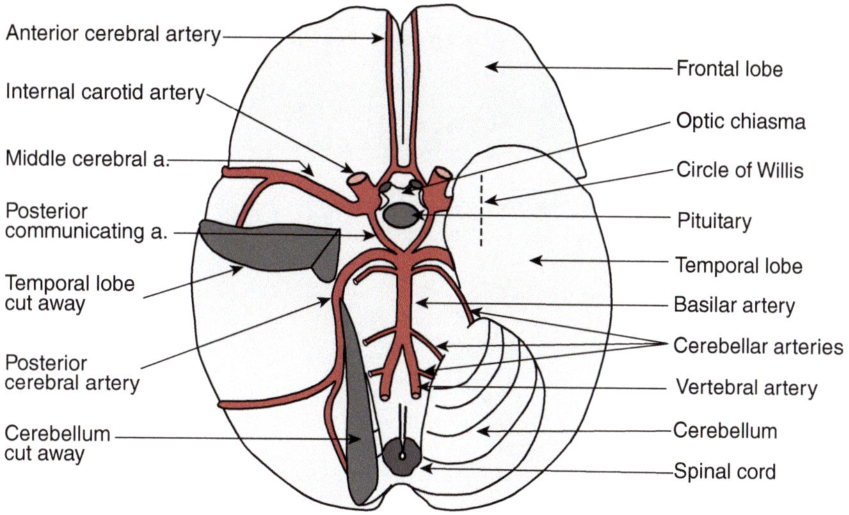

Figure 15.9 Circle of Willis and main cerebral arteries in man, viewed from the underside of the brain. The blood reaches the circle of Willis via the basilar artery and two internal carotid arteries. Middle cerebral artery territory includes motor and sensory cortex of central sulcus.

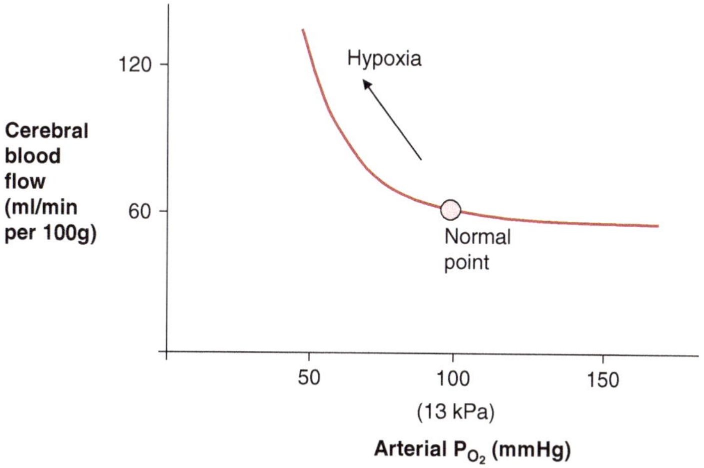

Figure 15.10 Effect of systemic hypoxia on total cerebral blood flow.

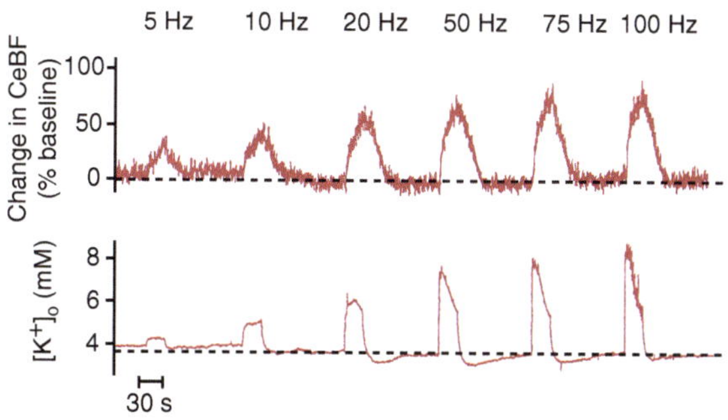

Figure 15.11 Effect of cerebellar neuron activity (stimulation rates, top row) on rat cerebellar blood flow (CeBF), monitored by laser Doppler. This is an example of metabolic hyperaemia. Concomitant rise in interstitial K^+ concentration $[K^+]_o$ is one of the vasodilator stimuli.

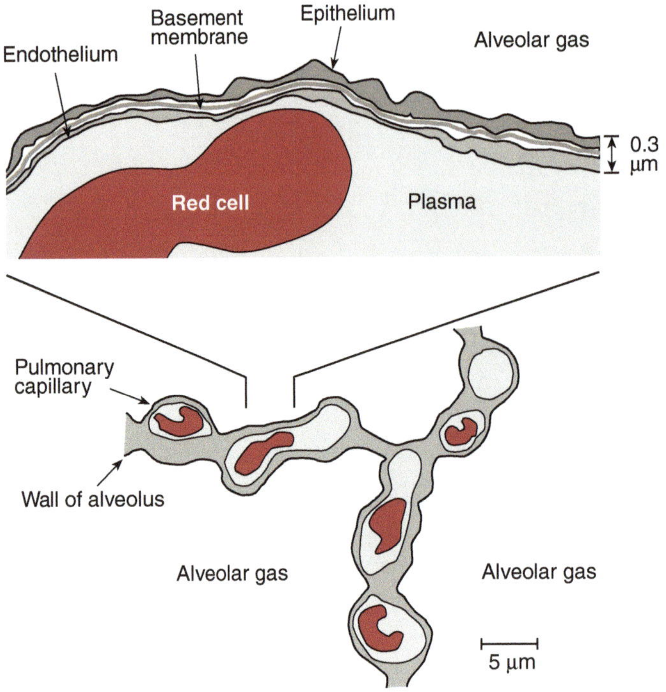

Figure 15.12 Ultrastructure of alveolar wall and pulmonary capillaries. Note high ratio of blood to tissue and extreme thinness of membrane separating plasma from alveolar gas, ~0.3 µm.

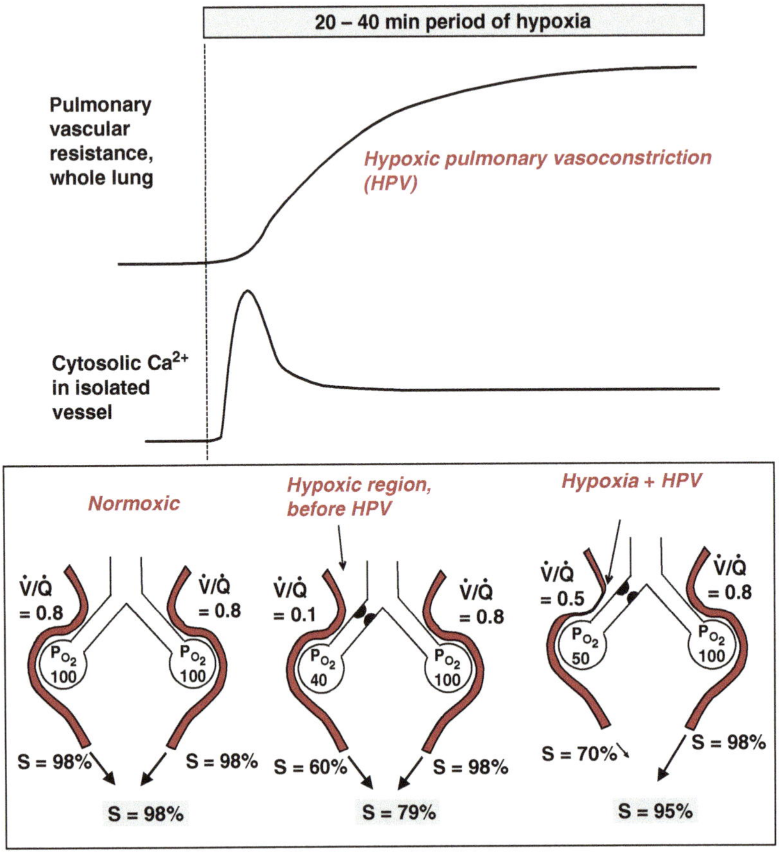

Figure 15.13 (*Top*) Hypoxic pulmonary vasoconstriction (HPV) in a perfused whole lung exposed to hypoxia. (*Middle*) Corresponding change in vascular myocyte cytosolic Ca^{2+} in an isolated rat pulmonary artery exposed to hypoxia. (*Bottom*) Effect of local alveolar hypoxia and HPV on gas exchange. HPV prevents extremely low ventilation/perfusion ratios, $\dot{V}/\dot{Q}$, and thus preserves the O_2 saturation (*S*) of mixed arterial blood. P_{O_2} in mmHg; arrow size indicates flow magnitude.

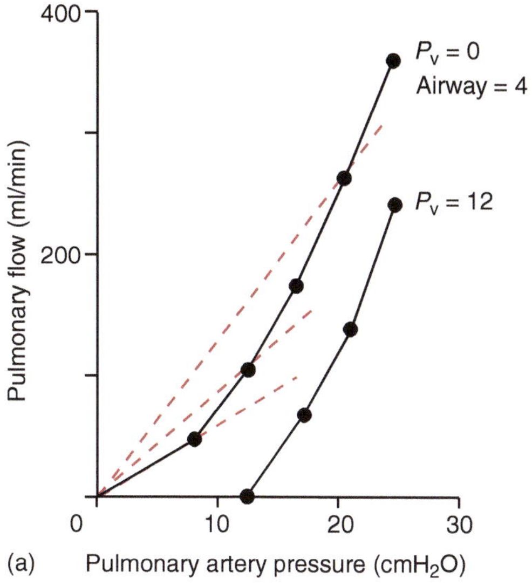

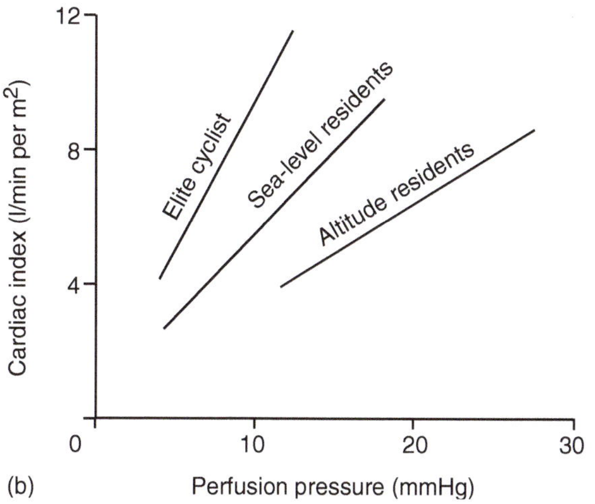

Figure 15.14 Pressure–flow relations in pulmonary circulation. (a) Isolated cat lung perfused with plasma, with venous pressure (P_v) set to zero or 12 cmH_2O; airway pressure 4 cmH_2O. Dashed lines are lines of constant conductance; pulmonary conductance increases as arterial pressure rises; so a 4× increase in right cardiac output requires less than a 4× increase in pressure. (b) Human curves during supine exercise. 'Perfusion pressure' is pulmonary artery pressure minus left atrial pressure (>0); airway pressure atmospheric.

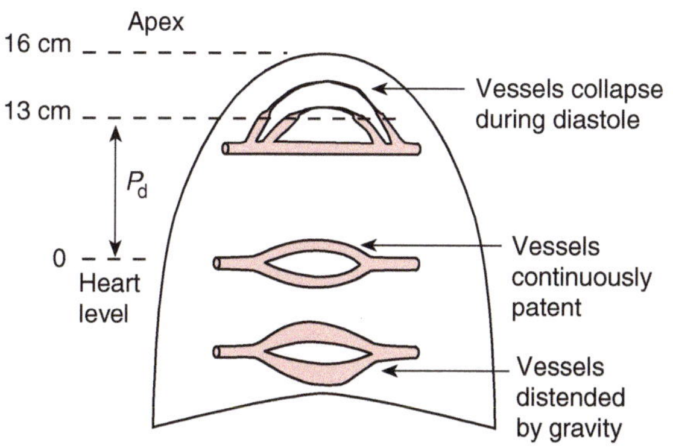

Figure 15.15 Gradient of perfusion in lung of a resting human in upright position. Scale shows vertical distance above heart. Diastolic artery pressure P_d is 13 cmH_2O (~9 mmHg) at heart level, falling to zero (atmospheric) 13 cm above heart. Vessels higher than this are only perfused during systole.

CHAPTER 16

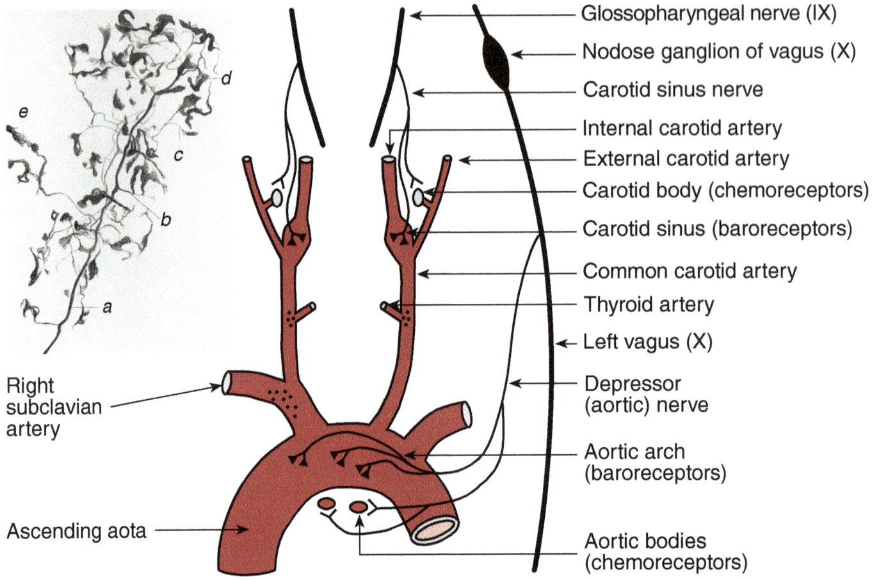

Figure 16.1 Main reflexogenic zones of arterial system; minor baroreceptor regions shown as dots. Right vagus not shown. *Inset*, single baroreceptor ending in human carotid sinus.

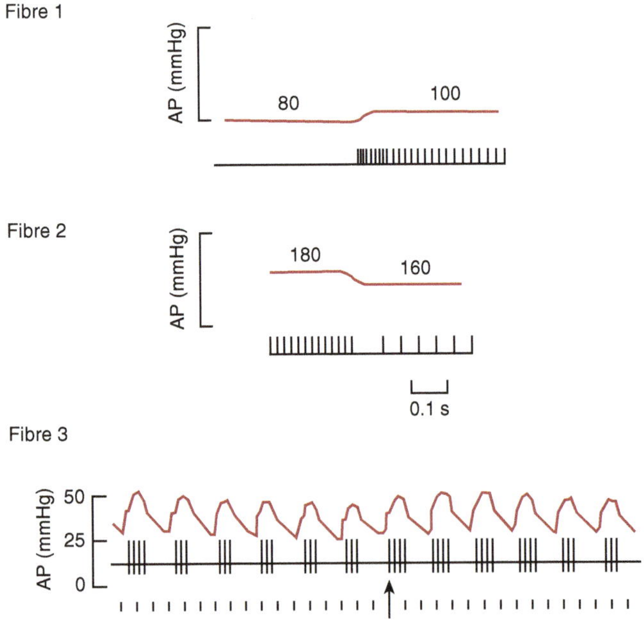

Figure 16.2 Firing characteristics of arterial baroreceptors. *Fibres 1–2*, Non-pulsatile arterial pressure (AP) was raised (fibre 1) or reduced (fibre 2). *Fibre 3*, Single baroreceptor fibre responding to a normal, pulsatile pressure. Note increased number of action potential per pulse when pulse pressure is high (arrow).

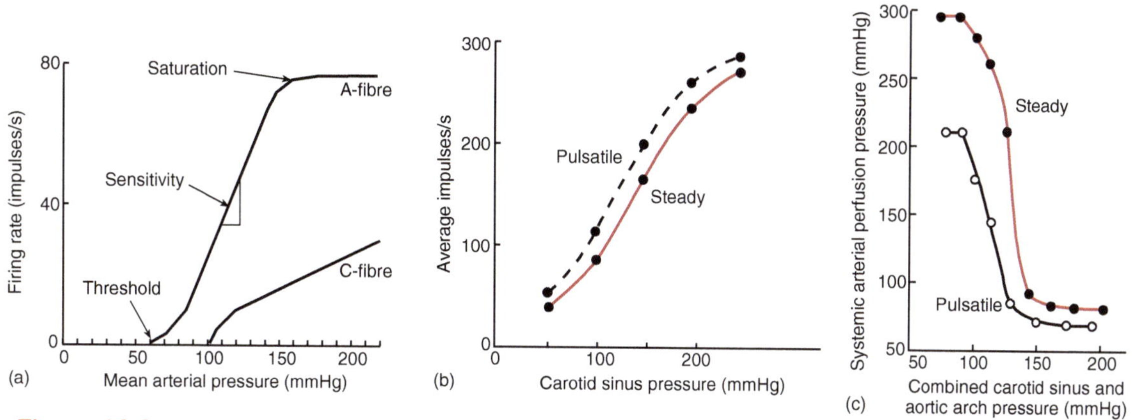

Figure 16.3 Baroreceptor types and the baroreflex. (a) Contrasting sensitivities and operating range of A-fibre and C-fibre baroreceptors. (b) Demonstration that a pulsatile pressure evoke higher baroreceptor activity than a steady pressure. (c) Raising pressure in a vascularly isolated, perfused baroreceptor region triggers a reflex fall in systemic arterial blood pressure, mediated by bradycardia and peripheral vasodilatation. Pulsatility strengthens the depressor reflex.

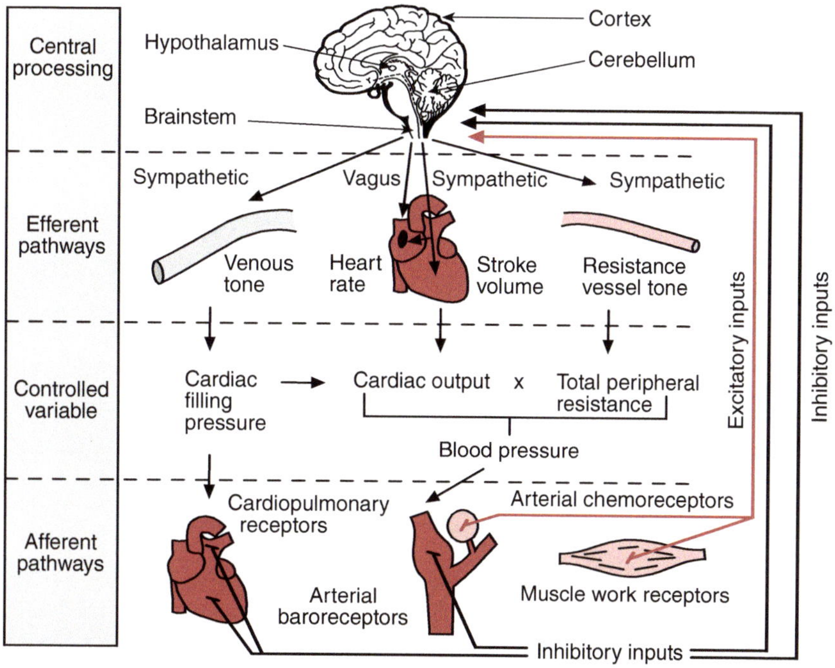

Figure 16.4 Overview of neural reflex control of the circulation; 'inhibitory' and 'excitatory' refer to net effect on cardiac output and blood pressure. Inhibitory reflexes are depressor, excitatory reflexes are pressor.

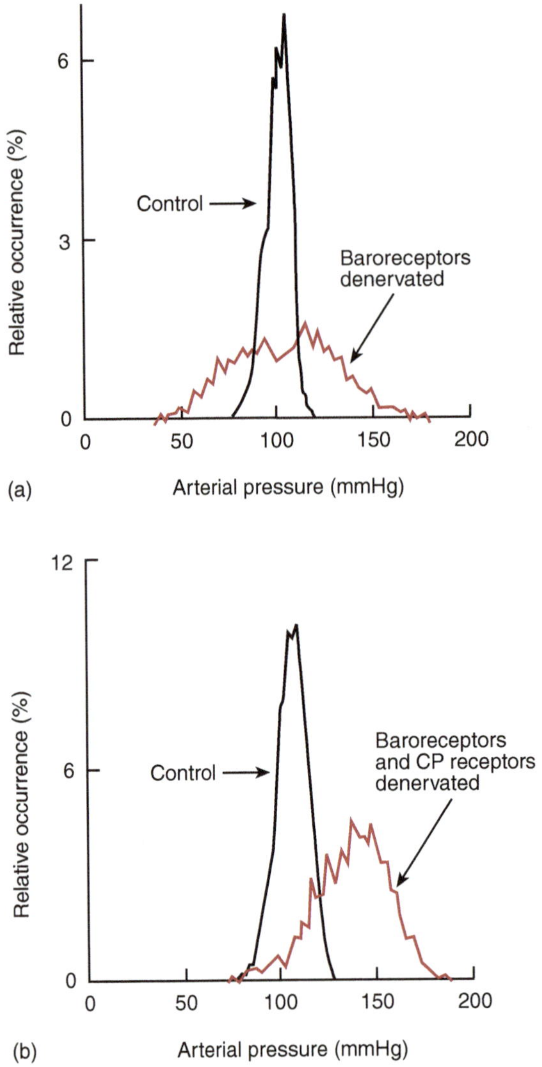

Figure 16.5 Baroreceptors stabilize arterial pressure. (a) In a normal dog, the variation in arterial pressure over time was narrow (control). Arterial baroreceptor denervation raised the mean pressure only moderately, but the fluctuation in pressure increased markedly. (b) After denervation of the cardiopulmonary receptors (CP) as well as arterial baroreceptors, there was a marked rise in mean pressure, as well as pressure instability.

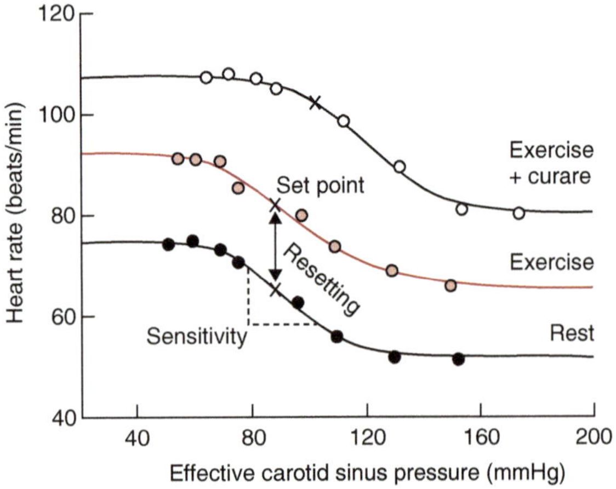

Figure 16.6 Resetting of human baroreflex during cycling (red line). After partial neuromuscular blockade by curare, a greater central command was needed to achieve the same level of exercise, and this reset the curve further. This shows that central command contributes to resetting during exercise.

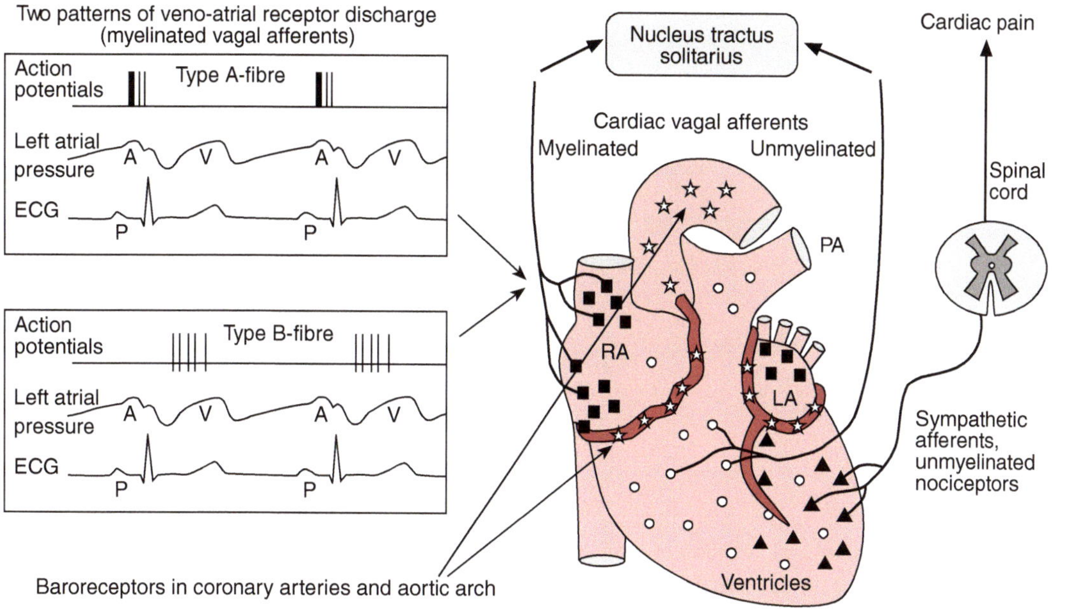

Figure 16.7 Cardiopulmonary afferent fibres. Squares, myelinated venoatrial stretch receptors; circles, unmyelinated mechanoreceptors; stars, arterial baroreceptors; triangles, nociceptive chemosensors; RA and LA, right and left atria, respectively; PA, pulmonary artery. Venoatrial receptor activity shown on left.

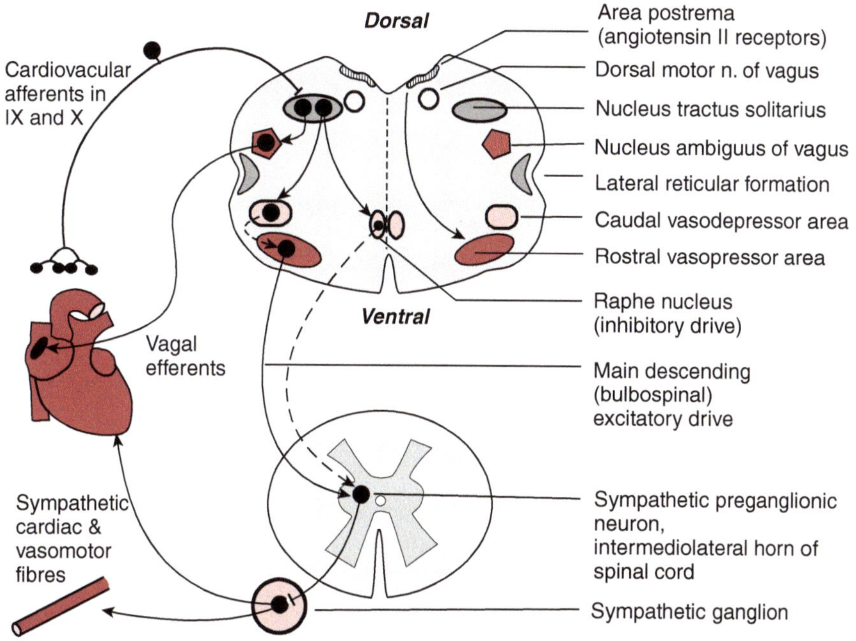

Figure 16.8 Transverse section of medulla, showing reflex pathways. Dashed lines indicate inhibitory pathways. The diagram is schematic: the various neuron groups occur at different rostrocaudal levels, so they would not in reality all be seen in a single section.

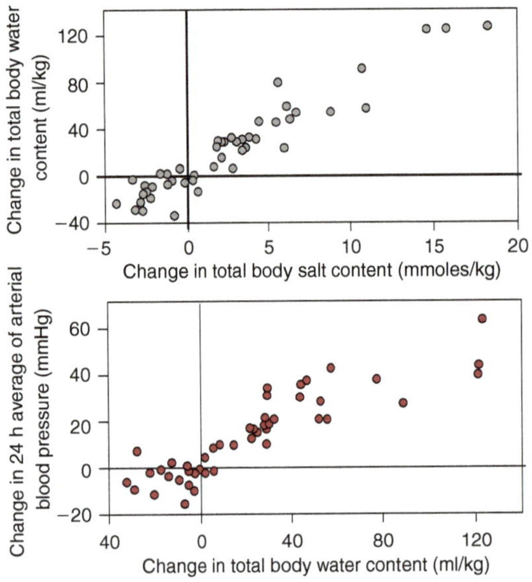

Figure 16.9 Effect of renal retention of salt and water on arterial blood pressure. (*Upper panel*) Water retention is closely coupled to salt retention (mainly Na^+, some K^+). (*Lower panel*) The rise in arterial blood pressure is closely coupled to the rise in body water, presumably via the Frank–Starling mechanism.

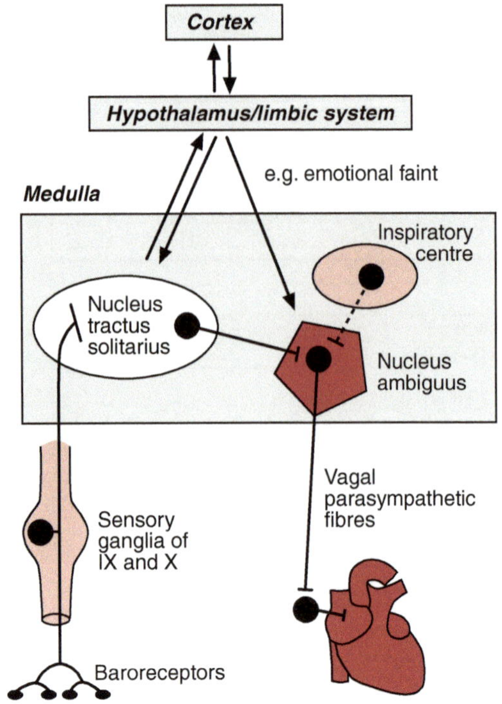

Figure 16.11 Central pathways for baroreflex regulation of vagal parasympathetic drive to heart. Inspiratory inhibition (dashed line) generates sinus arrhythmia.

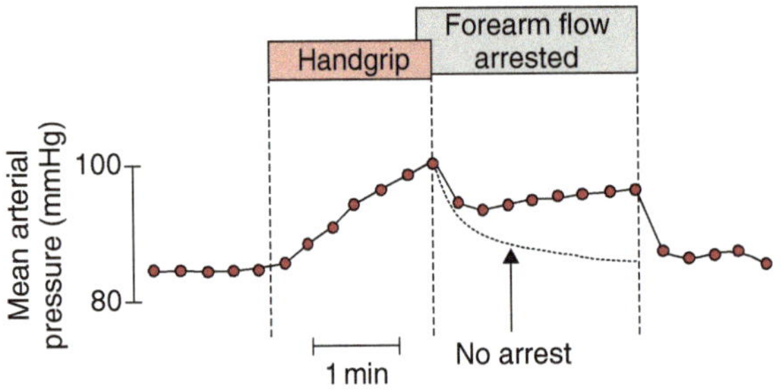

Figure 16.10 Classic proof that muscle metaboreceptors contribute to the human exercise pressor response. Isometric handgrip raises blood pressure. If blood is then trapped in the exercised arm by inflating a brachial cuff to supra-systolic pressure, the exercise pressor response is partly maintained, until the cuff is released.

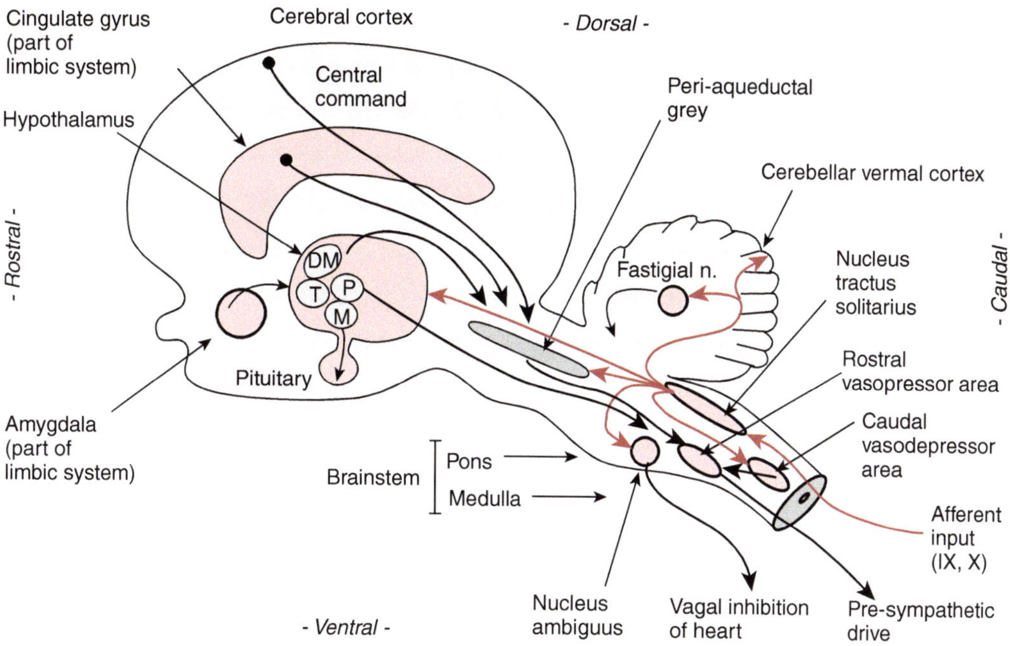

Figure 16.12 Longitudinal pathways for cardiovascular regulation in mammalian brain. DM, dorsomedial nucleus and peri-fornicular hypothalamus (alerting response); M, magnocellular neurons of supraoptic and paraventricular hypothalamic nuclei (synthesize vasopressin); P, parvocellular neurons of paraventricular nucleus (modulate sympathetic activity); T, temperature-regulating centre, anterior hypothalamus.

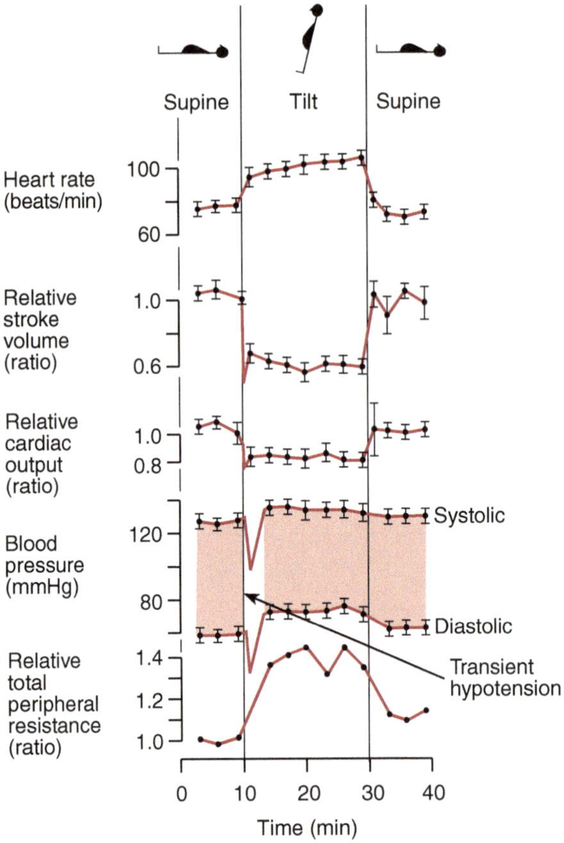

Figure 17.1 Response to a head-up tilt. Stroke volume, cardiac output and peripheral resistance are expressed as a fraction of the supine control values.

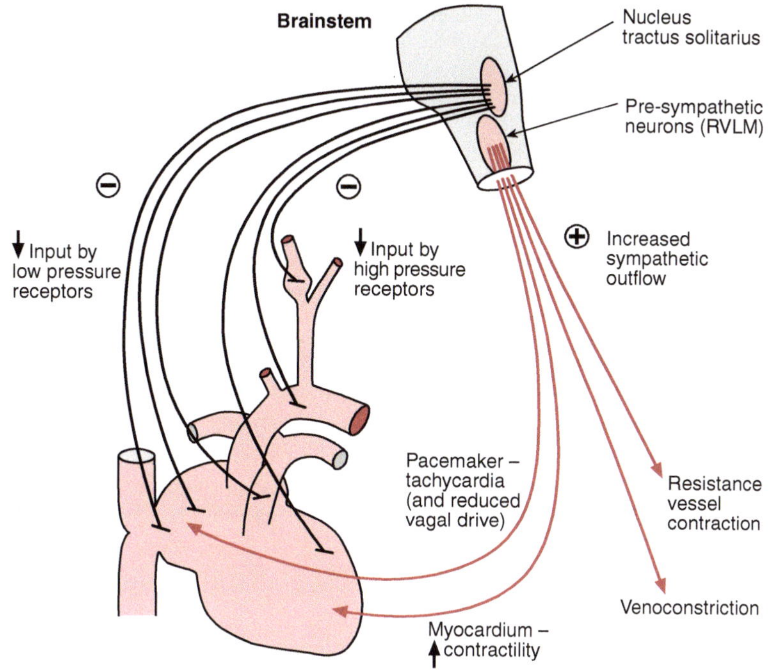

Figure 17.2 Reflex sympathetic response to orthostasis in humans. RVLM, rostroventrolateral medulla (site of rostral vasopressor area).

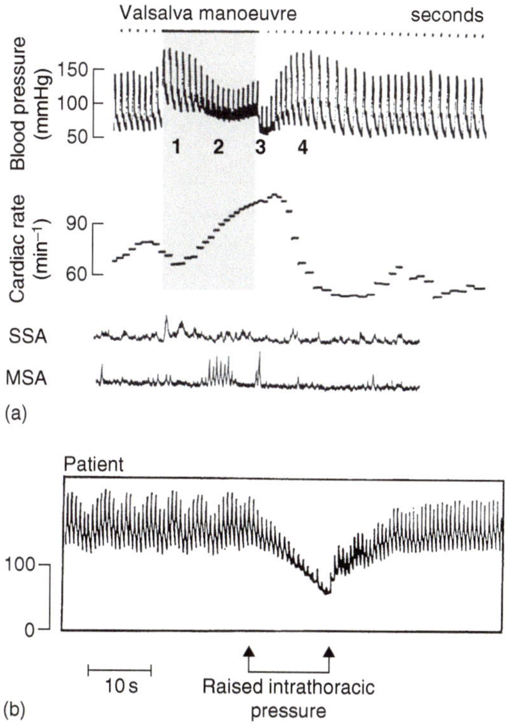

Figure 17.3 Effect of Valsalva manoeuvre on blood pressure and heart rate. (a) Normal subject. (b) Patient with idiopathic orthostatic hypotension, caused by an autonomic neuropathy. Pressure failed to stabilize in phase 2 and no reflex bradycardia in phase 4. SSA and MSA, skin and muscle sympathetic activity respectively.

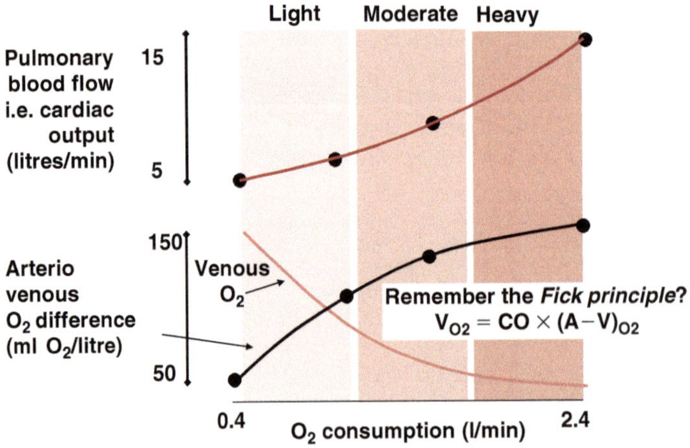

Figure 17.4 Relation between O_2 uptake $\dot{V}_{O_2}$ and pulmonary blood flow (cardiac output, CO). Graph also shows falling venous O_2 concentration, which increases the arteriovenous difference for O_2, $(A\text{-}V)_{O_2}$. The red cells are entering the lung emptier, but still leave it fully saturated.

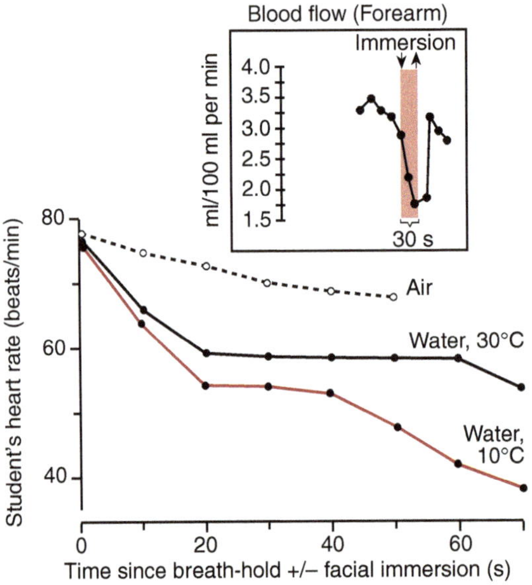

Figure 17.5 Diving response in a medical student; effect of breath-hold in air compared with facial immersion in cold water. (*Inset*) Concomitant vasoconstriction in forearm.

CHAPTER 18

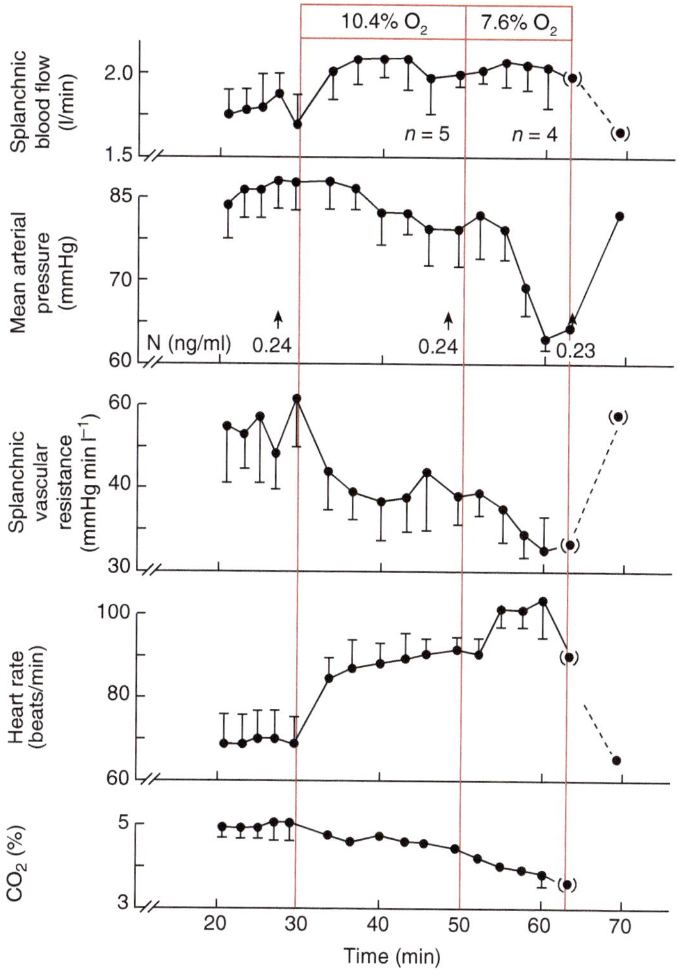

Figure 18.1 Response to hypoxaemia. Arterial P_{O_2} fell from 100 mmHg to 27 mmHg. Hyperventilation reduced alveolar CO_2. N, noradrenaline.

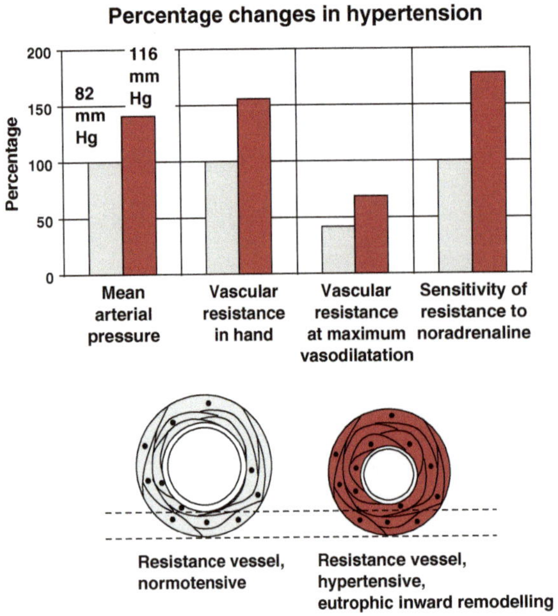

Figure 18.2 Changes in vascular resistance in hypertensive patients (red) compared with normal subjects (grey). (*Upper panel*) In the hypertensive patients, vascular resistance is raised at rest and after maximum vasodilatation; and the vasoconstrictor response to noradrenaline is increased. (*Lower panel*) Hypertension narrows the lumen and increases the wall thickness in small, resistance arteries.

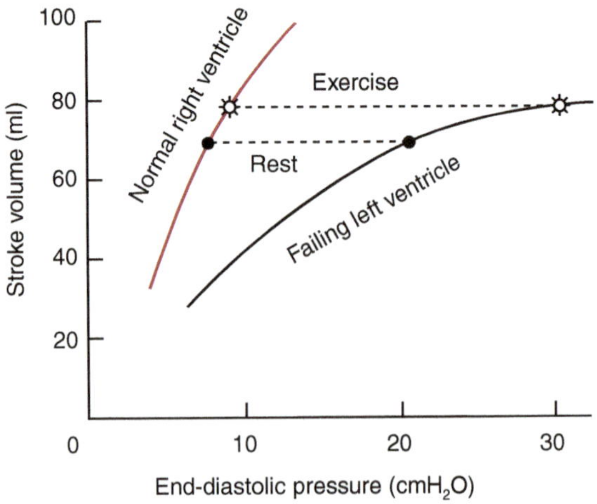

Figure 18.4 Operation of the Frank–Starling mechanism in a patient with a failing left ventricle, but as yet normal right ventricle. The left ventricle function curve is depressed (reduced contractility). At rest (filled circles), the left ventricle requires an elevated filling pressure to match the right ventricle stroke volume. During exercise (open symbols) the disparity in filling pressure becomes extreme, owing to the near-plateau on the function curve of the failing left ventricle. The attendant pulmonary congestion causes severe exertional dyspnoea.

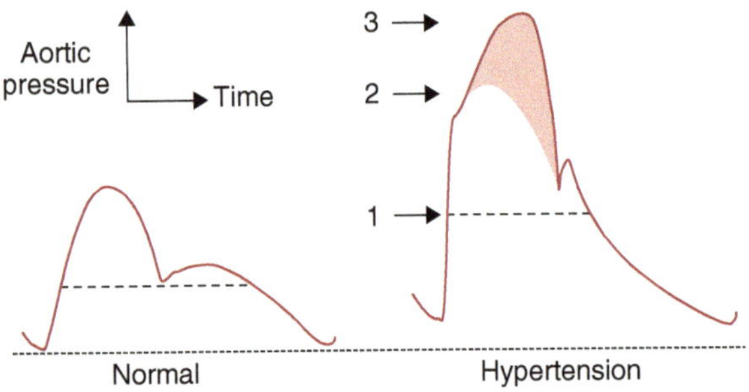

Figure 18.3 Changes in the aortic pressure wave in hypertension. Arrow 1 and dashed lines show the increase in mean pressure, caused by the increased resistance of small arterial vessels. Arrow 2 highlights the effect of reduced aortic compliance, namely a disproportionate increase in the systolic incident wave (clear area). Arrow 3 shows the augmentation of pressure in late systole by the early return of a large reflected wave (pink area).

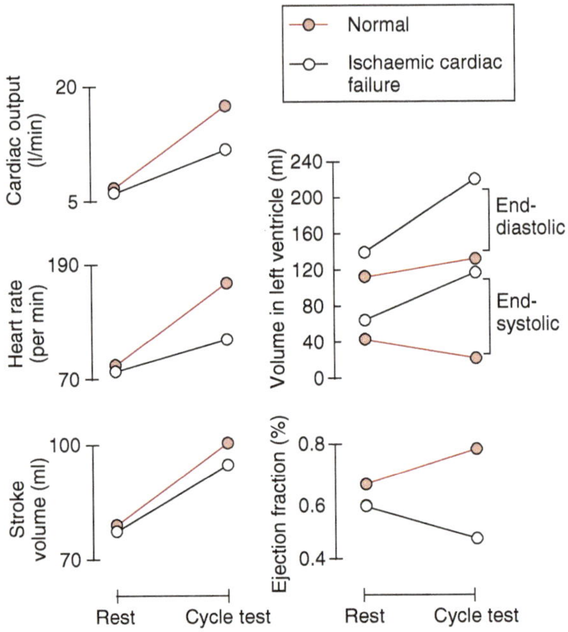

Figure 18.5 Effect of chronic cardiac failure on cardiac performance at rest and during a standard exercise test, namely submaximal bicycle ergometry.

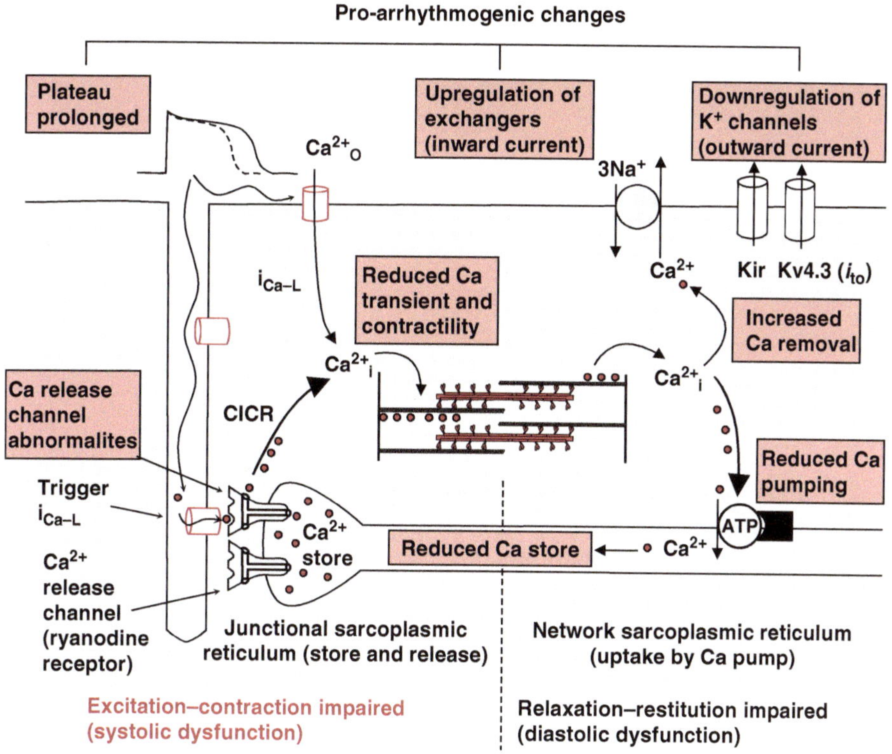

Figure 18.6 Changes in cardiac myocyte Ca^{2+} cycle, ionic currents and action potential in chronic heart failure. Dashed line is normal action potential. CICR, calcium-induced calcium release.

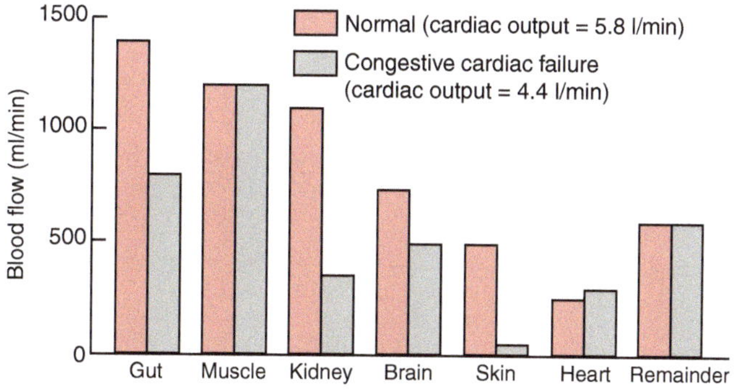

Figure 18.7 Redistribution of cardiac output in a resting patient with chronic cardiac failure and an output of 4.4 litre/min (grey columns). Note the reduced perfusion of the kidney, gut and skin, caused by a high sympathetic activity.

Figure acknowledgements

Figure 1.3 Data from Wade OL, Bishop JM. *Cardiac Output and Regional Flow*. Oxford: Blackwell, 1962.

Figure 2.2 After Noble MIM. *Circulation Research* 1968; **23**: 663–70.

Figure 2.4 Courtesy of Professor Horst Seller, University of Heidelberg.

Figure 3.7 After Myerburg RJ, Lazzara R. In: Fisch E (ed.). *Complex Electrocardiography*. Philadelphia, PA: Davis, 1973.

Figure 3.8 Adapted from Noble D. *The Initiation of the Heart Beat*. Oxford: Clarendon Press, 1979.

Figure 3.9 Records from Spurgeon *et al. American Journal of Physiology* 1990; **258**: H574–86.

Figure 3.10 Based on Noble D. The surprising heart. *Journal of Physiology* 1984; **353**: 1–50. With permission from Wiley-Blackwell.

Figure 3.13 Adapted from Sanguinetti MC, Keating MT. *News in Physiological Sciences*, 1997; **12**: 152–7. Copyright by American Physiological Society, with permission.

Figure 3.15 From Allen DG, Eisner DA, Smith GL, Wray S. *Journal of Physiology* 1985; **365**: 55P, with permission from Wiley-Blackwell.

Figure 3.16 Based on Benardeau *et al. American Journal of Physiology* 1996; **271**: H1151–61. Copyright by American Physiological Society, with permission.

Figure 4.2 After Bolter CP, Wallace DJ. and Hirst GDS. *Autonomic Neuroscience: Basic and Clinical* 2001 **94**, 93–101, with permission from Elsevier.

Figure 4.3 Records c–f are from Lewis' classic book, *The Mechanism and Graphic Registration of the Heart Beat*. London: Shaw and Sons, 1920.

Figure 4.4 Based on Petit-Jacques J *et al. News in Physiological Sciences* 1994; **9**: 77–9; copyright by American Physiological Society, with permission. And Noble D. In: Zipes DP, Jalife J (eds). *Cardiac Physiology from Cell to Bedside*. Philadelphia, PA: W.B. Saunders, 1995: 305–13.

Figure 4.6 From Hutter OF, Trautwein W. *Journal of General Physiology* 1956; **39**: 715–33. Copyright by Rockefeller University Press, with permission.

Figure 6.2 From Parker JD, Case RB. *Circulation* 1979; **60**: 4–12, by permission.

Figure 6.3 Based on concepts from Elzinga G, Westerhof N. *Circulation Research* 1979; **32**: 178–86; and Nichols WW, O'Rourke MF. *McDonald's Blood Flow in Arteries*, 5th edn. London: Arnold, 2005.

Figure 6.4 After Sonnenblick EH. *American Journal of Physiology* 1962; **202**: 931–9. Copyright by American Physiological Society, with permission.

Figure 6.5 Adapted from Fuchs F, Smith SS. *News in Physiological Science* 2001; **16**: 5–10. Copyright by American Physiological Society, with permission.

Figure 6.6 After Allen DG, Nichols CG, Smith GL. *Journal of Physiology* 1988; **406**: 359–70. With permission from Wiley-Blackwell.

Figure 6.9 After Gauer OH, Thron HL. In: Hamilton WF, Dow P (eds). *Handbook of Physiology, Circulation*, Vol. 3. Bethesda, MD: American Physiological Society, 1963: 2409–40.

Figure 6.10 From Amon KW, Crawford MH. *Journal of Clinical Ultrasound* 1979; **7**: 373–76.

Figure 6.11 From Sarnoff SJ, Mitchell JH. *Handbook of Physiology Cardiovascular Systems, Vol 1*. Baltimore, MD: American Physiological Society, 1962: 489–532, by permission.

Figure 6.12 Based in part on Burkhoff D, Mirsky I, Suga H *American Journal of Physiology* 2005; **289**: H501–12.

Figure 6.14 Based in part on Berne RM, Levy MN. *Cardiovascular Physiology*. St Louis, MO: Mosby, copyright Elsevier (1997), with permission.

Figure 6.15 After Rowell LB. *Human Circulation Regulation during Physical Stress*. New York: Oxford University Press, 1986.

Figure 6.16 Courtesy of Dr A Wilson, St George's Hospital, London.

Figure 6.19 Adapted from Linden RJ. *Anaesthesia* 1968; **23**: 566–84, with permission from Wiley-Blackwell.

Figure 6.20 From Berne RM, Rubio R. In: Berne RM, Sperekalis N (eds). *Handbook of Physiology, Cardiovascular System*, Vol. 1, The Heart. Bethesda, MD: American Physiological Society, 1979: 873–952, by permission.

Figure 6.21 Adapted from Simms AE, Paton JFR, Pickering AE. *Journal of Physiology* 2007; **579**: 473–86, with permission from Wiley-Blackwell.

Figure 6.22 Adapted from Innes JA, Simon TD, Murphy K, Guz A. *Quarterly Journal of Experimental Physiology* 1988; **73**: 323–41, with permission from Wiley-Blackwell.

Figure 6.23 Data from Stickland *et al. Journal of Physiology* 2004; **561**: 321–9.

Figure 7.1 From Innes JA, Simon TD, Murphy K, Guz A. *Quarterly Journal of Experimental Physiology* 1988; **73**: 323–41, by permission.

Figure 7.2 Based on Nichols WW, O'Rourke MF. *McDonald's Blood Flow in Arteries*, 5th edn. London: Arnold, 2005.

Figure 7.4 After Asmussen E, Nielsen M. *Acta Physiologica Scandinavica* 1953; **27**: 217. With permission from Wiley-Blackwell.

Figure 8.5 From Chien S, *Microvascular Research* 1992; **44**: 243–54, with permission from Elsevier.

Figure 8.6 After Gaetghens P. In: Gross DR, Wang NHC (eds). *The Rheology of Blood, Blood Vessels and Associated Tissues*. Amsterdam: Sijthoff and Noordhoff, with permission from Elsevier.

Figure 8.7 After Mills CJ, Gale IT, Gault JH *et al. Cardiovascular Research* 1970; **4**: 405; by permission of Oxford University Press, and Nichols WW, O'Rourke MF. *McDonald's Blood Flow in Arteries*, 5th edn. London: Arnold, 2005.

Figure 8.10 Based on Nichols WW, O'Rourke MF. *McDonald's Blood Flow in Arteries*. London: Arnold, 2005.

Figure 8.11 Adapted from Chien S. *Physiological Reviews* 1967; **47**: 214–88; (copyright by American Physiological Society, with permission), Jacobsen J, Sofelt S, Sheikh S, Warberg J, Secher NH. *Acta Physiologica Scandinavica* 1990; **138**: 167–73; and Länne T, Lundvall J. *Acta Physiologica Scandinavica* 1992; **146**: 299–306, with permission from Wiley-Blackwell.

Figure 8.12 After Nichols WW, O'Rourke MF. *McDonald's Blood Flow in Arteries*, 5th edn. London: Arnold, 2005.

Figure 8.13 After the classic experiment of Whittaker SRF, Winton FR. *Journal of Physiology* 1933; **78**: 339–69.

Figure 8.14 From Lind RA, McNicol GW. *Canadian Medical Association Journal* 1967; **96**: 706, by permission.

Figure 8.15 Public data from Department of Health National Statistics. *Health Survey for England 2003*, Vol 2 Risk Factors for Cardiovascular Disease.

Figure 8.16 From Hering. *Die Karotissinusreflexe auf Herz und Gefässe*. Dresden: T. Steinkopf, 1927.

Figure 8.18 After Snell RE, Clements JM, Patel DJ, Fry DL, Luchsinger PC. *Journal of Applied Physiology* 1965; **20**: 691. Copyright by American Physiological Society, with permission.

Figure 8.20 From Pappenheimer JR, Maes JP. *American Journal of Physiology* 1942; **137**: 187–99; and Stainsby WN, Renkin EM. *American Journal of Physiology* 1961; **201**: 117–22. Copyright by American Physiological Society, with permission.

Figure 8.26 Canine saphenous vein, from Vanhoutte PM, Leusen I. *Pfluger's Archiv* 1969; **306**: 341–53, with kind permission from Springer Science and Business Media.

Figure 9.1 From Bundgaard M. *Journal of Ultrastructural Research* 1984; **88**: 1–17, with permission from Elsevier.

Figure 9.3 Adapted using information from Drenckhahn D, Ness W. In Born GVR, Schwartz CJ (eds). *Vascular Endothelium*. Stuttgart: Schattauer, 1997; and Weinbaum S, Tarbell JM, Damiano ER. *Annual Review Biomedical Engineering* 2007; **9**: 121–67.

Figure 9.8 Redrawn from Freiman PC, Mitchell GC, Heistad DD *et al*. *Circulation Research* 1986. **58**: 783–9.

Figure 10.2 Redrawn from Adamson, Michel. *Journal of Physiology* 1993; **466**: 303–27. With permission from Wiley-Blackwell.

Figure 10.3 After Renkin EM, Curry FE. In: Giebisch G, Tosteson DC, Ussing HH (eds). *Membrane Transport in Biology*, Vol. IV. Berlin: Springer-Verlag, 1978: 1–45, with kind permission from Springer Science and Business Media.

Figure 10.6 Data of Renkin EM. In: Marchetti G, Taccardi B (eds). *International Symposium on Coronary Circulation*. Basel: Karger, 1967: 18–30.

Figure 10.8 From data of Blomstrand E, Saltin B. *Journal of Physiology* 1999; **514**: 293–302.

Figure 11.1 After Renkin EM. *American Journal of Physiology* 1986; **250**: H706–10. Copyright by American Physiological Society, with permission.

Figure 11.3(a) From Levick JR, Michel CC. *Journal of Physiology* 1978; **274**: 97–109; Bates DO *et al*. *Journal of Physiology* 1994; **477**: 355–63. With permission from Wiley-Blackwell.

Figure 11.3(b) Adapted from Levick JR. *Journal of Physiology* 2004; **557**: 704.

Figure 11.5 Drawn from data in Bates, Levick & Mortimer. *International Journal of Microcirculation Clinical & Experimental* 1992; **11**: 359–373, and Guyton, Taylor and Granger. *Circulation Physiology II; Dynamics and control of the Body Fluids.* WB Saunders: Philadelphia. 1975.

Figure 11.6 From Levick JR, Michel CC. *Journal of Physiology* 1978; **274**: 97–109, with permission from Wiley-Blackwell.

Figure 11.7 Data from Maspers M, Björnberg J, Mellander S. *Acta Physiologica Scandinavica* 1990; **140**: 73–83, by permission.

Figure 11.8 From the classic study of Krogh A, Landis EM, Turner AH. *Journal of Clinical Investigations* 1932; **11**: 63–95.

Figure 11.9 Adapted from Michel CC, Kendall S. *Journal of Physiology* 1997; **501**: 657–62, with permission from Wiley-Blackwell.

Figure 11.10 In: Renkin EM, Michel CC (eds). *Handbook of Physiology, Cardiovascular System, Vol. IV, Part II, Microcirculation*. Bethesda, MD: American Physiological Society, 1984: 309–74, by permission.

Figure 11.11 Data from many laboratories, reviewed in Levick JR, Mortimer PS. Fluid balance between microcirculation and interstitium in skin and other tissues; revision of classical filtration-reabsorption scheme. In: Messmer K (ed.). *Progress in Applied Microcirculation*. Basle: Karger, 1999: 42–62.

Figure 11.12 Adapted from Michel CC, Phillips ME. *Journal of Physiology* 1987; **388**: 421–35, with permission from Wiley-Blackwell.

Figure 11.14 Courtesy of Professor P Mortimer, Department of Dermatology, St. George's Hospital, London.

Figure 11.16 (a) From McHale N and colleagues. *Journal of Physiology* 1977; **272**: 33P–4P; and *Journal of Physiology* 1991; **438**: 168P, with permission from Wiley-Blackwell. (b) From Li B, Silver I, Szalai JP, Johnston MG. *Microvascular Research* 1998; **56**: 127–38, with permission from Elsevier.

Figure 11.17 After Taylor AE, Townsley MI. *News in Physiological Science* 1987; **2**: 48–52. Copyright by American Physiological Society, with permission.

Figure 11.18 Redrawn from work of He P, Zhang X, Curry FE. *American Journal of Physiology* 1996; **271**: H2377–87. Copyright by American Physiological Society, with permission.

Figure 12.1 Based partly on Gabella G. *Physiological Reviews* 1984; **64**: 455–77.

Figure 12.3 (a) and (b) From Golenhofen K, Hermstein N, Lammel E. *Microvascular Research* 1973; **5**: 73–80, with permission from Elsevier. (c) From Keatinge WR, Harman CM. *Local Mechanisms Controlling Blood Vessels*. London: Academic Press, 1980, with permission from Elsevier.

Figure 12.5 From Cheung DW. *Pfluger's Archiv* 1984; **400**: 335–7, with kind permission from Springer Science and Business Media.

Figure 12.7 Based on Ito T, Kajikuri J, Kurigama H. *Journal of Physiology* 1992; **457**: 297–314 with permission from Wiley-Blackwell; and Wier WG, Morgan KG. *Reviews of Physiology, Biochemistry and Pharmacology* 2003; **150**: 91–139, with permission from Springer Science and Business Media.

Figure 12.8 Courtesy of Professor WA Large, Department of Pharmacology, St. George's Hospital Medical School, London.

Figure 12.9 After Ushio-Fukai M *et al. Journal of Physiology* 1993; **462**: 679–96. With permission from Wiley-Blackwell.

Figure 12.10 After Sneddon P, Burnstock G. *European Journal of Pharmacology* 1984; **106**: 149–52, with permission from Elsevier.

Figure 12.12 Data from Siegel G *et al. Journal of Vascular Medicine and Biology* 1991; **3**: 140–9.

Figure 13.1 Data from Mellander S, Johansson B. *Pharmacological Reviews* 1968; **20**: 117–96, by permission.

Figure 13.2 Based on McCarron JG, Crichton CA, Langton PD, MacKenzie A, Smith GL. *Journal of Physiology* 1997; **498**: 371–9, with permission from Wiley-Blackwell; and Carlson BE, Secomb TW. *Microcirculation* 2005; **12**: 327–38, copyright Taylor & Francis Group, www.informaworld.com, reproduced with permission.

Figure 13.3 From Parkington HC, Tona MA, Coleman HA, Tare M. *Journal of Physiology* 1995; **484**: 469–80, with permission from Wiley-Blackwell.

Figure 13.4 From Walloe L, Wesche J. *Journal of Physiology* 1988; **405**: 257–73, with permission from Wiley-Blackwell.

Figure 13.5 (a) Drawn partly from data of Jones RD, Berne RM. Circulation Research 1964; 14: 126.

Figure 13.6 After Heistad DD, Kontos HA. In: Shepherd JT, Abboud FM (eds). *Handbook of Physiology, Cardiovascular System,* Vol. III, Part 1, Peripheral Circulation. Bethesda, MD: American Physiological Society, 1983: 137–81, by permission.

Figure 13.7 Adapted from Bruce J, Taggart M, Austin C. *Microvascular Research* 2004; **68**: 303–312, with permission from Elsevier.

Figure 13.8 Redrawn and modified using data from Altura B. *Microcirculation, Endothelium and Lymphatics* 1988; **4**: 97–110.

Figure 13.9 Data from Laird. In: Holland A, Noble M (eds). *Cardiac Metabolism*. Chichester: Wiley, 1983: 257–78.

Figure 13.10 Based in part on data from Wade OL, Bishop JM. *Cardiac Output and Regional Blood Flow*. Oxford: Blackwell, 1962.

Figure 13.11 Adapted with permission from Brown MD. In: Jordan D, Marshall J (eds). *Cardiovascular Regulation*. London: Portland Press, 1995: 113–26.

Figure 14.1 Adapted from Furness JB, Marshall JM. *Journal of Physiology* 1974; **239**: 75–88, with permission from Wiley-Blackwell.

Figure 14.2 After Hainsworth R, Karim F. *Journal of Physiology* 1976; **262**: 659–77, with permission from Wiley-Blackwell.

Figure 14.3 From Mellander S. *Acta Physiologica Scandinavica* 1960; **50** (Suppl.): 176, with permission from Wiley-Blackwell.

Figure 14.4 After Foreman JC. *Allergy* 1987; **42**: 1–11, with permission from Wiley-Blackwell.

Figure 14.5 From classic monograph, Barcroft H, Swan HJC. *Sympathetic Control of Human Blood Vessels*. London: Edward Arnold, 1953, by permission.

Figure 15.1 Data from Ingvar DH. *Brain Research* 1976; **107**: 188–97; and Lassen NA, Ingvar DH, Skinhoj E. *Scientific American* 1978; **239**: 50–9.

Figure 15.2 (a) After Greenfield ADM. In: Hamilton WF, Dow P (eds). *Handbook of Physiology, Cardiovascular System,* Vol. III, Part II, Peripheral Circulation. Bethesda, MD: American Physiological Society, 1963: 1325–52; (b) from Johnson JM, Rowell JB. *Journal of Applied Physiology* 1975; **39**: 920–4, copyright by American Physiological Society, with permission; (c) based on Van den Bande P, De Coninck A, Lievens P. *International Journal of Microcirculation* 1977; 55–60.

Figure 15.3 From Renkin EM. In: Marhetti G, Taccardi B (eds). *International Symposium on Coronary Circulation*. Basel: Karger, 1967: 18–30.

Figure 15.4 After Khouris EM, Gregg DE, Rayford CR. *Circulation Research* 1965; **17**: 427–37.

Figure 15.6 Redrawn from Deanfield JE, Shea M, Kensett M *et al. Lancet* 1984; **2**: 1001–5, with permission from Elsevier.

Figure 15.8 After Roddie IC. In: Shepherd JT, Abboud FM (eds). *Handbook of Physiology, Cardiovascular System*, Vol. III, Part 1, Peripheral Circulation. Bethesda, MD: American Physiological Society, 1983: 285–317.

Figure 15.11 From Caesar K, Akgören N, Mathiesen C, Lauritzen M. *Journal of Physiology* 1999; **520**: 281–92, by permission.

Figure 15.13 Based on Robertson TP, Aaronson PI, Ward JPT. *American Journal of Physiology* 1995; **268**: H301–7. Copyright by American Physiological Society, with permission.

Figure 15.14 (a) From Banister RJ, Torrance RW. *Quarterly Journal of Experimental Physiology* 1960; **45**: 352–7; (b) from Grover RF *et al*. Pulmonary circulation. In: Shepherd JT, Abboud FM (eds). *Handbook of Physiology, Cardiovascular System,* Vol III, Peripheral Circulation. Bethesda, MD: American Physiological Society, 1983: 103–36, by permission.

Figure 16.1 From Abraham A. *Microscopic Innervation of the Heart and Blood Vessels in Vertebrates Including Man*. Oxford: Pergamon Press, 1969, by permission.

Figure 16.2 Fibres 1 and 2 after Landgren S. *Acta Physiologica Scandinavica* 1952; **26**: 1–34; fibre 3 from Downing SE. *Journal of Physiology* 1960; **150**: 210–13, with permission from Wiley-Blackwell.

Figure 16.3 From (a) Coleridge HM, Coleridge JCG, Schultz HD. *Journal of Physiology* 1987; **394**: 291–313 with permission from Wiley-Blackwell; (b) Korner PI. *Physiological Reviews* 1971; **51**: 312–67, copyright by American Physiological Society, with permission; and (c) Angell-James JE, De Burgh Daly M. *Journal of Physiology* 1970; **209**: 257–93, with permission from Wiley-Blackwell.

Figure 16.5 (a) From Cowley AW, Liard JF, Guyton AC. *Circulation Research* 1973; **32**: 564–78; (b) Persson PB, Ehmke H, Kirchheim HR. *News in Physiological Sciences* 1989; **4**: 56–9. Copyright by American Physiological Society, with permission.

Figure 16.6 Based on Gallagher KM, Fadel, PJ, Strömstad M *et al. Journal of Physiology* 2001; **533**: 861–70, with permission from Wiley-Blackwell.

Figure 16.7 Based on Kappagoda CT, Linden RJ, Sivananthan N. *Journal of Physiology* 1979; **291**: 393–412, with permission from Wiley-Blackwell.

Figure 16.9 Data redrawn from Seeliger, Wronski, Ladwig *et al. Clinical and Experimental Pharmacology and Physiology* 2005; **32**: 394–9, with permission from Wiley-Blackwell.

Figure 16.10 Data from Rusch NJ, Shepherd JT, Webb RC, Vanhoutte PM. *Circulation Research* 1981; **48** (Suppl. 1): 118–25, by permission.

Figure 16.11 Based on Spyer KM. *Journal of Physiology* 1994; **474**: 1–19, with permission from Wiley-Blackwell.

Figure 17.1 From Smith JJ, Bush JE, Weideier VT, Tristani FE. *Journal of Applied Physiology* 1970; **29**: 133. Copyright by American Physiological Society, with permission.

Figure 17.3 (a) From Bannister Sir R. In: Sleight P (ed.). *Arterial Blood Pressure and Hypertension*. Oxford: Oxford University Press, 1980: 117–21; and Wallin BG, Elam M. *News in Physiological Sciences* 1994; **9**: 203–7; (b) from Johnson RH, Spalding JMK. *Disorders of the Autonomic Nervous System*. London: Blackwell, 1974, with permission from Wiley-Blackwell.

Figure 17.5 Courtesy of JR Henderson, unpublished. Inset from Heistad DD, Abboud FM, Eckstein JW. *Journal of Applied Physiology* 1968; **25**: 542–49. Copyright by American Physiological Society, with permission.

Figure 18.1 After Rowell LB. *Human Circulation Regulation during Physical Stress*. New York: Oxford University Press, 1986 (fig 12.9, p. 342); adapted from Rowell & Blackman. *American Journal of Physiology* 1986; **251**: H562–70. Copyright by American Physiological Society, with permission.

Figure 18.2 Results of Thybo NK, Stephens N, Cooper A, Aalkjaer C, Heagerty AM, Mulvany MJ. *Hypertension* 1995; **25**: 474–81.

Figure 18.3 Based on Nichols WW, O'Rourke MF. *McDonald's Blood Flow in Arteries*. London: Arnold, 2005.

Figure 18.6 Based on information in Sipido KR, Eisner D. *Cardiovascular Research* 2005; **68**: 167–74; and Bers DM. *Physiology* 2006; **21**: 380–7.

Figure 18.7 From Wade OL, Bishop JM. *Cardiac Output and Regional Flow*. Oxford: Blackwell, 1962, by permission.

All figures reproduced with permission of American Physiological Society are done so via Copyright Clearance Center.

All figures reproduced with permission of Rockefeller University Press are done so via Copyright Clearance Center.

CHAPTER 1

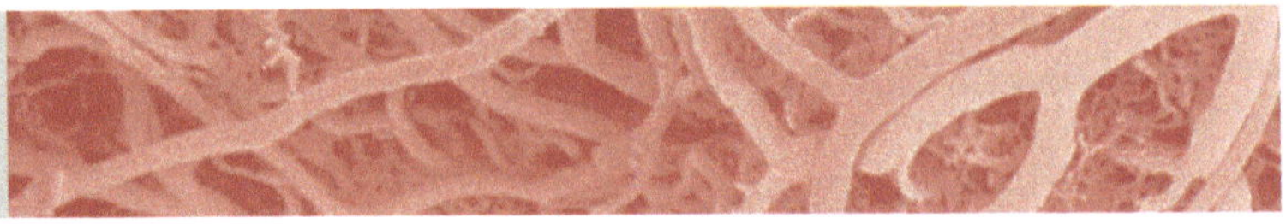

Table 1.1 Time taken for a glucose molecule to diffuse specified distance in one direction

Distance (*x*)	Time (*t*)[a]	Example *in vivo*
0.1 μm	0.000005 s	Neuromuscular gap
1.0 μm	0.0005 s	Capillary wall
10.0 μm	0.05 s	Capillary to cell
1 mm	9.26 min	Skin; artery wall
1 cm	15.4 h	Left ventricle wall

[a]Einstein's equation states $t = x^2/2D$, where D is solute diffusion coefficient (glucose, $0.9 \times 10^{-5} cm^2 s^{-1}$ at 37°C; oxygen in water, $3 \times 10^{-5} cm^2 s^{-1}$ at 37°C).
(Einstein A. *Theory of Brownian Movement* (translated by R Fürth and AD Cowper, 1956). New York: Dover Publications, 1905.)

Table 1.2 Composition of the blood vessel wall (%)

	Endothelium	Smooth muscle	Elastin tissue	Collagen
Elastic artery	5	25	40	27
Arteriole	10	60	10	20
Capillary	95	0	0	5 (basal lamina)
Venule	20	20	0	60

CHAPTER 2

Table 2.1 Mean pressures (mmHg) during cardiac cycle of a supine, resting human

	Right	Left
Atrium	3	8
Ventricle		
end of diastole	4	9
peak of systole	25	120

CHAPTER 3

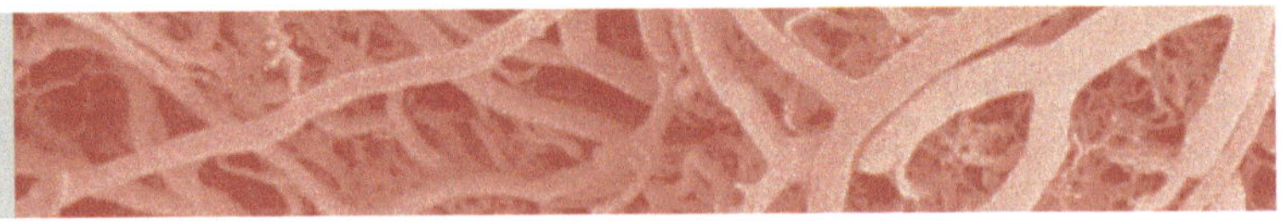

Table 3.1 Concentration of ions in resting cardiac myocytes

	Intracellular (mM)	Extracellular (mM)	Nernst equilibrium potential (mV)
K^+	140	4	−94
Na^+	10	140	+70
Ca^{2+}	0.0001[a]	1.2[b]	+124
Cl^-	30	120	−37
pH	7.0–7.1	7.4	–

[a]Value at rest.

[b]The total Ca^{2+} concentration in plasma is about double this, but only 1.2 mM is in ionic form.

CHAPTER 6

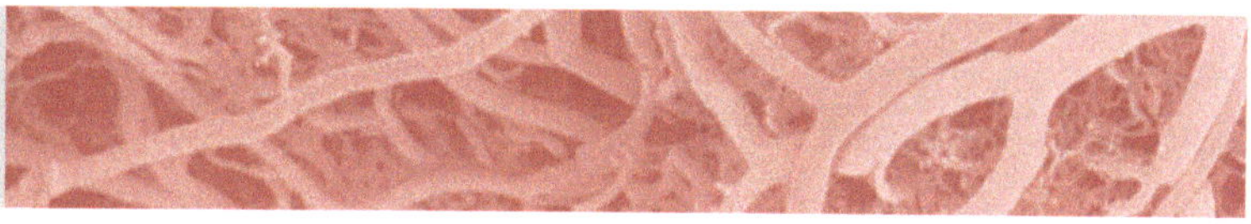

Table 6.1 Output of adult human heart in litres/min (mean and standard deviation)

	Rest	Exercise[a]
Normal adult	6.0 (1.3)	17.5 (6.0)
Coronary artery disease	5.7 (1.5)[b]	11.3 (4.3)

[a]At 85% of maximum heart rate or to onset of angina.
[b]Within the normal range at rest.

Table 6.2 Typical cardiac response to upright exercise in a non-athlete

	Rest	Hard exercise[a]
Oxygen consumption (l/min)	0.25	3.0
Cardiac output (l/min)	4.8	21.6
Heart rate (beats/min)	60.0	180.0
Stroke volume (ml)	80.0	120.0
End-diastolic volume (ml)	120.0	140.0
End-systolic residual volume (ml)	40.0	20.0
Ejection fraction	0.67	0.86
Cycle time (s)	1.0	0.33
Duration of systole (s)	0.35	0.2
Duration of diastole (s)	0.65	0.13

[a]85% of maximum increase in heart rate.

CHAPTER 14

Table 14.1 Pharmacology of adrenergic transmission

Receptor	Subtype	Principal location and effect	Agonists: relative potency	Antagonists	Therapeutic use of antagonists
α		Vascular myocytes: vasoconstriction	Noradrenaline (NA) and adrenaline (Ad) NA > Ad	Phentolamine, phenoxybenzamine	Raynaud's vasospasm Acute hypertension (phaeochromocytoma)
				Ergotamine	Migraine
	α_1	Post-junctional receptor on most vessels. Vasoconstriction via Gq, PLC, ↑ IP3 and DAG	NA > Ad, Phenylephrine	Prazosin, doxazosin, terazosin	Essential hypertension
	α_2	1. Autoreceptor of sympathetic varicosity: inhibits NA release. 2. Abundant post-junctional receptor in human skin vessels and muscle distal arterioles. Vasoconstriction via Gi, ↓ cAMP	Ad > NA Clonidine	Yohimbine, rauwolscine	–
β		1. SA node and myocardium: ↑ heart rate and contractility 2. Arterioles of heart, skeletal muscle and liver; vasodilatation	NA, Ad Isoprenaline	Propranolol, oxprenolol, alprenolol	Angina (↓ cardiac work) Hypertension
	β_1	SA node and myocardium: ↑ heart rate and contractility via Gs, adenylyl cyclase, ↑cAMP	NA > Ad Dobutamine (use; acute cardiac failure)	Atenolol, metroprolol, practolol (toxic)	Angina (↓ cardiac work) Hypertension (↓ cardiac output) Arrhythmias
	β_2	Arterioles of heart, skeletal muscle, liver Also bronchiole smooth muscle. Dilatation via Gs, ↑cAMP	Ad > NA Salbutamol, terbutaline		

CHAPTER 17

Table 17.1 Ventricular volume during upright, submaximal bicycle exercise in normal subjects and patients with multiple coronary artery disease

	Normal		Coronary disease	
	Rest	Exercise	Rest	Exercise
Cardiac output (litre/min)	6.0	17.5	5.7	11.3
Heart rate (beats/min)	81	170	75	119
Stroke volume (ml)[a]	76	102	76	96
End-diastolic volume (ml)[a]	116	128	138	216
End-systolic volume (ml)[a]	40	26	62	120
Ejection fraction[a]	0.66	0.8	0.6	0.46

[a]Left ventricle dimensions determined by radionuclide angiocardiography.
(After Rerych SK, Scholz PM, Newman GE et al. (1978) *Annals of Surgery*, **187**, 449–458.)

Table 17.2 Supine versus upright exercise at 30% of maximum O_2 consumption

	Stroke volume (ml)	Heart rate (beats/min)	Cardiac output (litre/min)
Supine			
Rest	111	60	6.4
Exercise	112	91	9.7
Upright			
Rest	76	76	5.6
Exercise	92	95	8.4

Index

Note: references in the form '2.4' denote the question and answer number. References to illustrations have been given in the same form but enclosed in brackets (e.g. '(2.4)'), usually following the question or answer which they are linked to, but sometimes on their own. Bracketed references in italics denote tables.